RECOVERY FROM
SCHIZOPHRENIA

RECOVERY FROM SCHIZOPHRENIA

EVIDENCE, HISTORY, AND HOPE

COURTENAY M. HARDING, PHD

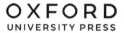

OXFORD
UNIVERSITY PRESS

Oxford University Press is a department of the University of Oxford. It furthers
the University's objective of excellence in research, scholarship, and education
by publishing worldwide. Oxford is a registered trade mark of Oxford University
Press in the UK and certain other countries.

Published in the United States of America by Oxford University Press
198 Madison Avenue, New York, NY 10016, United States of America.

Library of Congress Cataloging-in-Publication Data
Names: Harding, Courtenay, author.
Title: Recovery from schizophrenia : evidence, history, and hope / Courtenay M. Harding.
Description: New York, NY : Oxford University Press, [2024] |
Includes bibliographical references and index.
Identifiers: LCCN 2024013013 | ISBN 9780195380095 (hardback) |
ISBN 9780197783184 (epub) | ISBN 9780197783191 (ebook)
Subjects: LCSH: Schizophrenia—Vermont—History. |
Schizophrenia—Treatment—Vermont—History. |
Schizophrenics—Rehabilitation—Vermont—History.
Classification: LCC RC514 .H2966 2024 |
DDC 616.89/8009743—dc23/eng/20240405
LC record available at https://lccn.loc.gov/2024013013

DOI: 10.1093/oso/9780195380095.001.0001

Printed by Sheridan Books, Inc., United States of America

To my children: Robert, Brooke, and Ashley,
who contributed love, hugs, and ideas, and to the running of the
house, so their mother could go back to school do all this work,
and
To all the participants in these studies, who taught us critical
lessons about human persistence, rehabilitation, and the
possibilities of recovery, with implications for insisting on
biopsychosocial approaches and changing public policy.

Contents

PART THREE   SURPRISE DISCOVERIES

PART FOUR   NINE OTHER VERY-LONG-TERM STUDIES FROM ACROSS THE WORLD

PART FIVE   REHABILITATION PROGRAMS FOR RECOVERY

Tables

Foreword

It is highly unusual for two people to co-write a foreword for a book, but that is exactly what we wish to do. Both of us are senior community and university psychiatrists who live on opposite sides of the globe. We want to illustrate the impact of these stories about recovery and rehabilitation in persons from Vermont and Maine, in the United States, once diagnosed with schizophrenia and other serious and disabling forms of severe distress. Such research challenged the long-standing idea of marginal or down-hill levels of functioning as the only outcome possible and has thrown down the gauntlet to the fields of psychiatry, psychology, social work, and nursing.

I am Christian Beels, MD, living in New York City. I was one of the first in the nation to practice public and community psychiatry. In those early days of deinstitutionalization, my team and I, among many activities, set up a community mental health center in a defunct post office in the middle of the Bronx. We found an apartment building on the Lower West Side that gave people a place to live, and we also hired a chef to teach people skills so they could earn a living.

Most of my professional life has been divided between working in community institutions and the private office practice of psychiatry, and, in both places, the most challenging encounters were with families who had a young member just given a diagnosis of a serious mental illness. Schizophrenia was the prototype of these diagnoses, and the family wanted to know "What happens now? What do we do? What are the prospects for treatment, recovery, and for life?"

In addition to consultation with people like me, the family had a few options—mostly help from organizations of other such families, like the National Alliance on Mental Illness (NAMI) among many others. NAMI is a group of family members (many of them professionals) who became organized to help when the professional organizations mostly failed to do so. In New York, there were even some good outpatient programs. But, generally, the response to a situation like this—from the police to the emergency room—was uncertainty. Where to find a good doctor and a good hospital? How do you know? What is the next step? What is the long-term outcome?

Part of the problem is that American psychiatry has been stuck with the idea that there are two possible types of treatment for mental problems: psychotherapy, involving some kind of talk between a patient and a professional sitting in an office and mainly reserved for the well-off, and/or drugs or some other medical procedure brought forth by the neuroscientific establishment, especially for poorer people. Mostly, the number one treatment has been the immediate introduction of psychiatric medications. Most clinicians were not interested in the long-term effects of social learning in a supportive community. It's neither fast nor "scientific" or technical enough for us. And so we are unprepared for evidence from interventions and delivery systems that, in the end, produce the best results.

Fortunately, I met Courtenay Harding earlier in my career and read the papers produced by her team of National Institute of Mental Health (NIMH) investigators, so I knew some things that could be said to people in this situation. And, in my teaching responsibilities with psychiatric residents at Columbia and other professionals, I was able to present reviews of their work. But here, at last, in this book, we can read the whole story. It is a story that begins in a place—the state of Vermont—and makes clear that the place, the people who lived there, and how they were organized are all important ingredients in the process of recovery.

Professor Harding was trained in research psychology at the University of Vermont and continued following a patient cohort that began with the state's brave experiment in the social basis of recovery after many people tried and often discarded medication. Comparing her patients with a matched sample from the neighboring state of Maine working with the former director of the Maine State Bureau of Mental Health, Dr. Michael DeSisto, their teams produced a tour de force of epidemiological research to show that it really is the social environment that makes the difference over the long haul. She went on to Yale's Department of Psychiatry to work with John Strauss and his team and to learn clinical work at Connecticut Mental Health Center. After visiting other countries where similar experiments were in progress, she now brings the whole story together in this book, showing that there is another kind of science available to explain recovery from schizophrenia, even to American psychiatrists.

—C. Christian Beels, MD, New York, New York

I am Alan Rosen, a community and academic psychiatrist from Sidney, Australia. I have known Professor Courtenay Harding as an esteemed colleague for about 30 years. I have admired her immensely over that time for both her tenacity and persistence in swimming against the tide to complete two of the longest, most innovative, groundbreaking, and important cohort studies in our field.

I am a clinician and researcher in the field of community mental health services, working particularly with severe and persistent mental illness, early intervention programs, stigma, discrimination, human rights, and indigenous mental health. I have been involved intimately in the development of the Australian National Mental Health Service Standards and Strategy, functional measurement, and the Australian national mental health policy, and I am a co-author of its primary outcome evaluation tools. Professor Harding's studies helped us with all of these facets of mental health service development in Australia and New Zealand. Her results affirmed for us that there is something in community living per se that is inherently healing and that can be synergized by adequate community-based clinical care and support.

We met initially through international conferences on the course and clinical management of schizophrenia and related disorders. Since that time, my office has had the great pleasure of inviting and hosting Professor Harding at Mental Health Service (MHS) conferences in Australia and New Zealand and of being the recipient from time to time of her generous advice and comments in honing our academic, policy, and service development work relevant to her field.

Professor Harding is prominent among a small handful of clinician academics worldwide who are highly qualified and fully competent to address the full historical and current scope, trajectory, and horizons of research on recovery processes for individuals with severe mental illness. This is partly because (1) she has been a key player in this post-institutionalization and recovery journey history in Vermont to monitor the long-term effects of a pioneering initiative of systemic deinstitutionalization; (2) she has been a prominent researcher in the field, and her research work is still considered momentous and pioneering in our field; (3) she understands and exemplifies the important nexus between rigorous quantitative and qualitative research and the importance of ongoing ethical and humane engagement with informants; (4) the outcomes of her work were foundational and seminal in promoting to international prominence both the recovery movement and human rights agendas in mental health services; and (5) she is one of the most respected commentators of recent advances in this field, both academically and for the public.

Professor Harding and her teams had the patience and persistence to follow-up two matched cohorts of individuals with schizophrenia and other severe and debilitating disorders for more than three decades. Most outcome studies of this range of very long-term disorders are restricted to a year or to 5 years at the most. She is extremely capable, as her track record and our collective experience of her attests, as an innovative researcher, a teacher, a humane and acutely observant clinician, and as an academic and public communicator. She has consistently conveyed, over many years, a strong message of hope of recovery for individuals and their families who are living with schizophrenia. She has been increasingly backed by parallel evidence supporting the validity of her own groundbreaking studies while challenging the dominant prevailing expert consensus in psychiatry of "therapeutic pessimism" regarding the prognosis of schizophrenia.

This is a story which needs telling for multiple audiences: (1) for service-users, family caregivers, and service providers struggling with schizophrenia and trying to find evidence to back their conviction, often based on their experiences and intuitions, that working toward recovery in the community makes a huge difference in outcome; (2) for clinicians and researchers in the field, often disheartened by prevailing expert assumptions of pessimism and hopelessness regarding ultimate outcomes in schizophrenia; and (3) for young researchers generally, particularly if they also have to contend with the prejudicial and unwarranted life-long pathologizing of their clientele and the overvaluing of custodial care or biological treatments alone by academic elites. This view, virtually amounting to therapeutic nihilism, can lead researchers and clinicians to become overwhelmed by the initial negativity, deprivations, and domestic burdens carried by their clientele. The wide dissemination of this story of struggle and hopeful outcomes will encourage all these constituencies to continue their important work.

It is also a story of great professional and personal courage and persistence over many years working closely and continuously with one cohort. It may be worth noting in the context of the back-story of this volume that my first-ever live experience of Professor Harding was witnessing her giving an invited lecture at an international conference in Vancouver. She spoke in a calm tone and used modest terms, by no means over-claiming on the basis of her stated results. Her presentation was met with heckling by a vocal minority, uncharacteristic for such a formal academic setting. It included expressions of derision, personal invective, spiteful and snide comments, and unseemly rage on the part of certain senior academics and clinicians in the packed lecture halls whose assumptions of inevitable deterioration and ultimate poor outcomes in schizophrenia had obviously been challenged. Was there an element of misogyny behind this reaction also, considering that most of the protagonists were male and that emerging female academic stars in our field were less numerous in those days and perhaps considered easy targets? I really don't know because this intolerant behavior was not only directed at female academics, but also at the few other prominent researchers at that time who found glimmerings or even rich seams of evidence for therapeutic optimism, gradual healing, and recovery in community settings and who were still seen as heretical in the field of psychosis, and especially schizophrenia, in many quarters.

I was appalled by their behavior but later found out that this habitual, dogmatic, and incensed reaction was by no means uncommon and that both Dr. Harding and Professor John Strauss from Yale had to endure such public reactions for many years until mounting evidence gradually swamped such fiercely held prejudice. Even until recently, both speakers are still prone to evoke such reactions, even though the tide is now beginning to turn in our professions. I guess this is the nature of initial resistance to paradigm change in science.

The merit and rich substance of the central story is like mining a seam of gold. It is the history of early ground-breaking studies and researchers and of the patient amassing of evidence over many years relevant to illuminating recovery processes and pathways and the potential for more hopeful outcomes in severe psychiatric illnesses.

Professor Harding, along with Professor Larry Davidson (2005, 2006), has progressively reviewed the entire field during more recent years, and both are fully abreast of its outcomes and implications. This work will be invaluable for our clinical professionals and academics, patients and families, and others interested in the field. It will undoubtedly become a beacon to future generations of researchers and the embodiment of one of our most classic studies in the international annals of psychiatry and mental health services. It is also a story of the restorative power of resilience, buoyancy, and positive mental health in the face of the potential ravages of severe mental illness.

I have also been present when Professor Harding interacted informally with regional, national, and international networks, and I have found her to be an animated and wise contributor to conversations on many topics. She listens carefully and speaks as easily and respectfully to patients, families, and students as to seasoned researchers and clinicians. She is a softly spoken and mild-mannered person with wide intellectual and cultural interests and a most generous heart, with ample personal experience of heartache and overcoming it. Consequently, she is likely to continue to make a lively active contribution to the intellectual, social, emotional, and passionate community of scholars, service-providers, service-users and their families and advocates in the mental health movement.

—Professor Alan Rosen, AO, FRANZCP, MRCPsych,
MBBS, DPM, Grand Dip, PAS, Sydney, Australia

Acknowledgments

In the 19th century, the famous French physiologist Claude Bernard remarked, "Art is I; science is we." More than 135 people worked on the Vermont and Maine Studies. These were two three-decade investigations following 538 people once expected to grow old and die in their state hospitals—instead, 49–68%+ were able to reclaim their lives. I have tried to tell as many of their stories as possible in this book. My dissertation alone had 10 pages of acknowledgments, probably more than any other in academic world history!

As the stories indicate, I was smart enough to know how little I knew, and I hired an army of well-qualified and multidisciplinary professionals to get the job done. These included psychiatrists, psychologists, social workers, educational and rehab specialists, statisticians, and our study participants who had the lived experience and taught us all what we needed to know. It was a huge legacy that I have endeavored to pass on.

Some of the colleagues who mentored me and who made the research and the book possible were George Albee, Bill Anthony, Takamaru Ashikaga, Chris and Margaret Beels, Malcolm Bowers, Alan Breier, George Brooks, James Brooks, Luc Ciompi, Carmine Consalvo, Larry Davidson, William Deane, Patricia Deegan, Michael DeSisto, Joseph Fleiss, Alan Gelenberg, Byron and M. J. Good, Hisham Hafez, Michael Hogan, Gerard Hogarty, Su-Ting Hsu, Samuel Keith, Marsha Kincheloe, Paul Landerl, Peter Laqueur, Paul Lieberman, Brendan Maher, Ron Mandersheid, Dennis McCrory, Loren Mosher, Jane Murphy and Alexander Leighton, Richard Musty, Gordon Neligh, Marilyn Patton, Jaak Rakfeldt, Priscilla Ridgway, Jon Rolf, Alan and Viv Rosen, Phillip Saperia, Robert Shapiro, John Strauss, George Vaillant, Richard Warner, Edward Zigler, and Joseph Zubin. They provided so much specific support, plus their own thoughtful writings and encouragement across time. Without their guidance, their devotion to unraveling mysteries, and their quick perception that I could surely use all the help I could get, the book and all its antecedents might have been relegated to the dustbins of history.

Having a grandmother and a daughter who were once librarians, the list of acknowledgments also includes the University of Vermont and Yale med school librarians who, in the era before the proliferation of computers, were essential to any research. The local reference librarians at Tabb Library in Virginia saved the day on many occasions later in the writing of this book. Administrative assistants Andrea Pierce and Linda Clark really ran the show in each state, and Vi Graham typed the first grant application. Included were a few students who were learning by doing, just as the principal investigator was quietly doing as well. These hard workers are rarely mentioned, and, if they are, they are often listed last. For a complete list of our collaborators, see the end of any of our four primary papers.

People who are often taken for granted behind the scenes but who are critical to the process are friends and family. My parents were Robert and Eleanor Main. My father was, in actual fact, a rocket scientist who dreamed about going to the moon and helped to develop the prototype for the Apollo Project with the teams at NASA-Langley and Marshall Space Flight Center in Huntsville as early as 1958. The project was called the Arcturus and had a lunar lander, a lunar rover, and a multistage rocket with semi-liquid, semi-solid propellant. The U.S. government was uninterested in the work until the Soviets sent up Sputnik in 1957, but even then, it took a couple of years to get things rolling. He worked in secrecy, and none of us knew, until his untimely death in 1963 near Cape Canaveral, exactly what he had been working on until someone in the government wrote his obituary. All we knew was that he was excited by his work and that his children should also be excited by their own dreams and work hard to accomplish them. This is what I, too, have found, given that early efforts revealed that while many patients, especially those with schizophrenia, could get their lives back, it has taken 60–70 years to advance that finding and the funding of programs that encourage a real recovery process. Our mother, Eleanor, was seen by her children as the usual 1940s and 1950s housewife until our father died at age 47. Suddenly she took herself back to school and became a crackerjack elementary teacher. She joined the American International Schools, taught in Guam and Dubai, and traveled all over the rest of the world. So, when I lost my husband at age 32, she was also my new role model, and I went back to school myself and began the research outlined in this book.

It seems that one of my family's mottos was telling the world how to think differently about things. My sister Wingate Payne became a journalist and was a member of the editorial board for 18 years at the *Miami Herald* newspaper and sometimes a "talking head" on CNN. My brother Elliott Main became an obstetrician and researcher. He helped to change his field of maternal and child health as a Stanford professor, and our little sister Daphne Main became Associate Professor in the School of Business and Coordinator of Accounting at Loyola University in New Orleans. Her dissertation was on the problems with auditor decision-making under ambiguity. Their support and examples helped their big sister change from a housewife to a professor herself.

However, the most important contributors to their mother's welfare were my three children, who actually lived day by day with the Vermont project while growing up. Robert, Brooke, and Ashley pitched right in with the dishes, cooking, and pet care while still in elementary and middle school. We studied together around the dining room table, and they checked my report cards. I graduated with my doctorate the year before my son, Robert, graduated from Princeton. He wrote his Stanford dissertation in chemistry on non-equilibrium thermodynamics which he had to explain to me at least three times. Brooke became a computer-savvy librarian, who brought the famous Baltimore-based Enoch Pratt Free Library into the modern era, now a web application developer, and a private pilot. She has fielded many a frantic call from her mother when the book-writing computer rebelled and she proposed the title for this book. Ashley has a BA in Asian Art History from Mills College. She was one of the first group of students from the University of Colorado-Denver allowed to return to Kunming, China after the Tiananmen Square student protests. Ashley has been working as a senior paralegal for more than 25 years in the Washington, D.C. area, and has written briefs for the Fourth Circuit Court of Appeals as well as the Board of Appeals for immigration cases. I am so proud of all their accomplishments and of who they have become as adults.

Other wonderful family members are my granddaughters, Jessica, a new electrical engineer, and Caroline Harding becoming a nurse (treasures of my life), and Adrienne Harding, their own dear mother; Cliff Ellis, Brooke's partner, rebuilder of World War II and commercial airplanes; and Daphne's husband, Grant Butterbaugh, a neuropsychologist who was terrific to talk research with. They all expanded my horizons. Elliott's wife, Denise Main, another obstetrician and genetic counselor who attempted to explain some genetics to me, and Hilary Harding, who wrote technical manuals for the Department of Defense, are my sisters-in-law. Everyone has kept the lights burning, their families humming, and cheered me on—all the while hoping that I would eventually get this "darn book finished."

In addition, I have been surrounded by a faithful cheering squad of friends who are still incredibly important to me today, some of whom have been for decades. Of special note have been Camille and Bill Anthony, Peter Ashenden, Taka and Pam Ashikaga, Chris Beels and Margaret Newmark, Susan Childers, Caterina Corbascio, Betty Dahlquist and Paul Sherman, Art Dell Orto, David and Darragh Ellerson, Bob and Ann Elliott, Pat Feinberg, Alberto Fergusson, Mary Ellen Fortini, Frank Kirchner and David Nicholson, Paul Landerl, Martha Long, Jesse Kurtz Main, Tom and Ciri Malamud, Cathy and Bill McMains, Yvonne and Pete Moody, Judith Morse, Gina and Bob Nikkel, Joan Rapp, Trish Rone, Alan and Viv Rosen, Pat Russo, Margie Staker, Sandy Steingard, Jim and Joyce Stockdill, John Strauss, Linnea Taylor, Anne-Kari Torgalsbøen, Paul and Pam Troth, Phyllis Vine, Debbie Waldron, Yu-Mui Wan, Alan Weiss, and Jan and Stan Zisk.

Some are neighbors, such as Shirley and Tom White, Wes and Nina Thomas, Gary and Ann Cole. Marie and Ken Havener, Oscar and Susana Pimental, and Ron Foster, all of whom continue to provide cheer and much needed support, especially after I became a 77-year-old widow trying to finish a book with my devoted labradoodle. Katie by my side.

I am also indebted to my local editors who contributed so much to helping me write more clearly early on and keep my sanity. Linnea (who went the distance) Wingate, Yvonne, Phyllis, and Margaret have been godsends. Oxford's only instruction was that the book had to be for a wide audience and match their 61-page protocol. That was very tricky because my previous writing had been in academic journals. But I did appreciate Oxford's resilience while I struggled to get it done. Finally, I was assigned Executive Editor Sarah Harrington, at Oxford. Her support was unwavering, and she had an eagle eye toward replacing mundane words with elegant ones and convoluted phrasings with clarity and wisdom. I wish to also thank the unsung heroes of the Production crew: Sarah Ebel in NY, Divya Settu in Chennai and Annie Woy in PA. If the book is readable, interesting, and looks a lot more polished, it is because of everyone's guidance in NY and India, their generosity, skills, and endless patience.

I retired and moved to Virginia at age 71, to be with my new, but now late, husband, Everett Burton. He was a contractor working at NASA-Langley in the Analysis and Computational Section for more than 40 years. Although totally uninterested in problems with psychiatry and schizophrenia, he managed to support me when I periodically disappeared into my home office, cluttered high with boxes of scientific literature, in order to write while he created beautiful and peaceful gardens outside.

And last but not least, I would like to say how much I appreciated Stephen Deutsch, former chair of psychiatry at Eastern Virginia Medical School. He made me a visiting professor with access to the med school library—a real godsend.

In looking over this section of the book, it is clear that I am a most fortunate and grateful person and that there are many more helpful people not mentioned but much appreciated.

Introduction

This is a book about 11 worldwide long-term research studies, each of two to three decades long after first admission or long chronic hospitalizations. They provide evidence about the possibility of significant improvement and recovery from schizophrenia. Included are chapters about programs promoting forward movement as well as stories from the lives of patients, many of whom got their lives back, and the power of hope.

Since two of our own three-decade studies were completed in Vermont and Maine in the United States,[1-4] I have become fascinated that Northern New Englanders, like Alaskan native peoples, have more than 50 ways to describe snow (e.g., sleet, softly falling snow, powder, snowfall, drifting snow, slush, blizzards, flurries, hard pack, and blanket, etc.).[5] Each word helps to define a given—and often changing—situation and suggests how to cope with it. Like those many different types of snow, an older and outdated understanding of schizophrenia is slowly being replaced by the concept of Schizophrenia Spectrum Disorders,[6] reflecting a range of symptom presentations to the field of psychiatry, which also needs a broader array of strategies to understand and deal with these complex problems.

What is it about snow and becoming buried in it? Like an acute onset in schizophrenia, some skiers happily crisscross a slope in the high country away from commercial ski areas after a new snowfall. Suddenly and seemingly out of nowhere, an avalanche sweeps down, knocks skiers off their feet, and sends them tumbling under the snow. They have difficulty determining which way is up so they can try to dig out. If they are very lucky, trained people and dogs will find them. Many skiers will never ski in an unmarked area again, but some continue to do so at repeated risk, just like many first-episode patients will never have another episode (whereas many others will).

The slow onset of schizophrenia or other psychotic events is like drifting snow piling up. It can be difficult to tell at first if this is just a typical case

Recovery from Schizophrenia. Courtenay M. Harding, Oxford University Press. © Courtenay M. Harding 2024.
DOI: 10.1093/oso/9780195380095.001.0001

of a distressed young person withdrawing from friends and family, spending time alone on the computer or playing a guitar, forgetting hygiene, and becoming quite unpredictable. Thinking becomes muddled and emotions fluctuate. Then it can become terrifying when this person (and the family) cannot count on the usual strategies to pull out of the bad mood and behaviors. Panic replaces worry. Hallucinations and delusions try to make sense of a changeable world. Talking and behaviors become more and more disinhibited and disorienting. Months go by. Help is desperately sought, usually by others. The chaos and fear often become worse in a noisy, chaotic environment and simmer down in a quiet one. It is tough to dig out.

Blizzards of reduced visibility have affected the ideas put forth by psychiatry in the understanding and treatment of schizophrenia. For more than a century, a pessimistic stance toward schizophrenia maintained that it was basically not very treatable. Since the late 1800s, outcome was seen as marginal at best but mostly downhill.[7] Medications, introduced as miracles in the past 70 years, are seen as calming and suppressing some flamboyant symptoms and behaviors but neglecting important other ones, such as disorganized thinking, showing little emotion, and withdrawal from human interactions—all while piling on pharmacological side effects, but with no recovery or cure as hoped.[8]

For 125 years, schizophrenia spectrum was called "dementia praecox," then later renamed a "group of schizophrenias," and then just "schizophrenia" but divided into subtypes. Recently those subtypes were dropped as well. In addition, Asian psychiatry has started to rename and re-imagine schizophrenia.[9] Models have changed from illness to psychosocial to neurochemical (treated by medications) to biomedical (a brain disease)—none of which has provided any real understanding of what is going on, even though each model has declared it does. Tom Insel, who once ran the National Institute for Mental Health (NIMH), suggested that perhaps "schizophrenia" is similar to a term like "fever."[10] Fever is not considered an illness by itself but more of a symptom signal indicating the body is mostly coping with the possibility, in this example, of an infection of many different possible types. It appears that, in the case of schizophrenia, for instance, it may be a symptom signaling many unknown causes and pathways. However, decisions have been made to announce that the cause of schizophrenia is a brain disease/neurochemical disorder—yet without much really solid evidence that one of these might be the case. Instead, it is a current best-guess because the field has failed to produce brain scans, blood tests, or genetic markers diagnosable of and specific to schizophrenia as of 2024.[11] The assumption of brain disease has become frozen in place as *fact*, but challenges have surfaced and the snowplows are out.

Investigators from these 11 long-term studies followed people once diagnosed with schizophrenia over the course of two to three decades. All have all systematically found improvement and/or recovery over time in more than one-half to two-thirds of their combined cohorts of 2,700 people. Something is going on. Innovative clinicians have produced and researched a multitude of helpful programs. Many such programs are considered evidence-based by researchers, and others are shown to be actively successful. And all of them are still barely implemented due to policy and monetary constraints. Many people with the lived experiences of psychosis continue to provide significant evidence of and pathways toward recovery despite this unnecessary uphill climb,[12] but these innovative programs would help everyone still struggling.

One of the first possible thaws began 70 years ago, when a young psychiatrist named George Brooks, living and working in snowy Vermont, went looking for the people buried underneath the avalanche of schizophrenia in the state's only psychiatric hospital. Dr. Brooks and his staff (including his aides), along with his most profoundly disabled long-stay, back-ward patients, put their heads together to figure out why they were still profoundly struggling even after the introduction and use of chlorpromazine (Thorazine). These very chronic patients were expected to die in the hospital. Several early chapters of this book discuss the influences impacting this hospital and community program and how this extraordinary work evolved, work that was unlike anything ever done before.[13] It became world-famous and clinicians flocked to Vermont to understand how it happened. Contradictory to his biological training, Brooks found that by using this innovative program recovery and significant improvement were possible in his once profoundly disabled patients. Two-thirds of them reclaimed their lives! How this amazing feat was accomplished provides important direction for working with today's patients, insofar as most diagnosed people are still considered chronically ill even though most are trying to live in the community, and most with fairly minimal care. Brooks and his so-called hopeless cases laid the foundation of psychiatric rehabilitation, elaborated two decades later by Bill Anthony and the Boston University Center.[14]

Ninety-seven percent of Brooks's original cohort members were tracked for three decades after their first admission, with the help of NIMH and foundation funding and using comprehensive scientific protocols. We found that two-thirds of this group, which once were expected to grow old and die in the hospital, were able to make a decent life for themselves across time. What Brooks and these patients invented was an ingenious comprehensive program that is supremely relevant today. We have described the Vermont process carefully as it unfolded. During the past decades, more and more investigators have emerged reporting similar data worldwide. People with apparently permanent, chronic forms of schizophrenia and psychotic forms of major affective disorders can indeed significantly improve, and many fully recover.[15] How did this happen, and what are their strategies and ramifications?

I discovered this group in 1976, a year after the 20th anniversary of the program, quite by accident while looking for a small research project. Being intrigued by my pilot study results, I decided we needed to locate the rest of the original cohort ($N = 269$) and find out how they were doing. Thanks to significant funding by the NIMH and some from the Robert Wood Johnson Foundation, we were able to find 97% at an average of 32 years after their first hospital admissions. We ended up with one of the longest and most complete studies in the world literature.

The middle section of this book reveals how more than 100 senior multidisciplinary academic and clinical professionals from across the United States recognized how important it was to find out about this group, and they contributed their expertise to create a study with the toughest methodology and design possible. Field interviewers spent an average of 5 hours at kitchen tables across Vermont and elsewhere, armed with classic scales, schedules, and a Life Chart. Our medical records were especially comprehensive because the hospital had taken part in the original Thorazine trials during the early 1950s. All participants were rediagnosed using contemporary criteria. Our findings on continued significant improvement or recovery in these once long-stay patients with schizophrenia or chronic major affective disorders with psychotic features were exciting and showed us many new areas in recovery to consider. These findings continue to cause debates within the biomedical field.

Findings from our second long-term project (with participants averaging 36 years since first admission) was completed in Maine as a matched comparison study; these participants received minimal to no rehab programming. There, we found that there could also be a slow natural movement toward regaining health, a fact on which the Vermont rehab program was also building.

It turns out that nine other long-term studies of outcome from across the world revealed similar findings of improvement and recovery, and all had been mostly ignored by psychiatry as well. These studies are discussed and their findings described in later chapters.

Recovery as a possibility was finally recognized in the 1990s and is now acknowledged in the literature as well as in program and policy publications.[16,17] But programs and funding have basically remained almost the same as before, which means continued chronicity for so many people with these diagnoses. Programs continue to primarily consist of stabilization, maintenance, medications, and entitlements, with efforts at finding housing and learning to behave better socially. Rarely are such patients told that there might be a chance to recover and, critically, given some hope of doing so.

The last two chapters of the book discuss many other exciting programs in the United States and abroad with demonstrated effective and evidence-based results. All the inventors of these programs are thoughtful and creative innovators. Many programs did not cost much. Many were made in conjunction with or by people experiencing symptoms. Yet most of these programs are *still* not available to most struggling and disabled people. It is imperative that we change how we fund behavioral managed care and other community centers so that this rich trove of little-used strategies is available to all people struggling to get better. Otherwise, it is like saying to a cancer patient, "Yes, we have all these strategies and treatments but they are not available to you. Sorry."

Change includes rethinking the biomedical approach to bring social context, psychological functioning, and environmental impact into the mix as a comprehensive model. This integration shifts everything. Many more improvements and recoveries will happen. The power structure shifts from hierarchical to horizontal. This alteration will also mean that clinicians can find more joy in their practice by getting to know in depth the patients whom they serve, as whole persons with interesting lives, learning to reclaim their futures, walking the path together and teaching one another. Psychiatrists, patients, peer groups, families, rehab workers, psychologists, social workers, and multiple community players—everyone has something important to contribute by working together, growing together, solving problems together, and celebrating every inch forward toward improvement and recovery.

REFERENCES

1. Harding, C. M., Brooks, G. W., Ashikaga, T., Strauss, J. S., & Breier, A. (1987a). The Vermont longitudinal study of persons with severe mental illness: I. Methodology, study sample, and overall status 32 years later. *American Journal of Psychiatry*, *144*(6), 718–726.

2. Harding, C. M., Brooks, G. W., Ashikaga, T., Strauss, J. S., & Breier, A. (1987b). The Vermont longitudinal study: II. Long-term outcome of subjects who retrospectively met DSM-III criteria for schizophrenia. *American Journal of Psychiatry*, *144*(6), 727–735.

3. DeSisto, M. J., Harding, C. M., McCormick, R. V., Ashikaga, T., & Brooks, G. W. (1995a). The Maine-Vermont three-decade studies of serious mental illness: I. Matched comparison of cross-sectional outcome. *British Journal of Psychiatry*, *167*, 331–338.

4. DeSisto, M. J., Harding, C. M., McCormick, R. J., Ashikaga, T., & Brooks, G. W. (1995b). The Maine-Vermont three-decade studies of serious mental illness: II. Longitudinal course comparisons. *British Journal of Psychiatry*, *167*, 338–342.

5. https://www.washingtonpost.com/national/health-science/there-really-are-50-eskimo-words-for-snow/2013/01/14/e0e3f4e0-59a0-11e2-beee-6e38f52 15402_story.html

6. American Psychiatric Association. (2013). *Diagnostic and statistical manual of mental disorders – (5th ed.)* https://doi.org/10.1176/appi.books.9780890425596

7. Kraepelin, E. (1902). Dementia Praecox. In *Clinical psychiatry: A textbook for students and physicians* (6th ed.). (Trans. A. B. Diefendorf), Macmillan.

8. Steingard, S. (2019). Chapter 5: Clinical implications of the drug-centered approach. In: Sandra Steingard (Ed.), *Critical psychiatry: Controversies and clinical implications* (pp. 113–135). Springer.

9. Takahashi, H., Ideno, T., Okubo, S., Matsui, H., Takemura, K., Matsuura, M., Kato, M., & Okubo, Y. (2009). Impact of changing the Japanese term for "schizophrenia" for reasons of stereotypical beliefs of schizophrenia in Japanese youth. *Schizophrenia Research*, *112*(1-3), 149–152.

10. Insel, T. (2010). Rethinking schizophrenia. *Nature*. *468*(7321), 187–193. doi:10.1038/nature09552

11. van Os, J. (2016). Schizophrenia does not exist. *British Medical Journal*, 352–375. doi:https://doi.org/10.1136/bmj.i375

12. Vine, P. (2022). *Fighting for recovery: An activists' history of mental health reform*. Beacon Press.

13. Chittick, R. A., Brooks, G. W., Irons, F. S., & Deane, W. N. (1961). *The Vermont Story: Rehabilitation of chronic schizophrenic patients*. Queen City Printers, Out of Print.

14. Anthony W. A. (1993). Recovery from mental illness: The guiding vision of the mental health services system in the 1990s. *Psychiatric Rehabilitation Journal*, *16*, 11–24.

15. Harrow, M., Jobe, T. H., Faull, R. N., & Yang, J. (2017). A twenty-year multi-followup longitudinal study assessing whether antipsychotic medications contribute to work functioning in schizophrenia. *Psychiatry Research*, *256*, 267–274. doi:10.1016/psychres.2017.06069

16. Davidson, L., Harding, C. M., & Spaniol, L. (Eds.). (2005). *Research on Recovery from Severe Mental Illness: 30 years of Accumulating Evidence and Its Implications for Practice* (Vol. 1). Center for Psychiatric Rehabilitation, Boston University.

17. Davidson, L., Harding, C. M., & Spaniol, L. (Eds.). (2006). *Research on Recovery from Severe Mental Illness: 30 years of Accumulating Evidence and Its Implications for Practice* (Vol. 2). Center for Psychiatric Rehabilitation, Boston University.

PART ONE

Evolution of a
Revolution

I

Shocking Treatment in Colonial Vermont and Elsewhere

It seems to me that coping with the effects of what is called schizophrenia and with other devastating and debilitating mental health problems causes lives to be upended by metaphorical avalanches. The effect is compounded by traditional treatment and management approaches as people try to dig themselves out. Ineffective help is another avalanche to knock them down. People are left feeling diminished, denied, and ignored. The fact that much of the research in this book emanated from northern New England makes this metaphor seem doubly poignant because the winters there see an average of about 6–8 feet of snow plus a few avalanches each year.

To understand how remarkable the shift in care was in Vermont during the mid-1950s and early 1960s, which I will shortly describe, we need to understand what preceded those changes and why what happened in Vermont is still relevant to care today, 70 years later. What went on in New England starting in the 18th century reflected what was going on everywhere in early America as the nation grew in size and complexity. Knowing a little of this history will engender keen appreciation of how unusual the changes were that occurred in 1955 for the most chronic, demoralized, and dysfunctional patients, those diagnosed with schizophrenia and severe affective disorders. (And no, I am not talking about the advent of psychopharmacology because the patients under study who I describe had such a poor response to chlorpromazine [Thorazine] that they were unable to leave the hospital.)

Now, decades later, we need to rediscover Vermont's integrated components and philosophy of care, a model of care and treatment that brought

Recovery from Schizophrenia. Courtenay M. Harding, Oxford University Press. © Courtenay M. Harding 2024.
DOI: 10.1093/oso/9780195380095.003.0001

people from all over the world to come see for themselves. These revelations might restore hope and optimism among staff, patients, and families and encourage current programs around the world to start moving in the right direction.

"Care" in Early Vermont

In the 1790s, each small town in Vermont, as in many of the colonial regions, had an Overseer of the Poor, an official with absolute authority over those who were considered "poor, vagrant, idle and disorderly persons, idiots and lunatics."[1] The options for the disposition of such people were jails, almshouses, poor farms, or indentured servitude.

Early America, especially in rural areas, had few medically trained physicians. Those people filling the doctor's job "were often untrained apprentices who doubled as clergymen, barbers, civil officers, and plantation owners."[2,3] By 1824, houses for the poor in Burlington, Vermont, were thought to be "ridding the town of a worthless population," and Superintendents were authorized to "fetter, shackle, or whip" the Inmates.[4,5] Indeed, by 1850, there were 560 persons considered insane living in Vermont, out of a total population of 314,120.[6]

> For several decades the laws [of Vermont] were broad enough so that the overseer of the poor could auction off the poor and their families in a public place, he could bind them to an employer for many years, he could put them in jail or a miserable poor-house, etc. He was permitted to dispose of them separately with no regard for the family ties.[7,8,9]

The language of this job description is astonishing, especially for a state that latter prided itself on antislavery sentiments (Vermont was the first colony to outlaw slavery); these earlier actions and attitudes seem wildly contradictory.

Brief Thaws: The Era of Moral Treatment

In England, a new model of care had been proposed at the asylum known as the York Retreat. The Retreat based many of its ideas on the work of the Frenchman Philippe Pinel (1745–1826). Distressed by the suicide of a friend, Pinel, along with a trusted psychiatric aide, rescued a substantial number of people from the water-logged basement of Hospice de la Salpêtrière and from the disastrous biological treatments of the day (such as bleeding, purging, and blistering).[10] Instead, Pinel and his aide listened to these people and gave them access to the sunshine of the courtyard. Mental distress, Pinel believed, was the result of social and psychological factors and not moral failings (as was commonly held at the time). Pinel developed individualized approaches for treatment and studied diagnostic categories. He often hired recovered patients as staff and felt that "space, kindness, consolation, hope, and humor worked better" than common practices of the day.[11,12]

Like Pinel, William Tuke in England witnessed a good friend being brutalized at a local English asylum and, in 1796, decided to set up The Retreat, in York, open to members of the Quaker group, also known as the Society of Friends. Tuke deliberately avoided use of the term "hospital," which had become synonymous with the notorious Bethlem Hospital (the infamous asylum that came to be known as "Bedlam"). Tuke determined that treatment of patients with either melancholy (now called depression) or raving madness should involve the "elevation and reorganization of patients' mental processes," and he used philosophy, music, art, and literature to accomplish these goals.[13] This approach was in stark contrast to the usual treatments of the day for upper-class patients, which included laudanum (an opiate), leeches, and bloodletting. Meanwhile, the poorer patients in Bethlem were simply thrown in a cell and chained to the wall, often without clothes and only a blanket to cover themselves. Well-to-do people from town were allowed to come and stare.

In 1963, historian Samuel Bockhoven wrote a full and eloquent description of the helpful effects of Tuke's approach, known as Moral Treatment (borrowed from Pinel's *Traite de Morale*). The word "moral" was then defined quite differently from our current understanding of morality, which indicates the difference between right and wrong.[14] Into the 1840s, the word *moral* indicated "compassionate and understanding treatment of innocent sufferers," as was acknowledged to also impact "emotions and self-esteem."[15] Moral Treatment included a regular and organized schedule of physical and mental activities for the day, kind treatment with minimal or no use of restraints, and a relatively stress-free environment, an approach more similar to today's goals in rehabilitation.[16]

Tuke planted trees, orchards, flowers, and vegetable gardens so residents of his Retreat could be refreshed by nature. Each person had his or her own room with unbarred windows. There were sitting rooms where people could gather and talk. Patients were kept busy with work and considered to have "an innate core of goodness which could be restored to health by the proper environment and care."[17] The York Retreat still exists, is still Quaker, and treats patients, according to its website, with a focus on "equality and community, honesty and integrity, courage, peace, care for the environment, and hope."[18] However, in 2018, the government, in its wisdom, shut down the inpatient unit.[19]

Such ideas had also been tried centuries earlier in the mental health temples of ancient Greece and Rome, although when patients did not respond quickly enough, they were exiled.[20]

Vermont's Original Version of Moral Treatment

In 1834, the Vermont Asylum for the Insane in Brattleboro (now known as the Brattleboro Retreat) opened as a private hospital thanks to a $10,000 bequest (a remarkable sum in those days) from Anna Hunt Marsh, who lived at the intersection of Vermont, New Hampshire, and Massachusetts.[21] She was deeply distraught by the death of a young Brattleboro lawyer. He had been held under the icy cold "Bath of Surprise" until he lost consciousness and was then given a large dose of opium for "stupefaction of the senses," the preferred treatment of the time as espoused by Dr. James Brown of Edinburgh. Several years earlier, dismayed by the condition of a cousin at the State Lunatic Asylum at Worcester, Massachusetts, Mrs. Marsh had provided funds for that new hospital as well.[22]

The Vermont Asylum in Brattleboro had two classes of care and was originally designed to mimic the "moral management" theories of the day. This strategy was "to separate the distressed person from his or her family and worldly stressors, and to replace those relationships with a new family contained within the hospital."[23] "The patients, who, [according to its history], had been brought in to the Asylum as mad creatures chained in attics and huddling in hillside caves, quite naturally responded quickly and favorably to the support and love of their new family."[24]

Dorothea Dix From Maine

In 1840, along came social activist Dorothea Dix from Maine, who herself had grown up in an abusive household with an alcoholic father and a depressed and nonfunctional mother.[25] Having been exposed to the ideas of the York Retreat while staying in England, she began a 3-year, 10,000-mile trek across the United States, visiting "500 Almshouses, approximately 300 county jails, and an indeterminate number of hospitals."[26] She saw "miserable, wild, and stuporous men and women chained to walls and locked into pens—naked and filthy, brutalized, underfed, given no heat, sleeping on stone floors."[27] After assessing this appalling situation, she went to significant lengths to convince states of the need to build government-run hospitals.

To Dix, asylums in the truest sense of the word (meaning a place of safety, protection, sanctuary, and refuge) were ideally to be built in the rural countryside surrounded by nature and fresh air, outside of the rapidly expanding inner cities with their squalor, poverty, and pollution. Her efforts, and those of Dr. Thomas Kirkbride of Philadelphia, shifted the care and financial burden of suffering indigent persons from beleaguered families and communities to the state. During the same time, this strategy was advocated by the activist Horace Mann, who had shifted schools to state administration as well.[28]

In her lifetime, Dix saw 123 hospitals built and was instrumental in the founding of 32 of them.[29] The Kirkbride Plan for building hospitals included architectural blueprints designed to make the buildings themselves a therapeutic experience, with access to more fresh air and sunshine, separation of the sexes, and isolation of loud and disruptive people from better-functioning patients, as well as from the administrative offices of course.[30,31]

In 1846, Samuel Woodward, President of the Association of Medical Superintendents of American Institutions for the Insane (the forerunner of the American Psychiatric Association), read a paper before its annual meeting. Dr. Woodward said

> The abandonment of depletion, external irritants, drastic purges, and starvation, and the substitution of baths, narcotics and a generous diet, is not less to be appreciated than the change from manacles, chains, by locks, and confining chairs, to the present system of kindness, confidence, social intercourse, labor, religious teaching, and freedom from restraint. In this age of improvement, no class of mankind has felt its influence more favorably than the insane.[32]

Before the Vermont Asylum was built in 1834, only 4 of the 10 hospitals existing in the eastern states offered Moral Treatment, which by then had been rechristened as "Moral Management." Other hospitals included Bloomingdale Insane Asylum in New York (now The Haven at Westchester); the Connecticut Retreat for the Insane (now the Institute of Living in Hartford); McLean Asylum for the Insane, part of Massachusetts General in Belmont (known simply as McLean Hospital); and the Friends Asylum in the Frankford area of Philadelphia (now Friends Hospital). The Friends Asylum was originally begun in 1813, by Quakers, as the Asylum for the Relief of Persons Deprived of the Use of Their Reason and is the oldest hospital in the nation in continuous use.

The Asylum in Brattleboro attempted to copy much of the model of Moral Treatment, but, by 1873, it was found to have committed some sane individuals. A federal judge ordered an immediate investigation, which also found that some people had been incarcerated in basement cells. Other infractions against Moral Treatment were "the austerity of the wards, the barrenness of the closed yards, the total lack of religious services and cultural activities."[33]

How the Solution Became the Problem

Ironically, Dix's state hospital solution quickly became the next major public health problem as patients were simply custodialized in huge institutions without treatment.[34] Albert Deutsch, a 20th-century journalist and mental health advocate, also pointed out that "between 1840 and 1890, the general population of the United States increased from seventeen to nearly sixty-three million persons." The report went on to say that, during the same period, persons confined in American asylums grew from 2,561 in 1840 to 74,028 by 1890.[35] Hospitals had become dangerously overcrowded.

"Treatment" in state hospitals consisted of "three hots and a cot" (meaning three hot meals and a bed on which to sleep), generally in a large room with 50–60 other patients in facilities that had grown from the intended maximum of 250 beds to an overwhelming total of 15,000 in some institutions. Because patients might attempt or complete suicide with a belt or shoelaces, these were taken away from all, replaced with shapeless shifts and slippers. False teeth and eyeglasses were also removed for safety's sake. There was no privacy, significant abuses, no respect for individual needs or differences, no hope for improvement or recovery, and no expectations other than that staff and patients would grow old together. Few physicians were interested in the job of working in an asylum, so day-to-day care was primarily provided by aides with minimal training and little understanding of mental illness. In 1890, President of the American Psychiatric Association, William Godding, wrote

> The overcrowding goes on, cots are brought out at night and laid down on the corridor floors, at first one or two in nooks or alcoves that seem designed for this sort of thing, but the business grows, the special adaptation of recesses and alcoves becomes less apparent as the line of beds side by side stretches in lengthening vista down the hall. And still the floors fill up until one, two, three hundred are thus nightly—not accommodated but provided for. . . . Day by day, year by year, I have seen individualized treatment of special cases swamped by the rising tide of indiscriminate lunacy pouring through the wards, filling every crevice, rising higher and higher until gradually most distinctions and landmarks have been blotted out.[36]

"Treatments" at the turn of the 20th century again consisted of mechanical restraints such as camisoles, muffs, restraining sheets, even steel bed saddles, and hydrotherapy. Patients had no rights and were rarely reviewed for current symptom status after 2 years.[37]

The idea that living in a total institution itself could actually *cause* unusual behaviors did not take hold until Erving Goffman published his book *Asylums* in 1961.[38] In fact, by 1971, Arnold Ludwig wrote of accommodations made by patients to survive. He described a "good" patient as "dull, harmless, and inconspicuous, someone who being able to evade responsibility (sic), minimize stress, ignore others, to retain the right to behave unpredictably and have a certain diplomatic immunity."[39] Indeed, such patients abounded in these ever-increasing custodial institutions until they reached a population peak in 1955 of 559,000 individuals across the nation.[40]

Today state hospitals across America, with their large collections of multiple brick buildings and clusters of outbuildings, can be spotted from miles away. Many of these old hospitals have been converted to condos or have fallen into disrepair; some have completely disappeared. In some cases, former consumers of services have begun to rehabilitate the old weed-clogged cemeteries where deceased patients were buried beneath small, numbered stones—but which now carry names.[41]

The New Vermont State Asylum for the Insane

In 1888, the Vermont state government began to assume the responsibility and the cost of caring for people with serious mental illness. A new state hospital was funded and built in 1891, located in the very small town of Waterbury (population 2,232 then; now only about 3,200), 13 miles down the road from the state capital. The hospital sat in a lush green valley at the foot of Camels Hump, next to the Winooski River (a Native American word meaning "river of the onion," a vegetable known as *ramps or a garlic onion*). The hospital consisted of a cluster of buildings built like a French fortress, including round buildings with turrets.

A transfer of patients from the Asylum in Brattleboro began immediately with some forensic patients who had been deemed unfit for criminal proceedings. The Asylum had been experiencing increasingly overcrowded conditions, like most other hospitals in the country. In fact, every time the Asylum in Brattleboro added new buildings, the beds were immediately filled, eventually reaching a population of 400 people. Very soon, Brattleboro had sent most of its indigent patients to the new state hospital, whose population rose to 498 by 1896; the physical plant was severely taxed within 5 years.[42] Because the similar names of the hospitals caused confusion, the original hospital changed its name to the Brattleboro Retreat in 1892, and reverted to a private institution.[43]

By 1897, Vermont State Asylum Superintendent Dr. Frank W. Page had changed things dramatically. He had the facility cleaned from stem to stern; moved patients out of the cold, damp basement; removed mechanical restraints and seclusion; remodeled buildings; and landscaped the premises.[44] He also fired employees who were "inefficient and undisciplined" and introduced uniforms to provide some dignity to the retained staff members.[45] The name, Vermont State Asylum for the Insane, was changed in 1898 to Vermont State Hospital for the Insane (VSH), in the hopes that the shift would "rob the place of many of its terrors and remove the idea of abuses and inhumane treatment from the minds of the laity."[46] A pathology building was built then in the name of science, complete with a row of glass jars containing the brains of deceased patients awaiting investigation. A very large farm was acquired, and the early years saw a slaughter house, a piggery, a 250-chicken hennery, and a ball field built.[47] Many more buildings were added to the campus over the years.

In 1918, the worldwide influenza epidemic killed many patients and staff at VSH, including the superintendent. During this stressful time, many patients pitched in to help run the wards. There are many such stories from all over the world, with the common scenario of patients providing assistance whenever a calamity arose. By 1920, the hospital's population, despite the flu, had risen to 733. *Industrial therapy*, which essentially involved putting patients to work, began for male patients who took on janitorial work and manual labor within the hospital; women were taught "fancy work," basket-making, weaving, and rug-making.⁴⁸ Note that these activities were mainly considered to be therapy and not job skill building for the outside world.

There existed a traditional class system within VSH, as revealed in this description by sociologist William Deane of the facility's dining arrangements

> In the old dining room system . . . there were four dining areas: one for male patients, one for female patients, one for non-medical staff (including nurses), and the fourth for Professional Staff, the so-called "Doctors Dining Room." . . . [It] was [like] an unostentatious but dignified restaurant from an old section of Boston . . . such as Beacon Hill [whereas] the male dining room was considered to be like . . . the old Joliet, Illinois State Prison. The difference between these two menus was likened to 'the difference between the worst greasy spoon and Delmonico's [a fancy restaurant in New York City].' Further descriptions emphasized the 'social stiffness' of the Doctor's Dining Room with unwritten rules of where people sat, how much they would be served, and the extreme quietness required. Patients were the wait staff.⁴⁹

In their detailed 1988 book about the history of Vermont State Hospital, Marsha Kincheloe and Herbert Hunt describe events that occurred between 1925 and 1936.⁵⁰ In response to the surge in popularity of the American Eugenics Society, Vermont undertook a survey of all families who had a member or members with a history of legal entanglements, institutionalization, imprisonment, aboriginal background, delinquent or retarded children, or evidence of incest. The goal was "to purify and elevate the general population through widespread sterilization."⁵¹ Vermont was the only state, out of 22 in the union at that time, which refused to legalize mandatory sterilization (though some were still conducted). Such a project would be considered both illegal and shocking today. Fortunately, wiser heads prevailed, and the procedures were stopped. Eugenics proceeded in several other states and is still under periodic discussion today, believe it or not.⁵²

The Flood of 1927

According to Kincheloe and Hunt,[53] in October 1927, the rains came down and down. By early November, the Winooski River jumped its banks and began to flood the town of Waterbury and the hospital. The tunnels between buildings were filled, the electrical wires and heating pipes running through them shut down. As the water rose, 872 patients, 180 staff members, and all the hospital's records were moved to the second floor. There was no way of communicating between buildings. In one, everyone was forced to retreat to the attic. Livestock and one patient died, along with many residents of the village. Nearby citizens who were untouched by the flood began furiously to bake bread, fry doughnuts, and send water and milk to the villagers and hospital. The U.S. Army sent in "blankets, underwear, and medical supplies." It took 2 weeks to shovel out the mud.

> The reaction of the patients to their situation was remarkable. They did not seem to be in the least over-solicitous for their safety but rather seemed to have full confidence that the sturdy buildings would withstand almost any amount of flood and during the days immediately following there was a marked tendency to joke about the inconveniences and to make light of them.[54]

Overcrowding Continued

By 1936, 1,035 patients called the hospital home. More and more buildings and staff were added, but somehow it was never quite enough. Battles were waged between the superintendent, the state's governor, and members of the legislature. Politicians began to feel that state hospitals, like yachts, were a deep hole into which they poured money with little return. In 1948, Albert Deutsch published "The Shame of the States," which exposed the terrible conditions in state hospitals around the country.[55]

In 1944, a new superintendent, Rupert Chittick, took over. Upon his arrival he found twice as many patients as the buildings had been designed to accommodate, as well as an infestation of rats, roaches, and head lice. There were only two psychiatrists on staff. A third soon joined, but then one of the original physicians suddenly left in the middle of the night, leaving his keys on a table.[56] Chittick worked to develop his staff and relationships with the state's Department of Vocational Rehabilitation, social workers, and others to help solve some of the problems that the hospital was facing.

In 1947, George Brooks arrived as a new assistant physician, freshly discharged from the Army.

In the early to mid-1950s, there were 1,300 patients in Vermont State Hospital, but by then Brooks had already begun to instigate a revolution in the care of patients, and that is where this story really begins.[57]

2

The Evolution of a Vermont Country Doctor

Although I had worked with George Brooks for a couple of decades before he died, I found that I really didn't have the faintest idea why he had become a psychiatrist. Either I was not curious enough to ask enough questions, or he held much of his life close to his vest. Perhaps it was a little of both. So I rounded up his two sons one day and asked. Later, his brother Jim and I had many conversations over the phone. Much of George's early story came from the three of them, and I am retelling it here because I find many of the puzzle pieces of his life fit together in a remarkable way.

"Buddy, if you keep reading so many books, you'll end up in Waterbury someday," George was told, according to family lore. This prophecy of his mother's turned out to be true. "Waterbury" was code in Vermont for Vermont's only state hospital. "Buddy" was his mother's nickname for George W. Brooks, MD, who did end up working at the state hospital in Waterbury, as clinician, chief of research, and later as superintendent, for 37 years. We finally got him deinstitutionalized when he retired in 1984.

A Heritage That Affected Clinical Practice

Of the many mills run by the power of the Mad River in Warren, one of them belonged to Henry and Lena Brooks, George's parents. They made bobbins and bowling pins. Like many lumber mills, three of the Brooks's mills had burned down but they kept rebuilding. During the Great Depression, Henry was determined not to lay off his workers, so they kept making their products even though they were not being bought. These shaped and

Recovery from Schizophrenia. Courtenay M. Harding, Oxford University Press. © Courtenay M. Harding 2024.
DOI: 10.1093/oso/9780195380095.003.0002

painted wood pieces piled up and rotted in a shed. Henry borrowed about $40,000 to keep his workers on salary. When he couldn't pay it back, he slept for 3 days at the bank to get it to accept 2,500 acres of sugarbush and timberland as repayment. After all, a deal is a deal. Those acres are now part of a major ski mountain, the Sugarbush Resort, and are worth millions, much to the family's regret. But, as it turned out, the lessons of honesty and fair play were not lost on George.

Henry and Lena had a hobby of fixing up houses and selling them, so the family moved often, to different homes around the village. They had three children: a daughter, Arlie, and two sons, George and James. George was born in 1920, as the middle child. The children were born 7½ years apart so each was raised almost as if he or she was an only child. The family joke was that it took his parents "longer than elephants to have a child."

A Vermont Kind of Childhood

The village of Warren in the 1920s and 1930s was populated by 400 people of strong Yankee and French-Canadian traditions clustered within 36 square miles and nestled along the banks of the Mad River. As was, and still is, the case in many Vermont communities, everyone knew everyone else and their business. Children roamed freely, and all the adults watched over them. There was one general store with its wheel of cheddar cheese next to a choice of fishing tackle, and a one-room schoolhouse nearby that went to grade eight.

The family fondly described how George one day forgot to tie the family's Jersey cow to her rope and walked, his nose in a book, all the way to their pasture across the field near the mill pond. He had the rope but not the cow, being deeply lost in thought of other things. Eventually, as a psychiatrist, this remarkable ability to concentrate enabled George to listen earnestly to his patients without distraction, and he continued to read voluminously. These skills helped him change his profession.

Growing Up

George was a fragile child, prone to seizures and kidney problems. He much preferred to read than to run around. Following local folk wisdom, his parents had him sleep out on the porch under a pile of blankets to make him hardier. Given the frigid Vermont winters, it was a tough assignment. He slept so soundly that, when the dam on the Mad River broke with a loud crack during the infamous flood of 1927, he slept right through it. Everyone else rushed outside but George awoke the next morning to a new landscape, and this story became another family legend.

George attended the one-room schoolhouse and watched as other kids, who had come from impoverished households, struggled to make a life for themselves. Everyone was short of vitamins and showed symptoms of pre-pellagra and rickets. Cod liver oil was dished out from one spoon to 30 kids. As George became even more aware of the village's disabled and disadvantaged, he determined, by sophomore year in high school, that he would dedicate his life to helping people.

Another Warren boy was Kenneth J. Tillotson, MD, who later became well known as Psychiatrist-in-Chief at McLean Hospital of the Massachusetts General Hospital.[1] He became a family friend, role model, and mentor to young George. He later played an important role in George's career as a biological psychiatrist and psychopharmacologist.

George went on to high school in Montpelier, the state capital, 28 miles away. The first 18 miles was a dirt road, so, at age 13, he had to get a room in the city, becoming very self-reliant. Montpelier's population at the time was about 7,837 people, but, over seven decades later, the population hovered only around 7,484.[2]

Later, George attended the University of New Hampshire (Class of '41) because it was less expensive than the University of Vermont (UVM). His sleeping ability again became legendary: in 1938, he slept through a hurricane that ripped the roof off his dormitory.

George majored in pre-med but also became enamored of philosophy and wanted to switch majors. When he told his parents, they reportedly replied, "not with our money." So he went back to medicine. Much later, when Robert Spitzer, MD, and others sent a survey to US psychiatrists in the mid-1970s to find out which area of psychiatry was guiding their practices during the publication process of the third edition of the *Diagnostic and Statistical Manual of Mental Disorders* (DSM-III),[3] George was the only one who responded, "omnivorous," and indeed he was![4]

George went on to the UVM for his medical degree, then to an internship at the Mary Fletcher Hospital in Burlington. According to his family, he was reported by one of his professors as being "as smart as a whip." He shared an apartment with his younger brother, Jim, who was attending Burlington High School. Every weekend Jim would ride his bike 50 miles back home to Warren, a 5-hour trip. With his weekends free from a little brother, George met, courted, and married Jean Duncan, a red-haired nurse, during his second year of medical school. Brother Jim had to rent a room elsewhere.

The family found George to be fun-loving but serious and quick on his feet, because any family member could be cut to ribbons by the frequent sarcasm being dished out by all. George would come home and tell his mother everything he had just learned, and when she complained, he asked if "she wouldn't like to get her money's worth for his education?" George then went to serve in the US Army Medical Corps in 1944. During World War II, medical training was reduced in length.

How World War II Changed Everything

Back in Vermont, Dr. Rupert Chittick was appointed Superintendent at the state hospital during the same year, 1944. He had been trained at Harvard and worked as a psychiatrist at McLean Hospital. In Vermont, only two psychiatrists cared for more than 1,000 patients in an extremely over-crowded setting.[5] Many doctors and other staff members went off to war, but, fortunately, many of these patients had been trained to work in many roles throughout the hospital (such as working on the farm; housekeeping; working in the carpenter shop, food service, the mending room, and as office messengers). These "temporary workers" filled in for absent staff, and nurses even rode Morgan horses across Vermont to make house calls and care for a wide range of illnesses because of the extreme shortage of gasoline.

The military rejected for service more than 2 million men out of 15 million (13%) because of screening for psychiatric or neurological disorders.[6] When returning GIs came home in need of vocational training, many had psychiatric disabilities as well. In fact, 40% of medical military discharges were partially or fully due to psychiatric problems.[7]

The Vocational Rehabilitation Act was amended by Congress in 1943 to include and legitimize such services for psychiatric patients and thus began a new era of experimental rehabilitation efforts, including the efforts in Vermont undertaken during the mid-1950s and early 1960s.[8] However, it wasn't until early in the 1970s that a young psychologist, William Anthony, began to forge the new professional field of psychiatric rehabilitation in Boston. He developed comprehensive treatment strategies and workforce training to capture the national professional momentum toward providing services to those in need in the community.[9] In the meantime, the profession of psychiatry was beginning to swing toward the search for biological mechanisms of mental illness and to develop medications to cure it. Psychiatric rehabilitation was considered as only an ancillary treatment and, unfortunately, still is today in many sectors.

Making Mental Health a National Issue

Since the social problems brought into sharp relief by the Great Depression had begun to be addressed by the federal government starting in the 1930s, the country began moving in the direction of federal intervention for other problems as well. In 1945, the US Surgeon General asked the physicians Robert Felix, William Menninger, Francis Braceland, and Jack Ewalt to design a national institute for mental health. They also helped to initiate the Group for Advancement of Psychiatry (GAP), then considered a radical fringe group of the American Psychiatric Association and part of the Public Health Service. Around the same time, the National Advisory Mental Health Council issued a report calling for the closure of state hospitals.[10]

In 1946, Congress approved the National Mental Health Act, which established the National Institute of Mental Health (NIMH) but adjourned without funding it. Ironically, Felix had to seek foundation funding initially just to get the NIMH off the ground.[11]

In 1948, Albert Deutsch wrote his extraordinary exposé of conditions witnessed during his tour of state hospitals. In his book, *The Shame of States*, he wrote, "This writer heard state hospital doctors admit frankly that the animals of nearby piggeries were better fed, housed, and treated than many patients in their wards."[12] Given the resulting public outcry in 1949, congressional funding was finally approved and the NIMH moved out of the Mental Hygiene Division of the Public Health Service and under the umbrella of the National Institutes of Health (NIH) in the federal Department of Health, Education, and Welfare (HEW).

The NIMH mandate was research, training, and aiding states through grants and technical assistance. Felix became its first director and announced that 20th-century psychiatry would be "a revolution not an evolution."[13] And while I am sure that the advent of psychopharmacological interventions felt like a revolution, this turned out to be two steps forward for some people but one step back for many others. I think the step back was due to several factors: (1) the heavy toll of unexpected medication side effects; (2) the significant delays in actual care being available in the community; (3) the stabilization and maintenance approaches used once people were provided care there; (4) the relegation of psychosocial, psychodynamic, and other rehabilitation strategies to ancillary status; and (5) the relative lack of clear integration into the real community for many people.

The official agenda of the NIMH was to provide strong guidance in prevention, diagnosis, and treatment as well as to unofficially gain federal control of state hospital care, which was seen as reprehensible by the coalition of GAP members. Selected Congressional leaders (e.g., Senator Lister Hill and Representative John Fogarty), a couple of concerned philanthropists (e.g., Mary Lasker and Florence Mahoney), a newspaperman (Mike Gorman), and a psychiatric patient Mary Jane Ward (author of another exposé, the 1946 memoir *The Snake Pit*,[14] which was later made into a movie) were involved. This committee began to oversee the process of taking over state hospitals. These activists were joined by more consumers of services, and eventually they became known collectively in the media as the "Washington Health Syndicate."[15] They worked together for years to see that their agenda was successfully implemented. This was a new era of professional lobbying on Capitol Hill. The group's effort built strongly upon the work started by Clifford Beers and had been long anticipated by peer groups going back as far as 1908.[16]

The Professions Arise

Other than those practicing public policy at the national level, most psychiatrists were still heavily invested in psychoanalytic treatments for young, wealthy, and intelligent patients. Physicians in charge of state hospitals or practicing in them were on the lowest rung of the ladder of prestige in the profession. They often spoke little English, especially in big cities. It was within this mix of new ideas, policy changes, and the contradictory status of working in a state hospital that young George Brooks began his career in 1947, as an assistant physician in Vermont State Hospital (VSH), serving both the poor and the underserved, just as he had planned.

During and after the war, psychologists at the bachelor's and master's levels were working to assess recruit readiness, then dealing with postwar trauma in the Veterans Administration (VA) hospitals. The field had split into two cadres—academics versus practitioners—each of whom wanted a stronger voice; in the late 1940s, however, they reunited. Clinical training, which had been underwritten by VA hospitals, was sprouting up in academia, especially at Yale. Doctoral education, with its academic curriculum and traineeships (led by Catherine Cox Miles, Paul Muesner, and Norman Fishbach), along with its *deemphasis* on clinical practice, became a red-hot issue. A conference was held in Boulder, Colorado, in 1949, to define what it meant to be a "scientist-practitioner." The Boulder Model, as it has been known ever since, had been proposed throughout the late 1940s by David Shakow.[17] Later conferences, in 1955 and 1958, redesigned curricula and proposed postdoctoral programs to blend practice with a basic understanding of research and scientific knowledge.[18,19] However, it took the American Psychological Association, as late as 2019, to approve a certified graduate and postdoctoral program to especially train psychologists in the care of persons with serious and persistent mental health problems.[20]

Thus the 1950s saw a rapid increase in the number of university-based training programs with the goal of providing better care to neurotic patients. It was during these exciting times that a young psychologist, Donald Eldred, became the first in the field to work at VSH. As part of a team, he eventually studied members of the Vermont rehab cohort during Phase I and II of the Vermont Study in the 1950s and 1960s.[21]

Social work was established in the 19th century in England, with a focus on social injustice and care for the mentally ill, the poor, the homeless, and child labor. In the United States, the first social work course was taught at Columbia University more than 100 years ago. Within social work, professional models and analytic therapy quickly predominated, and the field increasingly embraced a private practice model throughout the 1950s and 1960s. At the same time, most community mental health centers and clinics were steadfastly directed by social workers, and have been for the past 50 years.[22]

It was not a social worker but a young sociologist (with a doctorate), William Deane, who, in the late 1940s, joined the staff at VSH and eventually helped to develop the Vermont rehabilitation program; Deane conducted the first follow-up study of those patients with Brooks.[23]

Psychiatric nurses, who had worked in state hospitals as "alienists" or "lunatic" nurses, became professionalized as well. The National League of Psychiatric Nurses met in Seattle, Washington, in 1943, to review and clarify nursing roles.[24] In 1950, Vera Hanks, Chief of Nurses at VSH, instituted a comprehensive training program for ward aides, who were certified then as psychiatric technicians. Their pay was raised, and their weekly hours cut back from 60 (!) to 48.[25] Barbara Curtis, another nurse, joined the original Vermont Study team in the mid-1950s.[26]

Treatment Strategies in the Late 1940s

As an assistant physician, one of Brooks's first jobs was to find and house, in one area, all the tuberculosis (TB) patients at the hospital. He discovered that the hospital contained more such patients than did the entire remainder of the state of Vermont at the time. In 1949, Brooks administered the last malaria treatment for syphilitic patients because penicillin had been found to be more effective.[27]

In the 1940s, VSH was a brick compound with a couple of large turreted round buildings connected to many others. It faced a large horseshoe-shaped driveway lined with old trees and a bounty of hydrangea bushes. Unlike other rural hospitals of its era, which were out in countryside pasturelands, this one sat near the end of Main Street in downtown Waterbury. Underneath many of the primary buildings, a warren of tunnels connected units and kept people going back and forth out of the snow and ice all winter.

Across the nation, as well as in Vermont, typical psychiatric treatments persisted, consisting of ice baths, gold salts injected into the subarachnoid space, insulin shock, and electroshock without relaxers, in addition to the use of restraining implements.[28] It is no wonder that pessimism about outcome continued to prevail.

Men and women were housed on separate wards, but apparently any savvy new superintendent could tell which was which by walking down the hallway outside because the women's units were much noisier. This observation appears to relate to differences in how males and females and their symptoms expressed themselves, but it often led to significant overmedication of women.[29]

George completed his residency in psychiatry in 1955, through the UVM, but he pursued a biological course influenced by his mentor Ken Tillotson's work in electroconvulsive therapy (ECT) and psychopharmacology. Although his family teased him about not completing his own analysis, he tucked his psychodynamic training into his multifaceted work with patients.

Patients' families during those years were told to grieve over their loved ones in the back wards "as if they had died and to get on living their own lives" because these patients would probably die in the hospital. It was also an era in which families were considered by many in psychiatry, especially psychoanalysts, to be the cause of illness.[30] Consequently, patients were disconnected from their families and communities, receiving few visits, letters, or packages from home. In fact, members of the Vermont staff thought they themselves would grow old and die shortly afterward as well, in retirement.

★★★

The story of VSH in the early 1950s was retold (though never replicated) across America and Europe. Brooks became known as "Mr. Rehabilitation." The plight of the "chronic patient" began to receive much attention.[31,32,33,34,35] Clinicians and researchers began to talk more and more about strategies to help, and George Brooks was included in many of these discussions. Although in the mid-1950s Brooks became board certified in psychiatry, at some point during the process he realized that both biological and analytical psychiatry had significant limits. Major changes were in the air.

3

A Puzzled Psychiatrist Became a Revolutionary With the Help of His Patients

And so it was that, in the middle of overcrowding and political battles, George Brooks, as one of the hospital's two psychiatrists, began to provide care for his patients. Vermont State Hospital (VSH) had become a town within a town, with continual overcrowding because many more patients were admitted than the hospital could accommodate. The smell of urine and infestations of bedbugs and roaches remained. VSH was not alone in facing these issues: the patient population in state hospitals across America reached its peak in the mid-1950s.[1]

Superintendent Rupert Chittick, MD, wanted many more buildings constructed or enlarged, and he spent a great deal of time dealing with political challenges to accomplishing his goals. Oversight of the hospital was transferred from the Department of Institutions and Corrections to the State Health Commission and continued to be moved from one state department to another for years. Officials at the Health Department decided the hospital was a political liability, and VSH was transferred back to the Department of Institutions. This action put VSH in competition for funds with all other institutions governed by the department. Vermont's governor, its legislature, and the hospital superintendent began to fight publicly.

In 1951, everything came to a head when a local radio news reporter broadcasted the following statement:

> I have to report that at Waterbury, I saw our fellow human beings, our fellow Vermonters, herded together closer than a Vermont farmer would think of keeping cattle in a barn. The hospital has had to take in 1300 patients in quarters only large enough for 982. This overcrowding is serious and delays the

Recovery from Schizophrenia. Courtenay M. Harding, Oxford University Press. © Courtenay M. Harding 2024.
DOI: 10.1093/oso/9780195380095.003.0003

recovery of patients. Under proper conditions, many more would recover. In many wards, the beds are less than a foot apart and beds line some of the corridors. Tiny rooms hardly large enough for one single bed, have two. There is no privacy and women are herded into a single bathroom facility which does nothing to maintain dignity and self-respect. Dr. Chittick feels that private bathroom facilities alone would contribute very considerably to the rehabilitation of the patients. Every precaution against fire is taken, but the hazards remain. The imagination of the listener can function better than any words of mine to visualize what a fire at the state hospital would mean.[2]

The governor, Lee Emerson, visited the hospital on the day after the broadcast, then referred the matter to a committee[3]—a classic gubernatorial delay tactic. But when the Waterbury Fire Chief estimated that "it would be lucky if 50% of the patients could get out in a bad fire," the Governor quickly decided to get new buildings funded.[4] Of course, one new building was named after the Commissioner of Institutions.

The Governor's committee was not completely inactive: it put out a report within 2 months of the radio broadcast recommending that not only should more buildings be built but also that the American Psychiatric Association (APA) should assess the hospital and make its own recommendations.[5] One of the suggestions made by the APA was to set up a residency training program, affiliated with the nearby medical school at the University of Vermont and later with its nursing school as well. All of these recommendations eventually came to fruition.

The New Age of Psychopharmacology

In the early 1950s, Brooks, emulating his mentor at McLean Hospital in Boston, Kenneth Tillotson, MD, and probably because of their friendship since boyhood, applied for and received one of the first SmithKline & French fellowships to study the effects of the "exciting new drug," chlorpromazine (Thorazine).[6] This drug was synthesized in 1950 and was originally used as a sedative for relieving apprehension and restlessness before surgery. Now it was given with great success, especially from the professional's point of view, to agitated patients who were considered combative and explosive with hyperactivity. Chlorpromazine caused huge excitement at all its test sites. For the first time, many profoundly ill patients seemed to get better, and many left the hospital.

Chlorpromazine is a broad-spectrum low-potency drug primarily affecting the D_2 dopamine receptor sites in the brain. Dopamine is both a hormone and a neurotransmitter, and its receptor sites are spread across the brain. The drug goes to where all the receptor sites are, even those *not* involved with psychiatric symptoms, and thus causes considerable side effects. Among the 94 possible side effects of chlorpromazine are drooling, cardiac problems, mask-like face, shuffling walk, sedation, hypotension, akathisia (urge to move constantly), pseudo-parkinsonism tremors, and tardive dyskinesia (TD).[7] TD is a very disabling condition that causes strange and "repetitive, involuntary, purposeless movements" of the arms, legs, and trunk."[8] It is a neurological syndrome and can cause the face to grimace, lips to smack, pucker, or purse, and eyes to blink rapidly.[9] For some people, especially older women, these side effects can be permanent. Imagine getting over your mental distress but not over the TD. In addition, because it made them photosensitive, patients were always seen wearing straw hats and bonnets, which made them stand out no matter where they were.

Another drug, released for use in 1954, was reserpine, which had been used for centuries in India for snakebite and insanity. Made from the dried root of the Rauwolfia serpentine plant, reserpine was developed further to help control high blood pressure and to relieve agitated states in schizophrenia, and it was used for some people who were unable to tolerate chlorpromazine. Reserpine's side effects, however, were depression, especially with suicidal thoughts, peptic ulcers, and ulcerative colitis, and it was not to be used in people undergoing electroconvulsive therapy (ECT).[10] In addition, reserpine could cause cardiovascular problems, nightmares, low blood pressure, nausea, vomiting, drowsiness, dizziness, general weakness, fatigue, erectile dysfunction, and obesity. Thus, using this drug came with major drawbacks. Today, reserpine is used primarily for high blood pressure control and as a sedative for horses on bed rest for injuries.[11,12]

Chlorpromazine Use at Vermont State Hospital

Nevertheless, the excitement of having a new strategy to help people rippled through psychiatry in much the same way as the discovery of new, atypical antipsychotics would in the 1980s and 1990s.[13,14] George Brooks went to his back wards and tried Thorazine on the most disabled patients. In the early

1980s, when I asked him why he tried to put nearly everyone on chlorpro-mazine, he replied, "That is what you do when you have so many hopeless cases; you try the newest approaches to see if one of them might work."[15]

Much to everyone's surprise, 178 people in the back wards suddenly be-came more functional and were able to be discharged. These findings had a significant impact on the staff as well.[16] After the introduction of chlor-promazine, the staff became excited and re-energized. They began to have a more optimistic sense of the possibilities for those left in the back wards, as well as for many of the newer patients entering the hospital. This was a highly significant breakthrough, one heralding an entirely new era in which primary treatment consisted of antipsychotics and a host of other drugs.

Who Was Left in the Back Wards After Chlorpromazine and Before Rehab?

After trying a therapeutic dosage range of chlorpromazine for 2½ years, some people had only a very modest response to the drug and not enough of a return to function that they could be released from the hospital. Later, in the 1980s, our Vermont Longitudinal Study sample was composed of those same poor and modest responders, the remaining back-ward patients. They were considered the worst cases and indeed this was one of the most profoundly ill and disabled groups ever studied in the long-term outcome world literature. The original sample did not include those older than 65 or those on legal mandates, nor those who were well enough to be considered for hospital re-lease or who already had resources upon which to rely in the community.[17]

The Group of Low Responders to Thorazine

Thus 269 remaining people who had responded poorly to Thorazine were selected for the Vermont rehab program in the 1950s. There were 144 women and 125 men. The average age was 40, but they ranged in age from 16 to 65 year.[18,19] The original *Diagnostic and Statistical Manual of Mental Disorders* (DSM-I)[20] diagnoses assigned to this group were 213 (79%) with schizophrenia, 34 (13%) with affective disorders, and 22 (8%) with co-occurring intellectual disabilities.[21]

It should be noted that in future follow-up studies of this cohort, the investigators had to re-examine each patient's diagnostic designation to make the diagnoses comparable to current diagnostic systems as they have evolved over time.[22] Using later criteria was an effort to provide evidence that the participants actually had contemporary versions of schizophrenia and other diagnoses. These efforts were particularly important because of a comparison study completed in the early 1970s examining differences between UK and US application of diagnoses. Those researchers found that the label of "schizophrenia" was handed out quite generously in the United States, while practitioners in the United Kingdom maintained a fairly narrow and more consistent application of the criteria.[23] We later found that the Vermont care team tended to practice more like British clinicians because, like those in Britain and in contrast to most US settings, they had more than sufficient time to observe symptoms and behaviors. And, in a direct comparison of DSM-I to DSM-III,[24,25] we later found that diagnostic reassignments made little difference in long-term outcome—a significant finding all by itself.[26]

For the past 120 years or so there has been a dictum, flatly stated by Emil Kraepelin in the late 1890s and early 1900s, that if you had dementia praecox (now called schizophrenia), you would either achieve only marginal levels of functioning or go downhill; if you were diagnosed with manic depression, you were likely to recover.[27,28] Table 3.1 provides a brief picture of how significantly disabled and disturbed this Vermont group had become.[29]

Table 3.2 presents this group's functional difficulties, some due to the results of psychiatric disorder and some due to long-term institutionalization.[30]

Table 3.1 Original clinical descriptions of the Vermont cohort

Bizarre delusions	Excessive guilt
Hallucinations	Disturbed sleep and eating patterns
Affective flattening	Loss of energy
Poverty of speech	Psychomotor retardation
Poverty of content of speech	Distractibility
Apathy	Grandiosity
Anhedonia	Flight of ideas
Problems with attention	Pressured speech
Hypo or hyperactivity	

From Chittick et al. (1961), 28.[27]

Table 3.2 Description of the functional disabilities displayed by the sample

16 years average duration of illness	44% with less than 9th-grade education
10 years being totally disabled (e.g., not being able to tell time, brush teeth, comb hair, or hold a fork)	Isolated from family and friends who had been told to grieve over them as if they had died and get on with their own lives
9-year average from first hospitalization, ranging up to 25 years for some	Slow, poor concentration
Middle-aged (average age 40 with a range of 15 to 65)	Impaired memory
62% were single	Touchy
	Suspicious
Impoverished (Hollingshead socioeconomic status levels of IV and V: the lowest two social classes)	Temperamental
	Unpredictable
	Medical history of drug and alcohol abuse
	Overly dependent on others to make minor decisions
	No goals or unrealistic ones

From Chittick et al. (1961), 29–30.[29]

The Vermont clinicians further described this group of Thorazine low responders as peculiar in their appearance, speech, and behaviors. Other problems were a constricted sense of time, space, and other people, as well as poor social judgment and little or no initiative. They also suffered from "a high incidence of chronic physical disease" and were also found to have prolonged psychomotor responses across a variety of tests. There was a high incidence of skin diseases, and some people developed additional disorders (such as tuberculosis and cancers); they had a critical need for dental care, visual corrections, and hearing aids.

"Reduction of Anxiety and Panic"

The following sections try to closely capture what the first years of this work were like, as reported in a very small booklet printed by the research team in 1961. This report of their research and findings, *The Vermont Story*, is a critical link to their work. There were only mimeograph machines at the hospital, and so they hired Queen City Printers, in Burlington, to handle the booklet's printing.[31] Its cover bears a picture of a person joyfully exiting from many doors into the world. The booklet is 9 × 6 inches and less than a ½-inch thick, and it is no longer in print. I believe the investigators printed it for their funders as well as for members of the legislature and the mental health community. It was printed only once, but the booklet's contents would be passed around extensively and would eventually become known worldwide.

The early Vermont team was well aware that "the sense of impending dissolution of the personality which accompanies the experience of fragmentation of the ego in schizophrenia is usually accompanied by a deep-seated sense of panic or overwhelming fear," as described by many patients and by Harry Stack Sullivan in 1953.[32] The team went on to describe the "sense of panic, horror, estrangement" experienced by people with schizophrenia when they became unable to count on thoughts and feelings that were once reliable.[33] To combat this nightmarish state and to help a person get on with adult development, the team set up what was described as "a kind, accepting, tolerant, permissive, but supporting and guiding social psychiatric program."[34]

The team also wrote in *The Vermont Story*, "Nine out of ten of our successful cases have had long experience (at least 2½ years or more) with neuroleptic treatment and are continuing treatment after rehabilitation."[35] (Ironically, the reverse happened over time. The most successful cases of recovery and many of the significantly improved cases eventually titrated themselves off drugs; some with clinical help and some without.[36])

The Vermont team was not the only group to prescribe chlorpromazine. From 1953 to 1963, it is estimated that the drug was administered to some 50 million patients, many of whom were forced to suffer its extreme side effects.[37] The Vermont team noted how these extrapyramidal syndromes (e.g., tremors, inability to sit still, involuntary facial movements, unintentional muscle contractions, or stiff muscles) interfered with patients' return to work and to the community. It is difficult to imagine how distressed and frustrated patients must have felt with these extra problems to overcome. Their clinicians worked hard by trial and error to pinpoint the lowest dose needed to improve functioning and with the fewest side effects. In general, these levels were 400 mg of chlorpromazine equivalents, which is considered today to be a low but often therapeutic dosage range. However, the team admitted that "This is sometimes a long and delicate process which has resulted in the use of a wide variety of dosage regimens of both so-called tranquilizers and anti-Parkinsonism drugs with very frequent changes."[38]

But it was this very same group of low responders that were provided rehabilitation and released from the hospital from 1955 to 1960 in Phase I; they were followed for the next 5 years, from 1960 to 1965 in Phase II; and were again followed-up in the early 1980s in Phase III—with 68% showing significant improvement and/or recovery! This same group taught us many important lessons about finding the real person hidden under the odd be-haviors and presenting symptoms, and showed us how capable they were of reclaiming their lives. The ongoing question is, "Why do we consistently and persistently continue to *underestimate* groups of similar people?"

Rehabilitation as a Collaborative Process Between Staff and Patients and Both Systems of Care

Donald Eldred, the first psychologist at VSH, was also a member of the Vermont Rehab team. He wrote about the Barden-LaFollette Act, which passed Congress in 1943[39] and which provided veterans returning from World War II access to physical rehabilitation; it also provided for those individuals who were considered "mentally handicapped" (now meaning those with intellectual disabilities), for the mentally ill, and even for those who were considered to have a "handicapping degree of emotional or per-sonality maladjustment."[40] The Act opened the door for hospitals across the nation to better prepare for the new influx of patients brought about by the war. By the time the original Vermont Study was initiated, the re-habilitation team had been working at VSH for a decade with these types of patients, but not much with people diagnosed with schizophrenia, bipolar disorder, or chronic forms of major depression.

In Vermont, the hospital superintendents (VSH [public] and The Brattleboro Retreat [private]) and some government officials put together a group called the Neuropsychiatric Advisory Committee in 1944.[41] This working group devised general policies and evaluation procedures to deal with returning veterans. Using the lingo of the day, most referred people were considered "psychoneurotic" and in need of getting back to work.

In the decade before 1955, the state's Director of Vocational Rehabilitation Francis Irons and psychiatrists at the state hospital had become increasingly aware of the possibilities of vocational rehabilitation for those returning from war, in addition to other patients who had been diagnosed with psychotic disorders. All vocational rehab workers became aware that not only job training was necessary, but that help with getting work and community adjustment were needed as well. "Indeed, the counselor, Barbara Curtis, R.N., [and member of the Vermont rehab team] found herself also involved with the personal problems, budgets of the patients and even marital aspirations"[42] as part of her work in one of the three newly established half-way rehabilitation houses located within a 40-mile radius of the hospital.

Combining Programs and Collaboration With Patients Because "My Ignorance Saved Me"

With all of this activity going on in the background, Brooks began to read two important, recently published books that strongly deviated from his traditional Freudian analytic training. This explains, at least partially, why he never completed his own analysis and what he did at the hospital after he finished reading.

The first book was a very small volume, published in 1953, and written by a British Army psychiatrist, Maxwell Jones, and six others. They wrote about setting up what they called "a therapeutic community," working with outpatient groups of people who were considered "both untreatable and unemployable."[43] Jones and his team also described an environment with a horizontal (rather than hierarchical) authority, one focused on education and work, shared decision-making, interdependence as a goal higher than independence, ex-patient clubs, and living-learning opportunities integrated into every social interaction and crisis.[44] While many contemporary community clinicians are under the impression that these approaches are new, Jones's work shows us that this is not the case. What is of great interest to me is that George Brooks used Jones's *outpatient* model for his inpatients, and with great success. In direct contrast, most of today's outpatients are living under an inpatient model of stabilization, maintenance, medications, and entitlements. It is no wonder many have become more chronic.

The second profoundly influential book was Harry Stack Sullivan's 1953 volume, *The Interpersonal Theory of Psychiatry*,[45] which suggested a 180-degree turn away from Freudian theory of internal drives and their formation of personality to an approach derived from social interaction and relationships. The publication of Sullivan's book caused a great deal of consternation among analysts. I was told that, in the early 1950s, physicians in training at the well-known Boston Psychopathic Hospital (later known as Massachusetts Mental Health Center) had to put Sullivan's book into a brown paper bag to carry it around campus in secret.

So, after 2½ years of prescribing chlorpromazine at the hospital, Brooks stopped thinking only as a biological psychiatrist and decided to introduce rehabilitation and a therapeutic community to the back ward at VSH, having found that medications alone did not much help these particular low-responding Thorazine patients to reclaim their lives.

Later, in its 1961 booklet *The Vermont Story*, the rehabilitation program emphasized that seven crucial factors laid the foundations for the development of modern rehabilitation. These were (1) relief of overcrowding, (2) the training program for psych aides, (3) better working conditions, (4) increases in professional staffing, (5) improvement in the physical plant, (6) the development of three rehabilitation houses, and (7) "therapeutic advances" with new drugs.[46]

Brooks relegated these factors to a collective second place many years later. He admitted to me, kind of sheepishly, that "my ignorance saved me!" He told me that he had had some exciting ideas gleaned from work being done in England about what to do next for his patients, but implementation was quite another matter. Furthermore, there was a lot of discussion but no comprehensive manuals in the United States providing guidance on how to treat chronic patients in state hospitals—after all, they were considered barely treatable and nearly all were still in custodial care in the early 1950s.

"What Do You Need to Get Out of Here Because I Don't Know"

Brooks did an astonishing but sensible thing. He went to the back wards, where patients were still running around with no clothes on while speaking animal gibberish and smearing feces on the walls. (Remember, this was after 2½ years of chlorpromazine, even at dosages considered today to be therapeutic.) He confessed that he had run out of ideas, and so asked patients, "What do you need to get out of here, because I don't know." This is noteworthy because, to this day, few physicians and other professionals in community mental health centers, clinics, and hospitals, ask this question: most assume they already know the answer. Brooks expected and received reasonable replies. His patients said, "Why should we get well? Nobody wants us. There is no place for us to go. We won't have any job. Where will we sleep? What will we eat?"[47] The gauntlet had been thrown down.

Devising a Model of Rehabilitation, Self-Sufficiency, and Community Integration

Thus, the target population was to be the same back ward patients described earlier who, in addition to their severe symptoms and behaviors, were still hospitalized because of the loss of vocational skills, additional symptoms of poor health, and the dissocializing effect of long-term hospitalization.[48] The staff's concern was not only with reducing hospital census but with helping this group find a decent and adequate life outside an institution and in the community. The model of the program emerged as *rehabilitation, self-sufficiency, and community integration*.[49] These aims are often described as central to today's community mental health center goals, but many if not most programs are focused primarily on stabilization, maintenance, medications, and entitlements, even though this will be vehemently denied.

Brooks began with a group of 12 women considered very paranoid. He asked them what they needed to get out of the hospital. They stared at him in disbelief. Slowly, they ventured to say that the food in the hospital was awful. Being also a closet behaviorist, Brooks went right to the kitchen and ordered up a Thanksgiving feast. The women were astonished that someone had actually listened to them and immediately responded. They were encouraged to be a little braver and to speak up on more serious matters. In the end, the project enrolled 269 back-ward patients.

Several very early papers by Vermont team clinicians present different enrollment numbers for a variety of reasons, including paper deadlines, deaths before release, and so on. For example, because the 1957 vocational rehabilitation grant (OVR 180) was specifically focused on getting people back to work, those who were at retirement age were not included in later publications. There also may have been an assumption that those older than 65 might not be possible to rehabilitate or employ—even though this has certainly been repeatedly proved not to be the case.

Moving Inch by Inch Toward Reclaiming Lives

By asking "What do you need next?" repeatedly, the clinical team and their patients began to assemble most of the components of basic psychiatric rehabilitation. Working collaboratively was the hallmark of the Vermont program and still is today in those programs considered to be "pockets of excellence."

Brooks admitted that he was best able to test out ideas while working together with the patients and staff in collaboration with the Department of Vocational Rehabilitation and while his boss (the Superintendent) and various state and federal oversight departments "left me alone." Such a "hands-off" environment is usually considered (correctly) to be impossible today given the many financial and legal constraints and structures imposed by governmental and managed care entities, which often trump core care values and creativity. However, some clinicians continue to successfully bring about change: Chapters 19 and 20 describe many contemporary innovations.

In addition to asking patients what they needed, another pivotal strategy of rehabilitation began with positive messages about the possibility of improvement, discharge, and shaping one's own future. "Shaping one's own future" meant figuring out what was meaningful to an individual and their sense of purpose. Both are critical characteristics of healthy and happy human beings. What is missing from rehabilitation in community systems today is a clear focus from the beginning on patients graduating out of the system, along with messages of excitement and preparation for doing so. Underlying this is the idea that people should not be defined by the problems they are trying to solve but by whatever hopes, dreams, skills, and talents they have or are about to discover—and that they can build lives around those ingredients.

Vermont pioneers developed major components of rehabilitation which should be considered essential today (see Table 3.3).[5,50] It must be remembered that the community mental health system for such patients did not formally exist in Vermont until the mid-1960s and only board and care homes. Therefore, the team had to take these patients out of the hospital and develop and provide comprehensive community supports for them, all while providing essential continuity of care. It took time to put the program together.

Table 3.3 Vermont rehabilitation components designed through collaborative effort

Drugs: Low but therapeutic doses of medications even though only modestly effective	**Activity therapy:** Graded group activities in occupational and recreational activities Write a play
Ward Care: Collaboration + level playing field + relaxed and noncustodial atmosphere Client driven + innovation	**Industrial therapy:** Using hospital plant as preliminary training opportunity in desired future job
Group therapy: Supportive and practical, solution-based Social skills training Classroom lectures on world topics Activities of daily living	**Vocational counseling:** Done by the Department of Vocational Rehabilitation (assessment, training, placement, and after-job and employer supports)
Graded privileges run by patient government Range of housing opportunities Positive messages about recovery	**Blurring the boundaries** between the hospital and community (e.g., peer support groups, "The Helping Hands," + outpatient clinics)

From Chittick et al. (1961), 31–34.[50]

Brooks admitted that some of these rehab components were really nothing very new, even at the time and even in inpatient settings. The big difference was that others had used them sparingly, one at a time. In Vermont, they were used together and in close collaboration with the patients themselves. The program was the first to utilize skills from another state agency, Vocational Rehabilitation, at a US state hospital in a combined psychological-educational-rehabilitation model.

Not Preparing Families for the Return Home Was a Mistake

Attempts to include and work with families turned out to be nearly a complete failure. Some families had not seen their loved one for years. In that era, families, especially mothers, were considered the cause of schizophrenia.[51] When many of these patients arrived home after having made great strides in their rehabilitation, families had no support, no psychoeducation, they had been taught no coping skills—nothing. In most cases, the return was a disaster. Patients returned to the hospital and later were discharged to halfway houses; they then had to establish their own independent situations within 2 years. Staff and patients believed that 2 years was enough time so that patients did not feel pressured or anxious. Some were able to re-establish family relationships with the help of siblings.

The Only State Hospital in Vermont

Again, it is important to remember that VSH is the only state hospital in Vermont (something most people have a hard time imagining). Anyone with a significant psychiatric problem (and sometimes not so significant) was typically brought in by a county sheriff or the State Police. Over time, some of these people were relegated to the back wards, while others returned to their lives. We must remember this because these studies reflect an entire state's population, while most other published studies only look at selected samples from one area, with all kinds of often unexplored variables impacting findings. As such, the Vermont findings may be more generalizable to long-stay people.

Working Creatively With Increased Money
But Still a Slender Budget

The superintendent reduced the overcrowded conditions, improved and expanded the physical plant, increased salaries for attendants, and reduced work hours from 60 to 45 while increasing the number of professional staff from two psychiatrists to seven and adding a psychologist, a dentist, social workers, and a Director of Nurses. The staff developed training and evaluation methods, increased scope, and used newly available drugs while keeping watch over side effects. They also developed a real working relationship with the Department of Vocational Rehabilitation, which opened three rebab houses as transition units. Of the 140 people in the study who used them, only 19 stayed for longer than a year.[52]

The patients each devised their own goals, picked whatever jobs they wished to learn and do, and chose where to live. When they left the hospital, many were reunited with their families through the bridging efforts of brothers or sisters. For many, this process was two steps forward and one step back, but they kept trying. If they became exhausted, Brooks let them come back for a short time to VSH as a "vacation," to rest and see friends, read a book from the patient library, or see a movie on campus. He met them in the Admissions Office with their discharge planning papers already in hand to show that this stay was only to be a brief respite.

The limited budget inspired great creativity, and this did not go unnoticed. In 1966, Gerald Caplan, a well-known authority on consultation to systems of care, wrote

> What I would like to see copied on a widespread scale is the pragmatic posture of the Vermont workers, who directly confront the day-to-day problems of the mentally disordered and then try to deal with them with their currently available resources. Their efforts are particularly marked by creative improvisation and enthusiastic hard work at the basic human relations level.[53]

Psychiatrist Hans Huessy wrote as an editorial comment in the same book that "Brooks challenges us not to fall for new oversimplification and models, but to maintain breadth and variety in our programs, to remember to meet the patient's needs rather than to force the patient to fit into our preconceived theory."[54]

4

Widening the Scope of Rehabilitation and Research

Why Present a 70-Year-Old Program?

It strikes me that readers may not understand why this book begins with a description of a program that was invented nearly 70 years ago, and why it might be good to know about such strategies in 2024 and beyond—especially since many people currently suffering from extreme distress are in community programs. The Vermont program's characteristics and philosophy are applicable to both hospital and community settings today, and, in many ways, its approach is still desperately needed. Although some of its components are now in place across the world, the Vermont program is still advanced compared to the way most other programs are implemented. It is *how* current programs are being applied today that causes so much frustration and disappointment; they unwittingly perpetuate more than 125 years of misplaced pessimism—the idea that schizophrenia and other serious diagnoses are life-long.

In the early Vermont Study, the participants were considered patients with the worst functioning: they had been long hospitalized and were not dissimilar to many trying to live independently in our communities today. Yet half to two-thirds of these disabled people retrieved their lives over time. The success rate of most modern programs of today can't hold a candle to this finding.

This chapter sheds light on what is missing from today's care system. I have endeavored to keep the emphasis on the critical aspects of the Vermont program by staying as close to the developers' own descriptions

Recovery from Schizophrenia. Courtenay M. Harding, Oxford University Press. © Courtenay M. Harding 2024.
DOI: 10.1093/oso/9780195380095.003.0004

as possible. What I continue to relay here is based on the hospital's original report, *The Vermont Story: Rehabilitation of Chronic Rehabilitation Patients*, the small booklet containing the report to the funding agency, Vocational Rehabilitation in Washington, DC, mentioned in the previous chapter that was only printed once in 1961 and has been long out of print.[1]

Widening the Scope of Rehabilitation and Research

At the Vermont State Hospital (VSH), Superintendent Rupert Chittick increased the number of attendants to 252, registered nurses to 20, and physicians to 7; he also added 3 social workers and 2 clinical psychologists. The hospital wisely decided to underpin the rehabilitation program with research. By 1957, George Brooks was also made director of research and secured a 3-year grant (OVR #180) from the federal Office of Vocational Rehabilitation (VR). The grant provided $30,000 per year (about $316,309 in 2022 dollars) with the goal of expanding the program and including those people struggling the most.

The Vermonters decided on a method called *participant observation research*,[2] which was derived from ethnographic studies in anthropology[3] and sociology.[4] Ethnographers live with and observe the culture of a group to learn what they have to teach us.[5] The research team felt guided by their values and that they were aligned with phenomenology principles[6] as well as with existential,[7] field,[8] and Gestalt psychology.[9] (Thus, Brooks managed to delve into philosophy after all, even though his parents had insisted that he pursue medicine instead.) For those of us who missed those courses, what fascinated him most were (1) the ingredients that make us human, (2) the study of social problems, (3) consciousness and direct experience, (4) what is it like to exist, (5) how people interact with others, and (6) seeing the whole rather than the parts.

The Vermont team employed many different research strategies: questionnaires, schedules, formal interviews of both staff and patients, and large wall charts graphing patterns and trends, as well as quiet observations of the therapeutic relationships built between the patients themselves.

This early innovative Vermont research approach included the following components:

- "The same personnel should conduct both research and therapy."[10]
- "One could express this as the need to measure change, i.e., progress of patients toward rehabilitation, while at the same time attempting to influence the change which one is attempting to measure."[11]
- "A sense of immediate need was always present requiring improvisation and direct action."[12]
- "Patients become not merely people to be studied but they become active participants in research."[13]

The values that researchers held and how they might have influenced study results were also willingly explored. Even today, these strategies are not often adopted by investigators in schizophrenia research enterprises.

The research team later made note of Rashkis's "Cognitive Restructuring: Why Research Is Therapy."[14] They felt that patients leading the way in the creation of new rehabilitation strategies was not only essential but also promoted a sense of empowerment on the road to recovery. In addition, the approach demanded that patients were part of planning, policy, and steering committee meetings, as well as the usual "suggestions and gripe sessions."[15] All findings were shared and reflected upon.

This mixture of qualitative and quantitative strategies was only halfway appropriate for such a pioneering enterprise, which they called *participatory observation research*. Without realizing it, the Vermont group ended up conducting their research using a related integrative approach now called participatory action research (PAR).[16]

Pioneering treatment research is equivalent to "bench research" in other sciences. As Einstein and Infeld once said, "To raise new questions, new possibilities, to regard old problems from a new angle, requires creative imagination and marks real advances in science."[17]

How Does Participant Observation Research Differ From Participatory Action Research?

Participant observation occurs when researchers choose a group of people to study; spend some time interacting with key informants, gatekeepers, and stakeholders; and use a variety of techniques such as interviews, observation, life histories, focus groups, and documents combining both quantitative and qualitative methods. Then they go away, analyze, and publish their findings. The goal ostensibly is to not disrupt normal activity, although in this writer's experience it seems difficult not to do so. In many cases, the research enterprise becomes part of the observed group's normal activity.

On the other hand, PAR is a dynamic process that develops from the unique needs, challenges, and learning experiences specific to a given group.[18] In PAR, everyone is an investigator, everyone is a collaborator, everyone is up to their elbows in the process. Change in behaviors and knowledge about the underlying processes are the goals that will benefit the whole group working together.

> The knowledge brought by the researcher and the knowledge of the people can then combine to help people understand and alter systems that were previously invisible or perceived as formidable or insurmountable barriers. . . . It is the implicitly empowering process in which a group of people become aware of the nature of their disenfranchisement, the mechanics through which inequity is perpetrated, and their ability to change their circumstances.[19]

As Kidd and Kral also point out, PAR "at its center, is a sharing of power."[20] In the end, I suspect that partaking in this kind of research did more than anything else to help these Vermonters (both patients and staff) leave behind their sense of hopelessness and helplessness in the face of serious and persistent disability, instead helping them to go forward to reclaim their lives and jobs.

What Else Did the Clinical Team Think Helped?

The group listed six more important components in *The Vermont Story*. These factors were thought to have played a key role in the program's success in addition to reducing patient anxiety and panic as described in the previous chapter.

1. Effective utilization and organization of ancillary personnel
2. Blending change with continuity and commitment
3. Reacquainting the patient with his world
4. Providing economic and social security for patients
5. Maintaining commitment of staff to patients and patients to staff
6. Compassionate relationships in a family(-type) setting[21]

I'll now delve more deeply into each of these components.

Effective Utilization and Organization of
Ancillary Personnel

The Vermont team of professionals involved in the project (a psychiatrist, a psychologist, a psychiatric nurse, a sociologist/anthropologist, and a vocational rehabilitation counselor) came to the startling conclusion that many good therapeutic relationships and work occurred with the nonprofessional staff. "[T]here are many roads open to work with the [patient] and not all these roads require the professional touch but all do require a human touch."[22] This finding was based not only on observation but also on what the patients told the professionals was helpful in their recovery process.[23]

The professionals also discovered that the ancillary staff of attendants who had been taking care of people in a traditional custodial manner and looked quite institutionalized themselves could and did adapt to a rehabilitation approach. As an example, Vera Hanks, eventually the Director of Nurses, began the process in 1950, with professional development classes and better conditions for nurses. Staff attitudes and behaviors were periodically measured by a structured scale as well as by observation.

The professional staff also worked hard to rid themselves of authoritarian tendencies and worked toward humanitarian ones, as suggested by Maxwell Jones (discussed in the previous chapter).[24] Staff also noted that working together as a well-functioning family permitted everyone to grow in a more positive direction and actually helped diffuse what is known as "transference phenomena"[25] because there were so many opportunities to interact with a wide variety of characters over time, not just one person.[26] (*Transference* is a psychological concept explaining why a person takes his or her positive, negative, or sexual emotions stemming from one relationship and transfers them onto another person; when a patient interacts with many people, the effect is diluted.) Just as patients needed time and space to evolve into ex-patients and fuller human beings, so the Vermont professionals also made room and opportunities for the nonprofessional staff to grow and change while supporting their anxious moments (e.g., "listening to problems and conveying confidence in the ability of the staff members to arrive at their own decisions"[27];"A patient government which does not have real power is no government; a ward meeting at which decisions are made for attendants, instead of by and with attendants, is useless").[28] These systematic leveling experiences were thought to "democratize the institution."[29]

Blending Change With Continuity and Commitment

The team tried to make sure that there was a sense of continuity in spite of all of the changes going on. Continuity was later deemed critical by a colleague of mine, Lee Bachrach,[30] and by others, but it is often overlooked in today's world. Important relationships were kept intact both in the hospital and after someone returned to the community. In fact, the same care team followed patients into the community because there was nothing else out there in terms of community mental health supports for formerly psychotic and profoundly ill patients. Therefore, out of necessity, the rehabilitation process continued in the "real world" and with the same faces.

The program staff considered the process of returning to the community to be gradual, and they tried "blurring the boundary between the hospital and the community."[31] And, all the while, the program continued to evolve in response to patient and staff needs and feedback, with constant creative activities such as "an extensive recreation program; weekend visits to the rehabilitation houses; extension of the occupational therapy program along 'university' lines which permit[ed] patients to enroll in 3 of 12 elective courses in seminars such as 'Social Problems in the United States' and 'Introduction to Sociology'; a series of other lectures; visits to the hospital by the 'Helping Hands,' the ex-patients' club; and day placement in employment situations within the community."[32] These approaches were certainly consistent with those of the moral treatment era that emerged 227 years earlier (described in Chapter 1) as well as with the approaches of other therapeutic communities. The staff were pleased that their methods of change and consistency were different from the concept of the "total push" programs of the 1950s, which "result[ed] in anxiety-panic produced by sudden change."[33]

Reacquainting the Patient With His or Her World

The patients involved in the early Vermont Study were considered "hopeless cases" and had been effectively isolated from their original families and communities; many had not been outside the hospital for 10–25 years, and there was no TV. The staff instituted a wide variety of educational programs to bring people up-to-date with what was going on in the world. These classes focused on topics such as national elections, the mechanics of electricity and plumbing in the very building in which people lived, activities of daily living, how banks worked, and voting. Many groups took part in writing a play about how the hospital was run and the different duties of the staff members. Expectations were outlined for patient responsibility as well. Other programs included activities overseen by general staff already present in the hospital, such as a vocational counselor, an occupational therapist, a group therapist, a nurse, a psychologist, and a psychiatrist. Graded privileges, such as freedom to explore the entire campus and going to town, were decided by the established patient government.[34]

Providing Economic and Social Security for Patients

Funds were sought to provide financial support for rehabilitation housing, which most people used as stepping-stones once they were out the hospital door. For every state vocational rehabilitation dollar spent, the federal government contributed $2 (or $21.09 today). This money was considered much more consistent and reliable than iffy support from foundations or community charities. Furthermore, clients who were unable to find work outside the hospital at first were provided $2 per week by the VR Department—again $21.09 in 2022 dollars. This support permitted them to buy a few items for themselves. The VR Department and the Knights of Columbus also provided such items as clothing and "eyeglasses, hearing aids, and braces etc." when needed.[35] When they began work, patients could build up a savings of $500 ($5,272 in 2022 dollars—a substantial sum) before being asked to contribute to room and board in the rehabilitation house. Budgeting classes were provided. All of this was designed to promote "economic self-respect."[36]

The early Vermont Team discussed the fact that subtle pressure could be put on patients who appeared to be taking advantage of their situation living in the house. Little by little, people began to realize that there were others waiting in the hospital to get out and that they had to take responsibility for themselves and move forward.[37]

After leaving the hospital, people were allowed to live in one of three rehabilitation houses for up to a year and a half if they wished. The clinical team felt that allowing patients a decent amount of time to adjust to the world enabled them to relax and begin to get their feet wet. Many people did not take so long to find work and other housing, but remarked that not having a 3- to 6-month deadline thrust upon them for accomplishing these goals was very helpful. Often clients who left would return to the rehabilitation houses for dinner once a month, to check in with friends. The clinicians noted that "the mean duration of stay in the houses is only 6 months, the median is 5 months, and the range is 1 to 24 months. Of 140 patients who have entered the rehabilitation houses, only 19 (14%) have remained there over 1 year."[38]

Today, when a person's level of functioning changes, for better or worse, they often must change residence, may lose friends, and may be forced to cope with new clinicians who do not know them or their capabilities. Vermont tried a different way. Patients lived in a home of their choice, with support staff coming to them when and if needed. This is now known as "supported housing."[39] In this way, Vermont was able to provide a stable environment as well as real continuity of care.

Maintaining Commitment of Staff to Patients and Patients to Staff

"We must stress that the rehabilitation of even a single patient is a long, slow, detailed, painful, and infinitely complex process."[40] The clinical team spoke about the "re-education, remotivation, and resocialization" efforts required and how these can take a toll on the hope and higher expectations of staff members.[41]

Of course, underlying all these rehabilitation strategies was the prescription of emerging first-generation antipsychotics, which continued to grow in usage, as well as other medications developed to try to offset side effects.[42] In Vermont, the dosage level continued to be a modest 400 mg chlorpromazine equivalents. For the first 10 years of the program, Brooks continued to prescribe and adjust dosages, and patients continued to take medications. Note that in the 1950s to the mid-1960s, the social distance in Vermont between physicians and farmers was significant. Doctors were universally admired, trusted, and often revered. Challenging prescriptions was rarely done. After people became more empowered and self-sufficient, and the team moved back into the hospital, increasing numbers of ex-patients withdrew from their medications. The Phase III study found that all of those who had recovered were off their psychotropics, and many of the significantly improved were, too.

During the Phase I and Phase II studies (the first rehab study and the 5-year follow-up) if patients became suicidal, homicidal, or very agitated, or needed medication recalibrated or physical care, the hospital by law was empowered to bring them back in because they had only been "released," not discharged. By the time Phase III occurred in the early 1980s, the law had changed. A person could only be brought to the hospital if he or she was a danger to self or others, much to the distress of family members, clinicians, the police, and sometimes to the patient him- or herself.

Later, the Vermont Study team explained that the "constant emergence of successes to balance failures," both across patients and within the same patient, "appeared to keep staff more hopeful than not."[43] The team described how, when patients relapsed and found that staff were still willing to help them try again for a second, third, or more time, more hope was engendered for all parties. Such striving toward recovering a life was accomplished by familiar staff who by now knew these individuals well. They had seen them at their best as well as at their worst. This experience of staff continuity was much easier than starting from scratch with a new staff person, as often happens in today's systems of care.

Compassionate Relationships in a Family-Type Setting

The clinical team wrote about the importance of a pleasant, homelike environment with decent food, clothing, and housing as well as having staff members who liked working with challenging patients. In fact, my Colorado colleague, Gordon Neligh, who was the director of the Program for Public Psychiatry in the 1990s on the old University of Colorado–Medical School's Denver Campus described to me such clinicians and other staff members as having the following attributes: "Warm, enthusiastic, high energy, hopefulness, commitment to client success, willing to take an active treatment stance, tenacity in the face of renewed symptoms, and sheer endurance."[44] In fact, active supervision was needed to keep staff from working too hard and to make certain that they, too, had a life outside the hospital from which to draw sustenance. Today, even supervisors themselves are exhausted, especially in underfunded settings, and they often end up with little life outside of work.

The Vermont Team described all sorts of challenges other than recurring symptoms. These problems included acting-out behaviors that offered corrective opportunities to disrupt the replay of old, unproductive, child–parent behaviors and interactions. Social and educational activities were seen to build on peoples' strengths and intelligence. In the end, the team declared that "the atmosphere in which rehabilitation and therapeutic work with hard-to-reach patients can develop, requires a sense of trust and commitment, realistic goals and optimism, and a compassionate concern."[45]

These findings appear to confirm what Manfred Bleuler said after 50 years of working with his patients and discovering that improvement and recovery could indeed happen.

> What is effective in the treatment of most schizophrenic patients is also effective, and decisive, in the development of the healthy individual; clear and steady personal relations; activity in accordance with one's talents, interests, and strengths; confrontation with responsibilities and even dangers; and, at the right time and in the right rhythm, rest and relaxation.[46]

Efforts in Setting Up Rehabilitation Housing in the Community: The NIMBY Encounters

The clinical team had to invent community mental health services for persons coming out of the hospital during the period just before John F. Kennedy's Community Mental Health Act of 1963.[47] Official community care for serious and persistent illness was not implemented broadly in Vermont until the 1970s. However, the Vermont team set up outpatient clinics, job opportunities, and supports, and they underwrote the peer support group known as Helping Hands. The first things people needed were places to live and a range of housing options. Rehabilitation houses were established in the Montpelier and Burlington areas. One city was the capital of the state and the other was the largest town in Vermont, with the hospital situated between them. Fights among community supporters and detractors soon emerged, including churches and nearby neighbors. NIMBY is an acronym for the fierce fighting stance of "not in my backyard" you won't![48] When rehabilitation houses were proposed, neighbors got upset and mounted campaigns against them. This behavior continues to this day.

Brooks recalled a time when he came back to a rehab house full of six little old ladies exhausted from such a fight within his own Episcopal church. He sank down quite discouraged, with a big sigh, into a comfortable chair.

One of the women patted him on the shoulder and said, "There, there, Dr. Brooks, we will just have to show them."[49]

Employment Programs

Employment is nature's best physician and is essential to human happiness.

—Galen (172 CE)[50]

I found Galen's saying, many years later, on the wall of the Irons Rehabilitation Center at the hospital. It appears that we have known about the healing aspect of work since early Rome. In the Vermont program, people had to go to work because there were no federal programs such as Social Security Income or Social Security Disability Income. They participated in an assessment of their interests, work histories, hopes, and dreams. Then they were provided with training specific to their desired goal, helped to obtain employment in their field of choice, and given after-employment supports (often forgotten these days).[51] They were placed usually with small employers (five or fewer employees) across Vermont. The employers had a "hotline" directly to Robert Lagor, the vocational rehabilitation counselor, who had worked with the patients directly during the assessment/training phase. The hotline could be used if an employer became concerned about the patient. Sometimes, 20 years later, an ex-patient who suddenly was out of a job would call Lagor, discouraged. Lagor would not reopen the case but would meet the person for coffee and discussion. That was all it would take to get them going again.

It should be noted that these once-disabled people were employed at the time of the 1958 recession that had spread across the country. Nevertheless, if patients had an episode, recession or not, it was often found that the employer had taken such an interest in them that they held their position open for them until they could return.

The Role of Peer Supports: "Helping Hands"

The first wave of people who left the hospital in the mid-1950s decided to form a peer support group called Helping Hands in the Montpelier-Burlington area.[52] This model of peers helping peers was similar to work that had already been going on at the program known as Fountain House in New York.[53] Helping Hands activity was not just for recently released patients themselves but also for their friends still in the hospital. The group's first step was to draft a document, "The Aims and Accomplishments of the Helping Hands."[54] They undertook this enterprise without the help of any staff member.

The manifesto laid out the ways in which the group could help with post-hospital adjustment. It established a bi-monthly meeting with the motto, "We help ourselves when we help others."[55] With this insight, the group hit upon the best therapeutic approach to foster recovery and tap into the real secret of rehabilitation. At these meetings, people felt accepted, and they participated in a wide range of social activities. Resocialization, education, helping others, and being accepted were key to the group's philosophy.

They enlarged their scope and began to visit people still in the hospital, telling them what the real world was like. They announced that "There are a lot of strange people out there who were never in the hospital." In 1980, Brooks told me this pronouncement turned out to be very helpful and empowering for people still on the inside because, once they were released, they might run into some of those characters. This amazing revelation allowed former patients to understand that a poor interaction with the postman, the pharmacist, or a man on the street just might not be due simply to having once been institutionalized. This piece of information helped to considerably reduce anxiety.

Helping Hands also produced a monthly newsletter. It was circulated not only to its 60 members but also to key members in the community, such as legislators, businessmen, ministers, and priests. Members felt the weight of being the first wave to rejoin the community, the responsibility to show others that they were capable and "ambassador[s] of good will."[56,57] They also went to Rutland to help ex-patients there set up a similar group.

The consumer advocate movement occurred inside the hospital as well. The stage play "Brighter Days Ahead" was produced by one of the therapy groups in the hospital and performed for patients still there.[58] The idea was originated by a member of the group reportedly in the throes of catatonic excitement. Writing a play about rehabilitation naturally became a sort of rehabilitation itself for the group. Working jointly with a therapist, week after week, the play began to take shape. Posters were created, and a cast party was held. The play started with "The Admission" and went on to introduce ways in which members of the staff worked with people (e.g., the occupational therapist, the work supervisor, the doctor and the patient, the students, social workers, and nurses).[59] The play addressed the effects of drugs, portrayed a vocational interview, showed how a group therapy session was conducted, and, finally, featured a farewell scene, which showed patients leaving the hospital with people shouting "Good luck!" and "Don't come back!" The play was an upbeat effort and was a forerunner of the educational efforts provided today in many peer and family support groups.

Another other major accomplishment of the group within the hospital was to itemize advice for others (such as staff, family, and members of the general public) about what to do—and, more importantly, what not to do—when dealing with "patients." Their advice is still useful today. Roughly paraphrased here and translated from a long and elegant set of suggestions is the essence of the first list.

"What We Would Like You to Do"

- Let us adjust to social gatherings in our own way and time.
- Don't watch us or ignore us. We want to be recognized as individuals who are able to function on our own and plan our lives.
- We are capable and expect to be given responsibility. When we are ready, we will get a job.
- Don't shield us from the public as if we have been a disgrace.
- Consider medication as an important component to our recovery process.
- Because of institutionalization, we may have some weird habits but we are not sick.
- Don't threaten us with rehospitalization to make us do what you wish.
- Don't send someone to go with us anywhere.
- Let us do things for ourselves, including picking our own friends.
- Don't keep talking about our appearance.
- It is OK for us to have a nice time and also if we are blue for a few days.
- Don't threaten anyone else with hospitalization like, "You'll end up in Waterbury someday." It undermines our experience.[60]

They went on to compose other lists, such as "What We Do That May Bother You" and also "What We'll Try to Do." These lists conveyed substantial wisdom and clarity. "What We Do That May Bother You" contained valuable expertise. For instance, what might seem like rigid behavior patterns are really acquired hospital habits such as rising before 6 AM and eating on a strict schedule, bathing and changing clothes less often than other people do because of hospital routines, and not talking to one another a lot because people were left alone. "What We'll Try to Do" was mainly about collaboration and trying to succeed.[61]

Reflection on How Their Problems Changed

In 1960, the clinicians interviewed in depth 78 people who once carried the label of chronic schizophrenia, asking some very interesting questions. The first was: "You seem to all of us to be much better. Do you feel that you are better?" Three of the 78 replied: "No, of course not. There never was anything wrong with me." Many people who had replied in the affirmative described the challenge of coping with a psychosis. "It was something like being in a nightmare all day and all night, all the time." "Nothing seemed real to me." "I didn't realize how things seemed until I got better." "I don't have words for it."[62] A few people did not want to discuss their experience at all. Many of these descriptions match those of people recovering from other life-threatening problems such as cancer or a heart attack.

When asked about factors that helped them feel better, almost half attributed their improvement to a relationship with another person or a group. The other half credited the drugs they had received, the new hospital atmosphere, or being able to work.

When asked if there was a "turning point" in the recovery process, almost everyone could pinpoint a time or an experience. Some of their comments, especially from those who had been diagnosed with catatonia or hebephrenia, were along the lines of "I woke up" or "I came to" or "I came alive again." Although some people with paranoid subtype also said such things, some also remarked on "getting a feeling for people again" or "getting over the suspicions."[63] Another common theme, that of "low turning points" or hitting rock bottom, was also written about by one of our Yale team members, Jaak Rakfeldt, in the 1980s.[64]

Everyone required a different length of time to recover. The team noted that "a great majority of these people are becoming self-supporting, apparently able to engage in satisfying relationships with other people in the community. Fourteen have been married, 4 engaged and 6 children born. Many others have girlfriends and boyfriends. They have developed firm, supporting relationships with each other."[65]

Exciting Results in the First Years

This is how George Brooks described the early outcome of this pioneering rehabilitation program in 1959.

> From the very beginning, there has been an air of optimism and, at times, a sort of awestruck wonder at the success of the whole thing. I recall particularly one party in which the clients at the Rehabilitation House gave for a group of rehabilitation candidates from the hospital. At one moment during the party, I stood aside to observe the festivities. I saw before me a group of about forty, well-dressed, attractive, self-confident women, ranging in age from twenty to fifty, who were all enjoying each other immensely. They were singing old songs, drinking coffee, and eating cake and cookies. They gathered at times into small groups sharing their experiences. In my mind's eye, I could see all but three or four of these as they appeared four years previously. Then, they were dilapidated derelicts on the disturbed and semi-disturbed wards of the hospital—denuditive, smearing walls of seclusion rooms. Some were completely withdrawn, apparently totally out of contact with any of the unpleasant reality about them. I was struck with great wonder of this transformation and [am] very thankful that I had been able to participate in it.[66]

At the time, the team compared their achievements to a recent report in the public health world about similar release rates for first admissions with schizophrenia, but of much younger people (20–45 years). "We are unable to suggest why our results with this new experience with a group of chronic, deteriorated, severely disabled patients should so parallel others' experience with more acute cases."[67]

It should be noted that after the Vermont results from the initial study were originally published in 1961, a national report, *Action for Mental Health*, was issued by the Joint Commission on Mental Illness and Health.[68] This effort was undertaken by members from the American Psychiatric

Association, the American Medical Association, the American Academy of Neurology, and the Department of Justice. They wrote,

> The fallacies of "total insanity," "hopelessness," and "incurability," should be attacked and the prospects of recovery and improvement through modern concepts of treatment and rehabilitation emphasized.

What Was Next in Vermont? Did All This Work Continue to Pay Off?

The early Vermont project continued for 10 years, from 1955 to 1965. Clinicians and administrators came from all over the globe to see the results for themselves. The last chapter of this section describes a modest follow-up in 1965 and its exciting, surprising, and challenging findings. The key question is: Did these findings hold up decades later?

5

Phase II

The 5-Year Follow-Up in 1965 and the Demise of Vermont State Hospital

From 1962 to 1965, Bill Deane (the sociologist on the team) and George Brooks conducted a 5-year follow-up of everyone who had entered the Vermont program's sample between January 1, 1955 and December 31, 1960.[1] These patients were originally profoundly ill, demoralized, and totally dysfunctional. Everyone had received the same (but unusual for the time) basic program consisting of drug treatment, open ward care, graded privileges, activity therapy, industrial therapy, vocational counseling, and other wide-ranging rehabilitation strategies described earlier—while also moving back and forth between the hospital and the community.[2] They lived in a unique environment that included these key ingredients: a horizontal organizational structure in which everyone had a vote; economic security; continuity of care, with the same providers in and out of hospital; expectations of both rights and responsibilities; a choice of residence; a sense of trust and commitment; and opportunities for social engagement.[3]

This group included 123 men and 140 women with an average age of 40 and an average of 9 years of education or less. In the original project, 213 (or 79%) of the participants were diagnosed with DSM-I schizophrenia,[4] (13%) with affective disorders, and 22 (8%) with mental retardation (now called intellectual disability).[5] All were rediagnosed with later criteria. Of the 269 original participants, 6 had died in the preceding 5 years (4 had died from natural causes in the hospital and 2, having been released, died as passengers in automobile accidents).[6] Nine other original participants were considered too disabled to participate and were not part of the follow-up.

Recovery from Schizophrenia. Courtenay M. Harding, Oxford University Press. © Courtenay M. Harding 2024.
DOI: 10.1093/oso/9780195380095.003.0005

Thus, for this follow-up study, 254 were available to complete short questionnaires. [7] There was much discussion in the field at the time about high suicide rates among such individuals, both inside hospitals and out in the community. For this reason, Deane and Brooks found the *absence* of suicide and homicide among their sample to be remarkable, especially since many in the cohort had been suicidal and/or homicidal prior to their first hospitalization. [8]

Given the funding shortfall for this study, only 113 people (42.9% of 263) were randomly selected to be interviewed. [9] This reduced Vermont sample was considered representative of all the back-ward patients who were referred to the rehab program and who were not older than 65 or on legal mandates, or who were "too well and nearing hospital release or already had resources upon which to rely out in the community." [10] General clinical and functional descriptions of the whole sample were discussed in Chapter 3.

An analysis of the interviewed sample ($n = 113$) versus the entire group ($n = 263$) revealed a slight over-selection of people diagnosed with schizophrenia (81 compared to 78). Table 5.1 [11] presents the comparison of the interviewed subsample and the entire original sample, revealing minimal differences between the two groups.

The investigators located and invited these 113 participants to the hospital for a set of small semi-structured interviews. The clinical team and

Table 5.1 Comparison of interviewed sample with full cohort for 5-year follow-up study

Variables	Interviewed sample (%)	Cohort (%)
Age	37.81	38.35
Education	9.44	9.7
Male	45.13	46.76
Female	54.86	53.23
Protestant	57.52	55.89
Catholic	41.59	42.96
Jewish	0.88	1.14
Schizophrenia	81.41	78.62
Other	18.58	21.67

others who knew these clients well were also interviewed, and data were also extracted from a large set of records generated from their hospital and rehab participation as well as from their original involvement in the clinical trials for Thorazine in the early 1950s.

Interviewees were paid $10 (equivalent to $95.82 in 2023) plus travel expenses. The interviewers regretted being unable to interview people in their own living spaces, but the team did not have the funding to do so. This problem was remedied later, in the Phase III long-term follow-up study, when we were able to interview in their homes members of this same group as well as many more from the entire cohort, no matter where they lived—even those who had left Vermont.

The Seven Major Research Inquiries

The seven major research questions posed in this phase of the 5-year follow-up were the following:

- Did the length of hospitalization affect post-hospital success?
- Did the assigned diagnosis play a role in level of success?
- Was the rehab house helpful compared to release directly to the community?
- Did patients' relationships with family change?
- Was there an optimal length of time in hospital and in the rehab program?
- Did the level of socialization change before and after hospitalization (e.g., employment, social activities, marriage, place of residence)?
- What was the continuing effect on the hospital of this rehab program?[12]

Data Collection

The questionnaires sent out in 1963, 1964, and 1965 had response rates of 90%, 86%, and 76%, respectively. This questionnaire consisted of a one-page inquiry asking about marital and employment status as well as community social relationships.[13] For 113 people, the one-page questionnaire was followed up with a semi-structured four-page interview close to the fifth anniversary of each person's referral to the rehab program. These questions focused on family composition, interactions with family and friends, participation in community organizations, feedback on the vocational training received, employment before and after hospitalization, interactions with other employers, and the participants' views on having been in the hospital or returning to the hospital.[14]

Outcome criteria[15] were the following:

1. Fully functional: Included full-time employment with evidence of an active social life
2. Partially functioning: Included full- or part-time employment with no evidence of an active social life, *or* an active social life with no employment
3. Not functioning: Included neither employed nor active socially

Strategies for Analyzing Data

This early Vermont research team used a variety of strategies to scrutinize these data. Large wall charts traced the evolution of people before and after the rehab program so that the team could visualize patterns and trends. I actually saw these colorful charts myself in 1976, 11 years later. The original team was also still in place at the hospital into the 1980s, during the later Phase III research. We found that they had tucked away all the data collected from the first and second phases of the Vermont Story studies. Even the VR counselor, Bob Lagor, who had been involved since 1955, had secreted the related VR records and clinical notes high up in the hospital attic. This would be considered ethically inappropriate today, but the early team suspected that someday someone might need these records again. They had sidestepped regular purging of old records as required by the state. Though these governmental stipulations are understandable to some, they are the bane of long-term investigators, and we were grateful that the files had been kept safe and secure and no one ever went up into the attic. It was a scary place.

Data analysis was conducted using 5 × 8-inch punch cards, called "McBee cards," which were employed in the era before computers became widely used.[16] Remember, I am talking about the 1960s here. These large cards had key variables punched in specific spots along the perimeter of each card through which actual knitting needles were passed, allowing the negative unpunched cards to fall out.[17] Today's investigators should feel some relief that technology has improved since then. I certainly did in the 1980s, after I was handed this same box of McBee cards and the knitting needles from the 1960s. It felt like they belonged in a museum—but then again, the computers and IBM punch cards that we used in the 1980s feel like tools from the Ice Age now in 2024! Chi-square statistical analyses by hand using 2 × 2 tables with one degree of freedom were used as well.

As early investigators, Deane and Brooks reflected on the many previously unanswered questions as they tried to understand the influences on outcome findings to be collected. For example:

- What was the impact of time in length of total institutionalization (e.g., counting time in a school for delinquents, other hospitals out of state—or, I would add, being kept in the home attic for 15 years)?
- How could researchers understand and chart the variable course of waxing and waning symptoms?
- Was time in the rehab house considered institutional or community?
- How could researchers understand the actual recovery process?
- What could researchers do with the fact that there were no common definitions of the concept of "recovery" and "relapse" (this is still a problem).[18]

Decisions were made to nail down clearer definitions relating to some of these questions. *Release from hospital* was defined as "out of hospital on the 15th day of two successive months" (which gave a minimum of 30–31 days out). Something less than that was considered a poor staff decision. *Duration of institutionalization* was broken down into three types: (1) length of continuous hospitalization before referral to rehab program, (2) total time in Vermont State Hospital (VSH) hospitalization across all admissions, and (3) total amount of time no matter which institution. *Protective setting* was defined as a participant not "fully economically or socially interdependent in any reasonable sense." This designation included sheltered workshops, board-and-care homes, or living at home without contributing to costs. The rehab houses were not included because of their "transitional and bridging function." *Family* was defined by older anthropological concepts as "family of orientation versus family of procreation."[19] These variables thus provided coding instructions for these innovative questions.

The Results of The 5-Year Follow-Up

Ten important findings emerged from the first follow-up study based on interviews and questionnaires. They reflect the enormous volume of hard work done by all parties. Table 5.2 presents the results.[20]

This project got a majority of people out of the hospital and into the community, with two-thirds finding jobs and achieving decent functional status. Given this cohort's general low education levels, the men were mostly single and worked as handymen and in maintenance jobs. They often liked to work in a general hospital, a nursing home, or for family. Women tended to work as housekeepers or caring for the elderly.[21] I believe the shift from being cared for to caring for others made a significant impact on these individuals' sense of self.

Many people stayed near VSH or the rehab houses in Burlington or Montpelier, familiar territory with friends and rehab counselors nearby. There was public transportation for visiting family, going to church, and making social calls. They went to the movies, listened to the radio, and

Table 5.2 Results from the 5-year follow-up study of *Vermont Story* participants

1. Two-thirds of this sample were maintained in the community at effective function and employment

2. Rehab workers continued to play key roles long after the official relationships ended

3. Relapses occurred frequently in the first 5 years, especially in one part of the group in the first 2 years

4. Rehab housing equilibrated the opportunities for people with very chronic histories to those with less chronicity

5. People with chronic forms of schizophrenia can do equally as well as those with chronic forms of other diagnoses

6. Essential to permanent success was vocational rehabilitation and counseling

7. Very long hospitalization (>7 years) made it tougher to stay in the community; however, more of the long-stay (5–7 years) people never came back to the hospital once out compared to those with shorter or very long stays

8. The response to rehabilitation in the first 2 years (especially in the first 6 months) was found to be the most predictive of longer successes

9. Such ongoing programs helped reduce numbers of long-stay patients in the hospital as well as get people who came back in to be released again

10. Aftercare workers became fatigued with the "constant renewal of roles and function" which put pressures on their own family relationships

watched TV. The rehab counselors admitted to helping patients find employment nearby because the counselors knew the area and its resources better.[22]

At the end of the first 10 years of rehabilitation efforts and research, however, everyone was exhausted, particularly staff, with a third of the patient group still struggling to make the transition. The most startling quote from this portion of the long-term work, after all the excitement and the creativity, was the following written by Deane and Brooks in 1967:

> Implicit in our findings is the fact that any plan for the rehabilitation of the chronic patient be conceived as long-term [*especially for this particular subset of the bottom third of the already poorest functioning bottom third of the entire hospital*], since all our evidence suggests that the commitment necessary to the chronic patient has no foreseeable end, and that unless constant attention be given to the chronic patient, the end result may be simply that he is out of the hospital operating at a high level of inadequacy and a low level of employment.[23]

It should be noted that sometimes clinicians and some families give up on ever seeing significant improvements, let alone full recovery. This message can have a dire effect on struggling people who may, as a result, settle into a perpetually medicated state—ironically, just as their problems may be lifting due to aging. This is why we need more government-funded long-term studies (not just 2- to 5-year projects), because *time* challenges many of the assumptions that we make about chronic disorders and disabilities. The classification of most illnesses as chronic is at least partially attributable to the severity of a subset of a cohort and exactly when investigators begin to assess them. Since the late 1800s, schizophrenia has generally been assumed to be a chronic illness at the outset.[24,25]

How Necessity Was the Mother of Invention

In 1965, when the first follow-up study was complete and the clinical and research teams had returned to the hospital full time, they still felt responsible for the well-being of all those patients with whom they had worked for the entire time they had been hospitalized and then when entering the community. The staff did not want to abandon them, something that often happens when sponsored projects end and funding evaporates. From the 1930s onward, locally funded "community counseling services," as community mental health services were called then, were tasked with providing prevention services for children and families, not for people with serious and persistent illness. Federally funded community mental health services in Vermont and elsewhere did not exist until after 1965, and even then often did not provide care for people with serious and persistent illnesses across the nation at large; this changed in the 1990s, when Public Law 99660 was instituted. Thus, in 1965, the clinical team was moved to seek out other community resources to which they could refer their clients.

If Mary was interested in singing, how about the church choir? If Joseph liked to play chess, how about the local chess club? If Laura made quilts, what about the nearest "sewing bee"? If Tom played sports, how about a league? If Susan loved to go to the movies, how about the local film club? This network of natural community supports turned out to be one more of Vermont's secrets. Such groups cost the mental health system nothing, and the people who joined found other members there with whom to make friends. Having friends with no history of mental illness widened ex-patients' social support systems, and, as a result, they became more deeply embedded in their communities rather than being socially isolated. Use of natural community entities was one more stroke of genius. This strategy was revealed to me in 1981, by Robert Lagor, from the Department of Vocational Rehabilitation, who was part of the original team.

Other Studies in the Same Early Era

The Vermont investigators had very little literature with which to compare their findings. Hardly anyone was doing research at state hospitals. Hardly anyone considered rehabilitation. However, at a few state hospitals, such as those in Stockton, California,[26] Warren, Pennsylvania,[27] and Boston, Massachusetts,[28] staff were conducting short research studies. California used the new "Total Push" approach, mentioned in the previous chapter, which advocated a rapid release for people who had been hospitalized. The Stockton study found that the experimental Total Push group, which had an average of 10 years of hospitalization with chronic forms of schizophrenia, had a similar "net release rate" to controls who did not participate in the program. Instead of becoming discouraged, this research team found that many therapeutic changes in the intervening years had occurred within the California system. The hospital that had served as an untreated control group now offered treatments and thus equilibrated the findings.[29]

From 1946 to 1950, while studying first admissions in 11 state hospital facilities across Pennsylvania, Goldstein and colleagues found a 70% release rate.[30] The Vermont investigators were dismayed to find that there was no evidence of what had happened to these chronic patients over time. In 1958, Freeman and Simmons tracked released low-functioning male patients and found an association between low levels of expectation and acceptance by families of the released person. Families needed help with coaching and skill-building.[31] Higher functioning returning patients who were married often returned to their spouses. In Deykin's small study, behaviors, appearance, and social skills all played a role in being accepted and supported.[32] These three characteristics appear to be true no matter the situation. Anne Evans and her group found that families often wanted discharge but remained realistic about their loved ones' capabilities.[33] Problems occurred if the house was short of space or income was unable to support an extra person or if the returning person was unable to get a job. Findings from other short follow-up studies began to trickle in from England and elsewhere in the United States.[34,35,36,37,38] They revealed that two-thirds of chronic patients could be released to the community but with marginal adjustment and high morbidity, unemployment, and readmission rates. Unfortunately, this pattern persists today in community systems, which have become almost custodial due to lack of adequate funding.

Now, in 2024, because of the lack of investment in broad-spectrum rehabilitation with its value-infused evidence-based practices, there are more than 57 million people with any kind of mental illness with less than half (47.2%) receiving any kind of care.[39] Of those, people with serious and persistent struggles in the United States alone account for 14.1 million and are languishing in community mental health centers and state hospitals, with 9.1 million not receiving any care in jails or prisons or out on the streets.[40]

What Else Happened to The *Vermont Story* Sample When the Funding Ran Out?

Everyone reading this chapter will have a good guess. Although the community mental health system developed in Vermont in the mid-1960s, its focus was like all others across the nation. High priorities were still families, couples, and children. Persons still struggling with severe problems were released from the hospital and were often relegated to board-and-care homes (in Vermont at least—unlike in many other states, where people ended up on the streets). But these Vermont board-and-care places (ironically referred to as "homes"), with few exceptions were no better than the nation's early state hospitals, with nothing for patients to do except sit around all day. They were unlicensed and not regulated in any way. In the mid-1970s, when I visited a large one near the hospital, I found 30 people using one medicine cup, unchanged gray sheets on the beds, and unclipped finger- and toenails. I reported this situation to the new CEO of the hospital, James Hunt, and the following year the legislature instituted licensing and many regulations. The large homes were then licensed and had to follow new regulations, such as shielded furnaces and outside stairs to second floors. That situation unfortunately meant the end of the smaller, better homes that also existed. Once again, two steps forward, one step back.

For those patients still in the hospital in 1965, Brooks sought and was awarded another federal grant, under a program known as the Hospital Improvement Project (HIP), for "educational therapy."[41] The goals were "more provision of rehabilitation, training, and re-education, for long-term patients; increased community contacts; and staff education."[42] Those patients not in the study and still in the hospital received all sorts of enrichment: excursions, remotivation programs, art workshops, and a whole host of other educational programs. This effort involved 2,300 women from church and Home Extension groups from across the state, and it provided such items as clothes for geriatric and adolescent patients, cheery curtains, and ward parties, in addition to birthday and Christmas gifts.[43] One can understand why unhappy, still poorly functioning but released patients wanted to come back!

Thirty percent of the original cohort were people now just sitting around in one of these care homes or walking the streets during the day but bored to tears and wishing to be back in the hospital. Brooks must have been heartbroken as well. In an interview in 1975, he described his recurrent nightmares of Dorothea Dix returning from the grave to declare that these ex-patients needed to be kept in a good hospital, an argument that gets periodically revived today.[44]

Driven by this concern, Brooks managed to acquire yet another federal grant, under the Improvement in Alternative Care (IMPAC) program, which lasted from 1971 to 1974.[45] It was focused on the boarding homes in the three counties close to the hospital (Washington, Chittenden, and Lamoille) as well as on a pair of smaller more rural ones. Although Vermont had placed people into protective housing rather than leaving them to the streets, it was not the kind of life that Brooks and those ex-patients had envisioned. The goal of the project was to unearth more community resources, such as church groups, that might provide a sort of a day hospital model, with activities and other initiatives, similar to programs today run by such groups for seniors and those with early dementia.[46]

Brooks also applied for and received yet another federal grant under the Rural Community Screening Program (RCSP), with its goal of reducing state hospital admissions from the three closest counties to the level of the more remote rural counties ($n = 1,122$ in 1973–1974 to 632 in 1976–1977).[47] At that time Vermont had a population of about 488,000, with more emerging community mental health centers scattered across the state. When ex-patients and others became upset about something, such as losing a job or a girlfriend, or some other crisis, they would come to the attention of the police, an employer, or a family member. Up until the screening grant, the unhappy person was often simply transported immediately to the state hospital. This new grant provided screening at the local level for Orange, Washington, and Lamoille counties. A concerned friend or family member called the local community mental health center, and the center referred the troubled person to highly trained screeners now positioned there as employees.[48] Community mental health clinics began learning how to be more helpful to people with complicated lives. Only 21% of all referred people were sent back to the hospital, primarily for suicidality; serious alcohol withdrawal symptoms, such as delirium tremens, seizures, and hallucinations; or significant problems with psychiatric medications. (This story was told to me by L. D. Taylor, the program evaluator, after I got my hands on the original report to the NIMH in 2020.)

How Vermont Became the State Without a State Hospital

Chittick retired as superintendent in 1968, and Brooks took over. In 1984, Brooks retired. We joked about the fact that it took 37 years for him to be deinstitutionalized himself. His dream was to be the last person to leave the hospital, locking the door behind him. Indeed, he almost achieved this: by 2011, the hospital census had plummeted from almost 1,300 in 1955 to 51.

Another severe flood occurred when Tropical Storm Irene arrived on August 26, 2011. Once again, as in 1927, everyone was moved out of the basements and first floors to the upper floors of the hospital buildings. The Medical Director, Dr. Batra, and the hospital teams spent all night making plans to triage people for moving the next day, either to a general hospital, a residential center, an empty unit in Corrections for forensic patients and other violent acting-out people, or to the Brattleboro Retreat, the private hospital on the southern border of the state.[49] The storm was so devastating that the state hospital was completely shut down. This disaster made Vermont the first US state without a state hospital.

There was considerable discussion about and planning for no longer having a state hospital, especially since the former patients who had been sent to residential centers managed to stay there without needing further hospital care.[50] Some people speculated that hospital staff had tended to be overly conservative about discharging patients prior to the storm. Perhaps, since the hospital had become decertified by Medicaid, staff members were also worried about their jobs. Although community mental health centers and a couple of general hospitals were willing to continue helping with patients in crisis, the general public was very concerned about not having a state hospital and pressed the legislature to build a new one. It was an era of changing leadership at the Department of Mental Health as well, and thus the original vision of managing without a state hospital was lost in the shuffle as told to me by W. D. McMains, MD, in 2020).

Eventually a new 25-bed hospital building was erected high on a hill in the little town of Berlin, across the street from Central Vermont Medical Center and a stone's throw from the capitol of Montpelier—and well away from any possible flooding.[51] Mother Nature had helped Brooks achieve his dream of closing the hospital, even if only for a short time.

The Unexpected Future of the
Vermont Story Cohort

What happened to all the people participating in the *Vermont Story* sample across the following years? In the following chapters, I will describe how as a nurse/psychology undergraduate student I inadvertently discovered this cohort as part of a small class project in 1976. Then I will describe how Brooks and I, with more than 125 other multidisciplinary investigators, clinicians, and statisticians from across the country, ended up designing and conducting a large project funded by the National Institute of Mental Health—with 97% of the entire original cohort found and accounted for. This project became one of the longest long-term follow-up studies (average of 32 years after first admission) of schizophrenia and major affective disorders with psychotic features in the world literature.[52,53]

PART TWO

New Team, New Study, Same Sample, Years Later

6

The Implausibility of Becoming a Phase III NIMH Principal Investigator

Shifting ahead to the mid-1970s, the chapters of Part Two retrace the decisions that were made on how to conduct a study of a rehabilitation program more than two decades after its start and three decades after the participants' first admission. More than 125 professors, researchers, and clinicians from a range of disciplines, along with people with lived experience, helped our National Institute of Mental Health (NIMH) grant proposals receive almost perfect scores. Publication of our results took the form of an unusual editorial and a dual set of papers in the *American Journal of Psychiatry*. Eventually papers from our Phase III studies would be referred to as "classics."[1,2,3,4]

This chapter reveals how I, who wanted to be a clinician in pediatrics before fate intervened, instead became a clinician and researcher in psychiatry thanks to George Brooks and Louise Davis (Chair of Nursing at Vermont College) before the Phase III study started. This is the case of a highly unusual career path, generous-hearted people, persistence, and plain old curiosity.

How a Housewife and Mother Became a Scientist

When I was 18 years old in 1958, I was allowed only 1 year of college before marriage. My parents expected me to find a "nice young man on the way up, be an executive's wife, and have kids." I had to fight for that year. My father, like many others in the post World War II era, thought that

Recovery from Schizophrenia. Courtenay M. Harding, Oxford University Press. © Courtenay M. Harding 2024.
DOI: 10.1093/oso/9780195380095.003.0006

education was "wasted on women" because we were expected to become "only" wives and mothers. Though I made the dean's list at college for the year I was there, I bought into this expectation myself.

During my 20s I happily spent time being a wife and mother. But in my early 30s I suddenly became a single mother with three young children. It was the early 1970s, and I had to decide quickly on a career that would pay the mortgage. Having had such a rewarding experience as a mother, I wanted to be in pediatrics, but becoming a pediatrician was not an option at the time if I wanted to remain an involved parent to my own children. A medical degree would have taken 3 more years of undergraduate study, 4 years in medical school, plus residency. My children would have been out of the house by then. What I did not know then was that I would eventually end up in a medical school—having entered through the proverbial back door—and that I would be a tenured professor—not in pediatrics but in psychiatry—for the next 40 years.

In 1973, after consultation with my friend and family pediatrician R. David Ellerson, I went to nursing school, determined to finish as quickly as possible and earn a living as a pediatric nurse practitioner, bachelor's and master's degrees in hand. At nearby Vermont College, the chair of nursing, Louise Davis, who had been trained at the famous Menninger Clinic,[5] immediately became determined to track me into psychiatric nursing. I persisted in the other direction, but she persisted even harder. And probably because I was more than a decade older than my classmates, Davis insisted on giving me cases with psychiatric complications, whether they were pediatric, medical/surgical, or geriatric patients. Nevertheless, pediatrics was still for me.

Learning from Psychiatric Patients

Eventually, as part of my studies, I ended up in the psych rotation at Vermont's only state hospital. I was petrified. The hospital met all my preconceived ideas, accumulated from the movies, about permanently institutionalized and scary patients. My instructor gave me one of the hospital's most well-known patients, whom I'll call Edward. I had recently read a paper (whose title and author I no longer recall) explaining that if a patient is anxious when meeting a new person, he or she will often revert to some delusional material. The paper suggested that if the person were allowed some time, he or she would eventually settle down and be able to carry on a conversation. Well, Edward had other plans. He was uninterruptible for our entire 1-hour meeting, naming every planet, flower, tree, and type of building in an encyclopedic list. I was totally flummoxed. When finished, he turned to a middle-aged woman sitting in a wheelchair who had come up beside him and asked, "Susan, are you ready for lunch? I'll wheel you in." It was a great first lesson for me because I saw that his tactics had kept me at arm's length, and he was much smarter than I have given him credit for.

Several years later, I saw Edward on the steps of the hospital and said hello. He started with the "sun and the moon and the stars. . . ."

I said, "Edward, when I was a nursing student, you said all that to me. You don't have to do that to me anymore."

"Oh," he said, "okay." And he never did it again, speaking instead in a coherent manner thereafter. From Edward I learned that staff expectations of non-illness behaviors from patients were important, as was behaving like adults ourselves.

I had other experiences at the hospital that shaped my professional life. I was assigned to "Abigail," a young woman of about 28, the following year. Abigail was another so-called notorious patient. She had infuriated the stern staff members, with their Yankee morality, by going into the tunnels under the hospital with any man who would offer her a cup of coffee. The staff had dubbed her Tunnel Abby, but my instructor had told me, "She needs a friend." I was affronted because, after all, I was working hard to become a professional, not a girlfriend.

But, of course, a friend was exactly what this young woman needed. During every visit we compared notes on our weight, looked in a big mirror, and talked about diets. When we went to the canteen, men would come and proposition Abigail right in front of me, so we began to talk about her ability to say no if she wanted to and how to practice safe sex. I took her downtown to a local café for her first off-campus outing in many years. I was caught off guard when she immediately propositioned a state trooper there in return for coffee. Fortunately, he knew about the hospital close by and did not take offense. We sat and had cups of tea and coffee and chatted about appropriate clothing and other "girl talk."

To write up Abigail's case for class, I decided to read through the 3-foot stack of papers constituting her records. Much to my shock, I discovered that she had been wrongly hospitalized at 18, having become hysterical after being hazed by a classmate. Sprinkled through her records were reports of her saying, "I am not crazy!" Every time she had escaped from the hospital in the subsequent 10 years, she had been returned and been either "snowed down" with Thorazine or provided electroconvulsive therapy (ECT). By the time I saw her, Abigail was looking and acting with behaviors that appeared to the staff as schizophrenia, with the subtype of hebephrenia (including behaviors such as constant giggles and inappropriate and provocative attire).

I submitted Abigail's life history paper on her wrongful commitment to the class. Unknown to me, the Chair of Nursing sent my paper to the Chief of Nurses at the hospital, and she disseminated it to the staff. Their animosity toward Abigail immediately turned to sympathy and a determination to get her out of the hospital. In 6 months, the staff managed to get her discharged and found her a board-and-care home near her family—out of kindness and, I suspect, with relief.

Abigail taught me to double-check the histories of my research study participants or clinical clients for wrongful hospitalizations and/or diagnoses. She also taught me about the vagaries of systems of care and about new ways to think about what a "professional" can be ... someone who also sees the person underneath the diagnostic label.

The Collision of Two Worlds on the 20th Anniversary of the Vermont Rehabilitation Program

I went back to the hospital as a temp RN for the summer of 1975, urgently needing the job before transferring to the University of Vermont (UVM) to secure my bachelor of science in nursing (BSN) degree. During the first week I attended a case conference. Clad in white uniforms, we interviewed a 26-year-old patient who was a puzzling case.

His psychiatrist thought he showed signs of Huntington's chorea but he was too young. The puzzle deepened because the patient said that his father had died of a heart attack and his mother of cancer. Huntington's disease is a rare genetic disorder which causes multiple movement, cognitive, and psychiatric disorders; if this young man had it, at least one of his parents would have had it as well. The list of possible symptoms is a mile long, and the illness comes from a mutation in just one inherited gene.[6]

The young man seemed very frightened coming into this interrogation. Superintendent George Brooks and the hospital staff peppered him with questions. Dr. Brooks asked him, "It says here that you are retarded, is that so?" I was appalled and furious. Later I fired off a letter to Brooks saying that this case conference and the manner in which the interview process had been conducted were ethically inappropriate, in my ever so humble opinion. Brooks, who by now was unused to being challenged, called me immediately into his office. We had a fierce fight, with neither of us giving an inch.

Brooks said, "In the past, patients never saw their records and never had a chance to correct them. Now I am giving them a chance to correct it!"

I retorted that the entire interview process could have been conducted completely differently (for instance, coaching the patient ahead of time about what to expect, not subjecting them to a roomful of starched and staring staff in white coats, asking questions in a different and softer style.) And perhaps the patient had rights of his own. Finally, I said that I would *prove* that this person did not have Huntington's. I flounced out of the office and probably shut the door a little harder than was necessary.

It is a wonder that I was not fired on the spot. In my spare time, I found unfortunately that the patient's *biological* mother had died in the same hospital of Huntington's disease. The family had at least four generations of the disease in its history, with cousins marrying first cousins; many had six out of eight children with it. Thinking back on this situation, I should have referred the family to Nancy Wexler and her sister, Alice, who were working hard to unravel the genetics and social history of this profound illness.[7] But I was unaware of their work then.

Although this outcome did not turn out as hoped, it moved Brooks to give me other patient mysteries confronting the staff. These small projects introduced me to the fun of research and the challenges that abound in clinical settings.

How Did I Learn to Speak Truth to Power?

Why in the world would a brand new RN get up on a high horse with Brooks a week into her job at the hospital? I had been primed for confrontation from an early age.

In 1958, when I was almost 18, I was unable to find a summer job because the country was in a significant recession. In desperation, I ended up working at a tobacco farm growing broadleaves for rolling cigars.

Every morning a rickety old bus came from Springfield, Massachusetts, down Route 75 and stopped at our federal-style house, called Fox Hill Farm. It was located in the pretty but small enclave of Suffield, Connecticut, just across the border and north of Hartford, the state capital. Out I would come at 5:45 AM, dressed in my preppy Bermuda shorts, hop on the bus, and off we would go to the fields. This happened 6 days a week, and I worked 12 hours a day. I was paid 50 cents an hour along with everyone else. My co-workers were a group of migrant workers, some of whom appeared to be over 70 years old.

Of course, my father, then chief of Missiles and Space Systems for United Aircraft, had announced to my mother when I was out of the room that he didn't think that I would last a week, having just graduated from an all-girls high school. Chances are that I probably would not have—if he had not made that pronouncement. I was kind of a quiet and naive person, but a stubborn teen. I thought I knew how the world worked and that I could handle it. I have always wondered whether my father said what he did so that I might hear it, just to see what I might do.

The big white tents were at 110° Fahrenheit while we planted small tobacco seedlings and ran string for them to wind their way up as they grew. For the first 3 weeks no one spoke to me, even if I tried to start a conversation. They pretended not to understand any English, and I only knew French. Eventually their curiosity got the better of them and they asked me why I was working with them. I told them that I was earning money for college, and suddenly they started speaking with me and relating their individual histories, filled with hardship and often tragedy. Their stories broke my heart and introduced me to the *real* real world. I received three offers of marriage, which made all of us women chuckle. Later in the summer, the men picked the leaves and the women used special sewing machines which took a pair of leaves and looped them by string in a line. Then, we would line a bunch on a wooden lath, and give it to the men to put dangerously high up in the barn for the air to dry the leaves. These descriptions reveal that the work was hot, hard, and dangerous. Near the end of the summer the boss took me off the line because I had had high school math, and he needed someone to fill in for his paymaster, who had quit. My migrant friends never spoke to me again.

That summer is when I learned about socioeconomics and "the inequities of power, status, and material privilege, which give members of a society widely different opportunities and alternatives."[8] The inequities made me angry and upset, and this changed my life. I learned to be fearless in confronting authority, and, later on, I was successful in changing some lives and systems when situations were grossly unfair. (And sometimes I made things worse.)

In my 20s, I simmered down and focused on my husband and three kids, as I had been brought up to do. In my 30s, challenging Superintendent Brooks was nothing new for me but probably startling to him. I speak softly but carry a big stick!

What started on that tobacco farm led to more than 40 years of conducting research, loving clinical work, teaching, writing academic papers, working in public policy, and speaking across the world. All of which was an effort to change things. Structures, systems, and America itself have come a long way, but they still have a long way to go. After years of experience, I learned that it's best to create an environment that encourages people to speak for themselves—then get out of the way. I have been taught by some of the most eloquent people with lived experiences dealing with severe distress and significant life challenges. George Brooks already knew all this in the late 1950s.

And it was John Strauss, Yale professor and well-known schizophrenia investigator, who modeled for me later how to have a helpful case conference. He was giving a Grand Rounds lecture at my original home department of psychiatry at the med school in Vermont. After the lecture, we went upstairs to the psych unit at the Mary Fletcher, a general hospital. He took a patient, a young man, aside, and told him what this meeting was all about, who was there, and that he could refuse the entire thing or refuse some of the questions. It was entirely up to him. Then Strauss proceeded to speak with him in front of the group, uncovering the person underneath the diagnostic label. He didn't jump right in with questions about symptoms. He found that the young man played the guitar, which he wished he had there in the hospital, and he was good on the computer. Over the course of the discussion, Strauss was able to discover some of the underlying problems and avenues for rehabilitation and care, none of which had been known to the treating team.

On my student rotation with a nearby visiting nurse association, we paid a call to a large board-and-care home full of former state hospital patients. I saw one medicine cup for more than 30 patients, soiled sheets, unwashed hair, and filthy fingernails. Later that day I went to lunch with the new CEO of the state hospital, Jim Hunt, and I told him what I had seen. He said that these care homes were not regulated and that the only thing he could do was to threaten the home's owners with not sending any more patients until they cleaned up their act. He made that call right after lunch. Then he became determined to work with the legislature to license all such homes in Vermont. It worked, and now they are licensed. Unfortunately, this legislated all the good small boarding places for one or two people right out of existence. These non-corporate homes were suddenly required to install firewalls around their furnaces, fire escapes from the second floor, and other prohibitively costly improvements. These were the unintended consequences of me and the state "riding in on a white horse." Sometimes good intentions don't turn out as we hope.

How a Nurse Tumbled Into Psychology

In the fall of 1975, after working at Vermont State Hospital, I had my uniforms and my books as I signed in at the UVM. For 2 years the dean of nursing and I had several conversations about my transfer as a senior from Vermont College. But on the day that I arrived I was called into the office by the *new* dean of nursing. She informed me that the old dean had been fired for over-accepting people into her classes; she had too many students and not enough clinical spots. To correct the situation, this new dean was requiring the seven older women who already had our RN licensures to wait for 4 more years to finish our senior years and earn our BSNs. (Of course, these were also the most dedicated women on her roster.) I had not a second to delay. I had to get out of school and go back to work at the end of the year. I asked to be transferred to the Psychology Department. The new Dean said that university policy required a student to be enrolled for a year in one college before transferring to another. I retorted that this was an unfair Catch 22.[9] After much persuading from a very upset me, she called the dean of arts and sciences, who said "Send her over!" He called Chair of

Psychology Richard Musty, who said "Send her over." The only person to disapprove of this transfer was the director of admissions, but it was quickly a fait accompli and too late for him to do anything about it.

When I arrived at his office, Musty immediately called the dean of nursing and read her the riot act for treating me the way she had. I was silently cheering and very grateful.

He proceeded to tell me, "Of course, you will lose all of your clinical credit hours and will need to do 42 classroom credit hours to get out of here."

I gulped. In the programs of the College of Arts and Sciences, clinical hours were not considered the same as academic credits.

He also said, "You will need to take freshman-, senior-, and graduate-level courses simultaneously. Therefore, I will waive the prerequisites and open any required classes which are now closed."

That is how I found myself suddenly a senior psychology student. Talk about total immersion! However, it left me with the unsettled feeling of having huge gaps in my education. I put on my roller skates and kept Musty as my faculty advisor.

How a Bachelor-Level Psychologist Became an NIMH Investigator

During a graduate-level course called Schizophrenia Research the next spring, taught by Professor Jon Rolf, I decided that the only way I could survive earning some of those 42 credit hours was to garner as many credit hours as possible doing research. Naturally I went back to Brooks to inquire what kind of *really small* project I could do. My goal was to get out of school and go back to pediatric nursing with a BA in psychology (although not with the BSN that I really wanted).

Brooks said something like, "Well, we have this going on in Unit A and this going on in Unit B, and *by the way*, I have an old research cohort with whom my clinical team worked in the late 1950s and early 1960s. This is the 20th anniversary of their program, and I have written to people to find out what they have been doing and how they are. They are writing letters back and perhaps you can do something with them."

Letters, I thought to myself, *great!* I said, "That would be easy. I can work on them at home." I never dreamed that I would be working on an expanded version of this project for the next 40 years.

The Seismic Shift

Just before I received my bachelor's degree in psychology that spring, a professor in the department, George Albee, heard me talk about having found 87% of Brooks's original rehab research cohort so far, after just one letter of inquiry. Albee had been interested in schizophrenia and IQ ever since a 1949 court case he was involved in, and he had also been a president of the American Psychological Association. His current field of interest was prevention. Other than Rolf lecturing on research in schizophrenia, no one in our psychology department was actually providing clinical care for patients diagnosed with schizophrenia. Many departments of psychology provided a general review course of abnormal psychology and/or conducted research. Albee alone recognized what we had found. For Brooks, these ex-patients were just his old cohort. For me in my total ignorance these people were just participants in the smallest study I could create. Albee suggested that I call Loren Mosher, Chief of the Schizophrenia Center at the NIMH, to see if they might be interested in funding a real study of this sample.

I picked up the phone and spoke to Mosher. He was enthusiastic but reminded me that I had only 7 days to submit a grant application for the next deadline. Both George Albee and George Brooks were leaving for vacations, and, as I recall, they said, "If you want this, kid, you write it."

Writing a federal grant is no mean feat. A NIMH grant proposal is full of complicated instructions, many different forms, budgets, and 25 required pages of formatted research protocol. They are often 5 to 10 inches thick or more! It's lucky I didn't know this at the time, and I would not have made it at all if Brooks hadn't left me his long-term secretary, Viola Graham. I also talked with the grants accounting office at the university on budgeting. I simply inserted into the protocol everything that I had learned in my one-semester course on schizophrenia research. I included studies done by William Carpenter and John Strauss, two preeminent schizophrenia investigators who had run the Washington Center for the World Health Organization (WHO) International Pilot Study.[10] I included their 14-item

Prognostic Scale and their four-item Outcome Scale in the proposal.[11,12] These were the only instruments I knew about at the time, and the fact that Brooks had been an investigator and grant reviewer himself certainly helped the review process. Little did I know that the race to meet grant deadlines would define the rest of my professional life.

Some Reasons Why Pilot Studies Are So Important

Brooks, who had served on NIMH review committees back in the 1960s, then made a very important move. He said that the grant committees were very interested in feasibility. Could I really gain access to these people, and would they agree to talk with me? Brooks hired me that summer to be a "research nurse" and find out. (Of course, there was no such state position, but he did it anyway.)

By that time, I had been taught by Professor Larry Gordon, my design and methodology teacher, that I should interview a "stratified subset." These 38 (15%) people needed to reflect key characteristics of the larger original 253-member sample (later found to be 269 people in Phase III). They were matched for age (within 10 years), residence (hospital, sheltered, or independent), and diagnosis (schizophrenia or not). There were 17 men and 21 women involved, with ages ranging from 39 to 80.[13]

Next, I set about making appointments and interviewing people. For diagnostic purposes I used a two-page draft instrument taken from one created at Rockland State Hospital in New York, called the Mental Status Examination Record (MSER), which used DIAGNO II, Version 2, and was computerized.[14] Although many investigators were working on instrument batteries, it was the only one that I knew about because our hospital had a computer link with Rockland. I believe that the instrument was a forerunner of the Structured Clinical Interview for the DSM-III-R (SCID). It was a psychological assessment for the *Diagnostic and Statistical Manual* (DSM),[15,16] which many psychiatrists used to make a diagnosis. The DSM eventually became a massive clinical guide, developed and retooled over the succeeding years by New York State Psychiatric Institute at Columbia University and many other psychiatrists across the country, for the American Psychiatric Association.

I made appointments to see people, and they all let me in the door because I represented Brooks and the original team with whom they had worked so long and hard many years ago. In the years since leaving Brooks's program, almost half of this small sample had achieved independent living, with many having a couple of readmissions early on after their initial release. Only one person was found to be in the hospital, and the remaining people were living in sheltered settings, including those in their 70s and 80s who were now in nursing homes. Employment had increased, with full-time employment rising to 40% and part-time to about 25%. Nine women had 27 children among them to care for. Fewer than half of the sample was considered to be free of the signs and symptoms of schizophrenia, although all said that they were receiving medications at local clinics.[17] Later we discovered that this was not the case. Many had given up the use of psychotropics but hadn't told their doctors. Disruptive and unlawful behaviors were nonexistent. By and large we had a very brief glimpse of the possible range of clinical, occupational, functional, and personal outcomes for this group. Perhaps all those collaborative efforts at rehabilitation might have been productive after all for many of these very-long-stay patients.

At the end of the summer, Brooks said, as I recall, "I need to fill your state position as nurse on one of my units now." As a thankless wretch, I turned him down, left town, and went to Boston to work in the Neurosurgical Intensive Care Unit at Children's Hospital—back to pediatrics, back to nursing as I had planned. During the fall, I dutifully hand-calculated simple percentages based on the summer's interviews. I wrote up the small Pilot Report, sent it in to the Initial Review Group (IRG) at the NIMH, and continued on in nursing.

A Most Unusual Site Visit

The following spring, I heard that Brooks and I would host a site visit during which several investigators who were members of the Initial Review Group (IRG) would observe, first-hand, the grant applicants and their working environments. Although rarely done these days, this usually meant a serious intention to fund the proposal. For us, those visitors were Loren Mosher and Jack Maser from the Schizophrenia Center at NIMH; along with Professor John Strauss himself, then working in Rochester, New

York; and Professor Malcolm Bowers, Vice Chair at Yale's Department of Psychiatry.

I bundled my three children and two Newfoundland dogs into our station wagon and went back to Vermont. We stayed with our former pediatrician and his family. I fell asleep reading over the grant proposal the night we arrived. All I had was a cardboard box full of data and no real idea what a site visit would be like.

The next day Brooks and I snickered as we watched these four city slickers plow through tall banks of snow in their raincoats and galoshes, even though Strauss was from two other infamous snow-covered places (Rochester, New York and Erie, Pennsylvania). We met in the superintendent's office, and it soon became clear to these visitors that I was actually the principal investigator (PI) and that Brooks was my back-up technical support person. They didn't blink. I did not know that NIMH grant applicants were supposed to already have their terminal degrees (a PhD or an MD), so I did not blink either.

The visitors went on rounds with Brooks, who was dressed casually in an old V-neck sweater. But they were impressed because he knew the names and histories of each patient. They asked to see the clinical records and found that they were some of the best available anywhere, with full occupational, family, social, medical, and drug histories. Remember that our proposed study patients had participated in the original Thorazine trials as well. In addition, their Vermont records had been augmented with others collected from hospitals outside the state when they were admitted elsewhere. Furthermore, there were whole conversations recorded between clinicians and their patients. And down another hallway were their vocational rehabilitation records as well. The visitors seemed entranced.

They kindly said to me, in a most diplomatic manner, "Courtenay, we know that you only had 7 days to produce the application. We suggest that you stay in Boston, quit your job, and we'll provide you with seed money to rewrite the application after you consult with people down there. This study seems like a diamond in the rough."

Together we figured out a budget that included a salary for me, consultation money, and ad hoc secretarial services. They ran the money through the appointment that Brooks had at UVM Psychiatry and put me on their roster. It took months for me to appreciate that this was a vastly atypical site visit and that these four individuals were probably the only ones in the field who would have taken such a chance on a complete rookie.

I asked Malcolm Bowers, many years later, why he took the risk and he said something like, "The NIMH had funded many big names in the past whose studies had not produced much, so why not try an unknown?" John Strauss replied, "Well, you were so damned enthusiastic. We figured you'd get the job done." These guys had just called my big bluff.

7

Learning About Research, the Generosity of the Field, and Politics in Science

Scrambling to Cover My Big Bluff With a University-Without-Walls

I quit my job at Children's Hospital, with its security and pension plan. I was able to find a carrel office at Countway Medical Library at the Harvard Medical School, located right next door to where I had been working.

On my very first day I went over to Mass Mental Health Center across campus to participate in a grand rounds lecture given by a well-known Harvard professor. At the end of the lecture, I summoned up enough courage to raise my hand during the Q&A session. The response was the classic Harvard put-down; I was basically told that the question was not worth answering. I was furious because, 40 years later, I still believe it to be an interesting one.

I went home and, after the kids were in bed, I wrote in very large letters on a piece of paper about my frustration and anger. I declared to myself that I wanted the opportunity to provide a slice of knowledge and to be part of the action. That declaration was a revelation to me and actually very helpful across the long haul. I went back the following week and dared to ask another question. This time the speaker was the renowned behavioral psychologist, B. F. Skinner. I asked a question about his newly republished book, *Walden II*.[1] He came down off the podium and walked to where I was sitting and took 20 minutes to answer. From that time forward I knew that there would be both helpful and not so helpful people in my world.

Recovery from Schizophrenia. Courtenay M. Harding, Oxford University Press. © Courtenay M. Harding 2024.
DOI: 10.1093/oso/9780195380095.003.0007

Attending a University-Without-Walls

I started reviewing the schizophrenia literature in earnest. Albee had suggested that I speak to his friend and colleague, Brendan Maher, then chair
at Harvard's Department of Psychology and later to become the dean of its
graduate school of arts and sciences. At a time when psychiatry was generally focusing on descriptive studies, Maher had been encouraging the use of
experimental methodology and designs developed by psychology.[2,3] Maher
agreed to meet with me every Friday afternoon at Kirkland Hall to consult
on these issues for my study. He did it for 18 months and never took any
consultation fees. When I asked why, he replied, rubbing his hands together
with glee, "I love to do work that is of practical significance."

He also taught me how to change a challenge into a strength for the grant
proposal. It was his work in developing an elegant design and methodology
that has supported the study findings to this day. This well-designed study
would eventually overcome some of the skepticism of academic nay-sayers
who did not believe that such once seriously and profoundly disabled people could reclaim their lives.

More Consultation on Longitudinal Questions

Whenever Maher felt that we needed further consultation, he would have
me speak with other colleagues around the country. To deal with longitudinal questions, I met with Jane Murphy, PhD, a professor at the Harvard
School of Public Health. She is a renowned anthropologist and an epidemiologist who was working on her own 40-year population study of depression in Nova Scotia, known as the Stirling County Studies.[4]

Murphy suggested that I look at a monograph that had been written
by her husband, Alexander Leighton, MD, a cross-cultural psychiatrist and
leading Harvard epidemiologist, with his first wife, Dorothea, when both
worked at Johns Hopkins. I went over to the Peabody Anthropological
Museum at Harvard. A staff member brought up from the basement a very
dusty old manuscript wrapped in brown paper and string. It was called
"Gregorio, the Hand-Trembler,"[5] and was a story about a Navajo shaman,
written in 1949, when there was a great academic interest in understanding

Native Americans. Leighton had been a student of Adolf Meyer, chair of psychiatry at Johns Hopkins early in the century. Leighton had added more social context to Meyer's 1919 model of psychobiology, creating a mechanism known as a Life Chart in the quest for understanding schizophrenia and other illnesses.[6]

The morning after I read this document, I awoke excited from a dawn daydream and called Brooks in Vermont at 7 AM (after all, he had grown up on a farm, and must be up by then). What I saw in my reverie was a way to collect the life history material that I needed to answer the burning question: "How did these people get where they are today?"

Most studies only looked at "How they are today." I saw my team interviewing people around their kitchen tables with a big chart and template, working backward from today across 10 domains of function (i.e., working, residence, hospitalizations, significant others, life events, etc.).[7] Brooks liked the idea because it was a joint effort on the part of the person and the interviewer, and, indeed, it worked very well. He reminded me that the act of a researcher holding his writing close to his or her vest while interviewing a subject can spark some paranoia.

When he was the chief medical officer of the early, famous clinical and rehabilitation center of The Village-ISA in Long Beach, California, Mark Ragins, MD, actually showed the person he was interviewing the history he had just taken and asked, "So, did I get it right?"[8] He then handed the person a menu of possible programs for them to try. How often do clinicians do that?

The Search for Control or Comparison Samples

Murphy and I began to talk about control group issues, and she had me call another well-known professor, Lee Robins, in St. Louis, to discuss these as well. We explored all sorts of ideas, such as matching to other people on the ward not participating in the rehabilitation program, matching to a same-sex 5th-grade classmate as a normative life match, or matching to a person of the same age and sex without a mental health history living nearby. Each strategy would ask and answer a different comparison question.

I began to understand that there really wasn't an absolute "gold standard" for a perfect research protocol—in our case it really depended on what the real world would allow. Having experts discuss the pros and cons of each idea provided me with a wonderful education. For example, we found that there was no one left on the unit who did *not* participate in the rehabilitation program (other than those older than 65 or on legal mandates), that many people were old enough that their school records no longer existed in Vermont, and, ironically, that the National Institute of Mental Health (NIMH) was not interested at the time in studying so-called normal people in the community as a match. Eventually we decided on a matched comparison of patients at another hospital from the same time period but who did not receive any rehabilitation. That study, known as the Maine-Vermont Comparison Study, is described in later chapters.[9,10]

Robins had written a book, *Deviant Children Grown Up*,[11] in which she discussed what worked and what did not for her research protocol (also her dissertation). Many other investigators do not want others to know how the proverbial sausages are made—how much is serendipity, how often luck plays a role. I benefitted from her book, and I am following her example here, in laying out the pros and cons of our research for the benefit of future investigators.

Maher then sent me to Bonnie Spring, a professor in the Harvard Psychology Department, to work with her on the measurement of psychopathology. She had also worked with Joseph Zubin, PhD, former Chief of Psychiatric Research and founder of the Biometrics Research Department at the New located at the Psychiatric Institute at Columbia, on their well-known "stress-vulnerability hypothesis."[12] I was thrilled to have so many female mentors. It was rare in those days in psychiatry and psychology although much improved today.

How We Lose Validity with Academic English in Our Instruments

I also worked every week with Professor Robert Shapiro, who was the head of inpatient services at Massachusetts Mental Health Center, where Brooks had trained briefly years earlier. Shapiro and I met once a week at the end of his long working day at his lovely home office in the suburbs. He would rush in, gobble down dinner with his family, and spend an hour or so with me. We reviewed various instruments that he knew about when he was the site director in Denmark for the International Pilot Study of Schizophrenia,[13] run by the World Health Organization (WHO) at nine sites across the world. Because Shapiro was such an experienced clinical investigator, he helped me select 15 current scales and schedules, which were structured and could hold up to the rigors of *reliability* and perhaps *validity*. (Simply stated, being *reliable* means that using an instrument time after time under the similar conditions will generally yield the same answer and raters need to rate the same answer in the same way. *Validity* means that the instrument really measures what it was intended to measure in the real world. This is much more difficult. One can be very reliable but not very valid.) We also utilized the WHO Psychiatric History instrument for record reviews revised into segments and described later.[14]

What I learned in looking at the questions in some of these instruments was how often the English represented a highly educated approach. The language in the instruments certainly appealed to some in the field and read very smoothly and intelligently. But it was clear to me that many interviewees would be put off by questions such as, "How do you meet your expenses?" and would prefer and better understand, "Where do you get the money to pay your bills?" Thus, we asked some questions in terms we felt most patients could better understand.

Finding a Statistician and Not Just Any Statistician

Brendan Maher then sent me down to New York to visit Professor Joseph Fleiss, one of the most highly regarded statisticians in the country and later head of the Division of Biostatistics at the Columbia University Mailman School of Public Health.[15] Fleiss said with a laugh when I called, "If Harvard says I am the best, come on down!" I was nervous because I had only a year's worth of freshmen statistics at that point. On the plane from Boston to New York, I read a paperback book that featured jelly beans on the cover just so that I could nod in the right places.

I got to Fleiss's office a little bit early and struck up a conversation with his secretary, a small older woman with a heavy Brooklyn accent. Fleiss arrived in haste and went directly into his office and shut the door. He started yelling at whoever was in there. I asked his secretary if he always yelled at people. Fleiss had said that if I arrived at noon he would take me to lunch. I had managed to arrive just in time and Fleiss came rushing out of his office. His secretary said to him, "She just asked me if you always yell at people?" I wanted to crawl under her desk, but he simply laughed and declared that the person in his office was partially deaf.

I scarcely managed to keep up with Fleiss, with his white coat tails flying, as we raced down four flights of stairs, then up Broadway to a local deli. He walked up to the counter and in great New York style belted out, "A corned beef on rye and celery soda. What do you want, Courtenay?" Then we ran back to his building and up those same four flights. He pulled out the sliding shelf from his desk and plunked the food down, and we began our negotiation regarding his participation in the study.

We had an interesting discussion about ways to measure social class status in a society that lived beyond its slender means by bartering services— something not measured by traditional scales. At that point in time, Vermont was 36th in the nation for income, and yet New Yorkers were flocking to the state because of the lifestyle. Within half an hour Fleiss said, "I give you permission to put my name on the grant as your statistician. I'll send you a letter. So many people have put my name on their grants without my permission." He stood up, and I went to the airport. I flew home simply amazed by the whole trip.

Helping to Pioneer the Protection of Human Subjects

One of the key requirements of any protocol is to protect human subjects. Believe it or not, this idea was just coming into focus in the 1970s. Many breaches of protection had occurred across the history of research, and we wanted to avoid that at all costs. I was very fortunate to have met one of the best lawyers in the field on a plane back from Washington, DC. His seat turned out to be next to mine. His name was Stanley J. Herr, JD, DPhil,[16] then at Harvard Law School; he specialized in fair play with disadvantaged and underserved populations, such as persons with intellectual disabilities. (I later introduced him as "Horton," from the Dr. Seuss book *Horton Hears a Who*,[17] to the Fellows at the center now known as the Edward Zigler Center for Child Development and Social Policy at Yale. In that story, Horton is an elephant advocating for tiny creatures living in Whoville, a world drawn no bigger than a dandelion puffball with neighbors who denied their existence; Dr. Herr successfully argued landmark cases for the civil rights of children who were "out of sight and out of mind," such as those institutionalized for intellectual disabilities [e.g., the infamous Willowbrook case] and many others.)

With Herr's help, we drafted a covenant with our study participants stating our commitment to protect their basic rights of informed consent, their right to confidentiality, their right to privacy, and their right to refuse participation without consequences (as well as the right to refuse to answer a question or to stop at any time). Participants also knew who the director of the project was and to whom to complain if needed. They were told what would happen to their data, which would have no name identifier and which would be kept in a locked cabinet. We now take these rights for granted but, even as late as the 1970s, many notorious studies were still in progress breaching all patient protections and eventually resulting in government intervention.[18]

If we happened to speak to spouses or other family members in the course of setting up appointments, we presented ourselves as researchers from the University of Vermont (UVM) conducting a study of older Vermonters. We used a post office box at the university on our stationery and deleted all references to the Department of Psychiatry, the state hospital, or the Department of Vocational Rehabilitation. When we approached a person for an actual interview sequence, each interviewer had multiple sets of identification cards from the university, the hospital, and the vocational rehabilitation office. Because we were able to speak with most of the original research team members, we were able to identify which original clinical team member had a significant working relationship with each of the original cohort members. Making appointments under each appropriate umbrella contributed to the success rate. Since this was the late 1970s, believe it or not, we were pioneering.

Later, Herr also provided advice about permission to obtain and use photographs when we found that the faces of our participants revealed human dignity, determination, health, and liveliness. Many people gave us permission to show their faces on slides to professionals at scientific meetings. These were the first psychiatric photographs widely circulated since the late 1800s, when a book on long-term hospitalized patients showed people looking disheveled and vacant. Those pictures had contributed to much of the stigma attached to mental illness today.[19] Showing healthy people astonished many professionals.

Beautifully taken by Paul Landerl, one of our field interviewers, with permission I carried the 8 × 10-inch black-and-white photos down to the NIMH. I spread them out on a huge conference table and scientists streamed in from the Institute to see real people in a real mental health system. Ordinarily, these hard-working government employees only see people reduced to statistical numbers on volumes of white paper. We wanted so much to produce a book with these wonderful Vermont faces. Although the participants were willing, their families were not, and so the book with healthy faces is lost to time.

The Second Grant Proposal as Promised

When it was time to write the new grant application, I shifted the dining room table to the picture window in the living room looking out on the garden. I drew a cartoon showing a liter Pepsi bottle strung up to an IV stand next to me, and I began to try to write a much more complicated protocol. It had a cross-sectional segment ("How are you today and in the past month?"). It had a longitudinal section ("What did you do with your life before and after the rehabilitation program?") and a multilayered record review. It also had a matched comparison study as well as a follow-up of the children and grandchildren of the sample. Remember that this was before ubiquitous home computers. I lived on caffeine.

Second Site Visit: A Very Different Kettle of Fish!

We received word that the NIMH was sending seven people for the next site visit. This time I had encouraged Brooks to wear a three-piece suit instead of his old sweater. I had read more of the literature. We had a conference room and alternate budgets. We had high-powered consultants. This was a very good thing, especially because both Strauss and Bowers had cycled off the Initial Review Group. The people who came included Mosher, Chief of the Schizophrenia Center and now a declared friend-of-the-grant; Jack Maser at the Center; and five mid-level investigators, plus the highly regarded Professor of Psychiatry Gerard (Jerry) Hogarty, MSW, from the University of Pittsburgh, as the outside reviewer. The site reviewers nitpicked everything. They nitpicked and nitpicked until I thought I would lose my own mind.

I was so frustrated when they left that I went to a classroom and covered all the blackboards with lists. There were lists of what the field and my mentors said were now important. There were lists of questions that I felt strongly about, and there were lists of what the site visitors had stripped out. These mid-level visitors had said,

"No need to rediagnose these subjects. We all know they are old chronic schizophrenics!"

"Drop the longitudinal piece because you can't possibly get enough data to track it."

"Don't do any cost-benefit analysis because knowing that one of your subjects makes 12 free shirts for needy children in her community every year is not our idea of items to include in cost-benefits."

I was furious. I made a command decision to leave everything in except the cost-benefit analysis because we didn't have an economist on the team. Later I found that the NIMH did not really care if an investigator does twice as much work for the same dollar—and I am happy to say that my instincts actually paid off, as the reader will learn in ensuing chapters. I now tell students to trust their own instincts and stick up for them.

I also found out later that these mid-level site reviewers were upset that I did not have my terminal degree and about the amount of money I had requested. Mosher later admitted that he had said to them in executive session that we had accomplished so much more than anyone had expected. They were "kind of shamed into funding us," and they gave us a nearly perfect score of 104, with 100 being perfect, and the range up to 500 being totally unacceptable.

Starting the Study and Graduate School Simultaneously

With the grant in place, I packed up my family again and moved back to Vermont. In the meantime, Hogarty had written to me and strongly encouraged me to get my doctorate. He said that, in the current era, he himself would not have become a professor of psychiatry with his MSW even with his well-known series of studies, though I knew that the field considered them to be truly elegant.[20] If I wanted a job after the grant was over, I would need a PhD. He also wrote in this letter some lyrical prose. He spoke about the thrill of being able to put a little sliver of knowledge into the field's understanding of such complex processes involved in schizophrenia and how tough it was to be constantly peer-reviewed. He ended with a joke—being Hogarty—about how his own letter looked like he, himself, was applying, to graduate school. So I was forewarned about what I was getting myself into.

I had assumed that with an estimated 100-hour-a-week job and three middle-sized children, I would not be able to get my doctorate. Further, the UVM Department of Psychology was a traditional place and really didn't like part-time students. But, given Hogarty's insistence, I went back to Rik Musty, my old chair and advisor. I told him I could only take a couple of classes a semester and he said, "Well, you do have your dissertation in hand." So suddenly I was in graduate school on one end of campus and also on the faculty of psychiatry on the other.

The Department of Psychiatry did not know what to do with me because I had more money for research than anyone else at the time. They made up a faculty position title because I did not meet any of the criteria for formal positions without my terminal degree. The head of grants and contracts for the university was upset, saying, "You can't have that salary level because it is greater than the dean of nursing." But since I was not within the university salary structure and with an oddball title, he was unable to change it.

Musty broke the rules again and let me specialize early and generalize late. This meant that I took courses highly relevant to my day-to-day challenges in getting the study off the ground and could take foundational courses, such as child development, later. To be taught a subject that one immediately applies to real life turned out for me to be the very best way to learn.

Not Letting Anyone Take Over the Study

Before I left for Vermont, I received a letter from a world-famous neuro-scientist and geneticist at Harvard, Seymour Kety, who had been the first scientific director of the intramural research programs at the NIMH, among other positions. He asked me to consult on his new Danish Study on how to recognize independent versus dependent life events. I had recently been only a lowly recorder of a lively discussion at a recent NIMH meeting about these issues, with experts such as George Brown of England, Joseph Zubin, and Bruce Dohrenwend discussing the nuances. I realized that I had only minimal expertise on his particular question, but I dutifully wrote out what I knew from the aforementioned discussion in a one-page letter and sent it back. I realized later that I should have sent a bill for consulting, but I was too naïve.

Boston is a small city, and, before long, word was out that I had a very big research project on schizophrenia in the works. I received an invitation to have lunch and tour the grounds from Shervert Frazier, Psychiatrist-in-Chief of Harvard's famous McLean Hospital. Although I was perplexed, it was a nice opportunity, and the conversation was actually very helpful. He spoke about a female patient who had just been interviewed with the newest very early trial version of the Structured Clinical Interview for the DSM-III-R (SCID)[21] mentioned earlier. Three psychiatrists had watched the interview from behind a one-way mirror. I was told that these three clinicians had about 125 years of experience among them. During the interview, the patient had said "no" to several questions about alcohol use, and so the skip pattern was done (meaning the remaining questions on that topic were skipped), with the final diagnosis designated as schizophrenia. However, Frazier went on to say that one of the observing physicians had later met the woman on the unit and conducted a clinical interview with her. She admitted that she actually had a habit of drinking large quantities of vodka over many years and had lied in response to the alcohol questions earlier. This psychiatrist thought that she was probably suffering from Korsakoff's syndrome instead.[22] Frazier spoke about the importance of combining clinical expertise with our new structured interviews. The Vermont team took his advice to heart and combined both approaches in our interviews.

Later in the afternoon I was bundled into a golf cart and taken over to the Mailman Research Center, where Seymour Kety held sway.[23] I did not meet him but an assistant suddenly brought me a seven-page contract without any previous discussion. It outlined terms stating that Kety would have first authorship on the first paper on the study, and I was to have first authorship on the second paper. The list went on and on, outlining future papers. In exchange for this "honor," I was to let his team follow our interviewers and conduct a battery of biological measures on the Vermont Longitudinal Study participants. I was stunned and practically speechless, a state unusual for me.

I thought to myself, "For heaven's sake, I have teams of people that I have worked with for months. Furthermore, how could I explain this request to people who had been told during the rehab program in the 1950s that it was quite possible they could recover and feel like 'normal' people again. How could I ask, 'By the way, we need your urine, blood samples, and eye tests?'" Wouldn't they feel like guinea pigs and not really normal and our consultants after all? Still dumbfounded, I simply blurted out "Well, we just don't do things that way in Vermont!" Not a terribly brilliant reply nor explanation.

The Dark Side of Science

Shortly thereafter, in a hushed auditorium at the UVM and after flowery introductions were made, Kety stood at the podium to present an important colloquium on his newest research. His first words, addressed to faculties of both psychology and psychiatry, were, "Courtenay Harding is a foolish young woman impeding the progress of science!" They are etched, crystal clearly, in my mind.

This was my first introduction to the darker side of science. This was Science, with a capital S (the politicized kind), and the experience revealed the existence of different kinds of academic tribes.[24] Indeed, the exclusive nature of Science later played out in the review by geneticists of another of my grant proposals. Further, the tribe showed up again in the refusal to publish the Maine-Vermont long-term matched comparison study of 35 years in the *New England Journal of Medicine*—even though the matching protocol was published in the *American Journal of Psychiatry* as two lead articles, and the Maine counterpart also had nearly a perfect NIMH score. We went to the *British Journal of Psychiatry* instead. Memories are very long. I was shocked. I am glad to report that, in general, people in the scientific fields of psychology and psychiatry can be particularly generous-hearted (see this book's Acknowledgements, thanking even more than the 125 people who contributed key components to the third and fourth phases of the study in the base papers).

Fortunately, my chair in psychology, Rik Musty jumped to my defense and stood up for me, for which I shall be eternally grateful. It was a challenging way to begin one's career. Later, I discovered that being yelled at has its advantages as well, although I did not really appreciate it at the time.

Loren Mosher at the NIMH Schizophrenia Center seemed pleased that I had resisted all the glory apparently inherent in focusing on biological issues and working with Kety. In all probability, I would have wound up as a handmaiden in the big-time biogenetic Harvard machinery long before it would produce anything helpful in psychiatry. Instead, I became kind of a mascot of the NIMH for the next 5 years, a walking example that the Institute could be human and support such a rookie. It was one of the best decisions that I made during the project, although it didn't make my career easier, with Dark Science lurking around every corner—and with a very long memory. I knew that the Vermont participants would have indeed felt strange and like patients again if we had asked for those measures. I felt very loyal to them and to Brooks and to our team. Everyone would have rightly rebelled and been hurt.

Not Dismissing Biological Interactions

All the same I must add that now, as a nurse, a psychologist, and a professor of psychiatry and rehabilitation, I strongly believe that any extreme state has biopsychosocial antecedents because probably *everything* does, minute to minute. *Biopsychosocial* means a mixture of three important components (biology, psychological, and social interactions) reacting together. It also seems to me that recovery is possible because of the interactions between these improved components as well, as simple-minded as this may sound. Under different circumstances I would always like to have measurements across the spectrum because they might teach us important things about such interactions. However, Kety's was not the way. Forty years later, those biological measures proposed by his team have done little to explain schizophrenia. So, in the end, I did not actually "impede the progress of science" after all, much to my relief. It might be said that what we learned in Vermont and Maine actually moved the field forward.

Living Well Is the Best Revenge

In my dissertation, I gratefully wrote up 10 full pages of acknowledgments thanking all the people who had participated in our NIMH follow-up studies. Their generosity in sharing their expertise and wisdom is truly a tribute to the caring professions. Furthermore, none of them asked for consultation fees!

That small research project of letters, which I finished to get out of college so that I could go back to pediatric nursing, later turned into one of the longest studies of schizophrenia in the world literature (av. 32 years) and the longest study of deinstitutionalized patients in the United States (25 years). Talk about serendipity. It would change my life forever, and I ended up in psychiatry just as the original chair of nursing at Vermont College had predicted all along.

Furthermore, this "foolish young woman" has received 47 honors and awards across her career on behalf of all the participants and team members. One of the ones that I treasure most was from the foundation arm of the American Psychological Association. It was the Alexander Gralnick 2004–2005 Investigator Award "recognizing exceptional contributions to the study of schizophrenia and other serious mental illness and for mentoring a new generation of researchers." Passing the baton by sharing what my mentors taught me has been an enduring pleasure. The next chapters will show how we put all that advice to work and what we found.

8

How We Measured a Life Lived

Preparation Is Worth All the Effort

There was still so much *more* work to do to prepare to conduct our research project. It was frustrating, not being able to rush into the field
after all the time spent studying the literature, deciding on the questions to
be asked, meeting with consultants, selecting the instruments, writing the
grant proposal, surviving site visits, having one's bluff called, hiring staff,
and upending one's life. But the groundwork is essential and pays off with
major benefits down the road. In fact, our early undivided attention to design and methodology made all the difference in the eventual acceptance
of our findings, especially because we ended up challenging 125 years of
thinking about the long-term outcome of schizophrenia and other serious
and persistent psychiatric problems.

I dubbed our project the "Vermont Longitudinal Research Project," also
known as VLRP. (It sounded like "slurp" with a "v." My children fantasized
that it was akin to SMERSH,[1] the devious organization in the James Bond
movies, (and they still joke about it.) Now that the National Institute of
Mental Health (NIMH) had called my bluff, I had to move my family back
to Burlington, Vermont. I started graduate school and began to learn how
to run a very large study. Being a mother seemed to help because my kids
pitched in and cheered me on.

Recovery from Schizophrenia. Courtenay M. Harding, Oxford University Press. © Courtenay M. Harding 2024.
DOI: 10.1093/oso/9780195380095.003.0008

The Cost and Benefits of Working
Across Disciplines

I maintained a very careful balance between being a graduate student at one end of campus and being a new faculty member in the Department of Psychiatry on the other end, at the School of Medicine. I had decided to run my NIMH grant through the Psychiatry Department, for the very practical reason that academic psychology (at the time) rarely had much to do with treating serious and persistent mental illness, especially schizophrenia until 2019.[2] There are, of course, a few excellent exceptions, of both people and programs.

Professor Albee was the one who recognized that Brooks and I might have a special cohort to study, and he suggested we find out if the NIMH might be interested. He was also a past president of the American Psychological Association and was understandably quite furious that I had put the grant through psychiatry. I still believe that it was a good decision, although this cross-disciplinary stance has over time made me feel somewhat like the outsider in both professions. On the other hand, neither was I caught within each profession's narrow silo of knowledge. This "outsidership" allowed me to be exposed to the richness of thinking in both fields, as well as to those of nursing and social work, without being blinded by the self-imposed limitations of each field. In 1966, Thomas Kuhn remarked

> The scientific community consists . . . of members of a scientific specialty . . . who have undergone similar educations and professional initiations; in the process they have absorbed the same technical literature and drawn many of the same lessons from it.[3]

The narrowness Kuhn was talking about also helps to explain why paradigms are so difficult to change and why science becomes politicized. My son majored in physics at Princeton and eventually trained as a theoretical and catalytic chemist at Stanford. He informed me that the so-called hard sciences were just as politicized, and their protocols just as biased by subjective decision-making, as were the so-called soft sciences. This was a revelation to me.

The compound exposure of psychiatry and psychology as well as the significant gaps in my education due to my unusual career path allowed me to ask questions in the Vermont protocol which might not otherwise have been considered, let alone asked, in that era. Working with multiple disciplines across time has always been exceedingly rewarding, and I believe this is critical to improved understanding of human behavior and schizophrenia. If I had been trained as a psychiatrist alone, chances are that I would have focused primarily on symptoms, diagnosis, and medication adherence; if I had been trained only as a psychologist, I might have targeted behaviors, personality, and neuropsychological status. If I had trained as a nurse, I might have assessed functioning and health behaviors; if I had trained only in social work, I might have paid primary attention to family systems and the community environment. But by putting all of these perspectives together, I aimed to describe the whole person in his or her context. At the time, I confess, most of my questions were driven simply by profound curiosity. Some of my questions were, "Just who are these people?" "Why did they end up in the hospital?" "How come they stayed there? "What is rehabilitation?" "What were their lives like after the rehab program?" "What do they think helped or hindered them along the way?"

Recognizing Significant Limitations

I ended up becoming a jack of all trades and a master of none. To build our team, I began looking for people who were highly skilled and much more experienced than I. In retrospect, I believe that the NIMH actually got a better study from us than it would have following the usual routine, in which the professor is awarded the grant and hires his or her students to collect the data. Instead, the NIMH funded a graduate student who hired professor-level and other professionals to collect the data and analyze it.

To begin, I hired Carmine Consalvo, MEd, and Paul Landerl, LCSW, as interviewers. They had been working as front-line clinicians, with teaching and social work backgrounds, for many years in public outpatient settings, with people who had serious and persistent problems. At the time, they both felt somewhat burned out and discouraged by prospects of improvement for the people they were working with and were fleeing to research for a breather. They were intelligent, creative, very keen observers of human beings and full of good humor.

Landerl and Consalvo also taught me how to be a better boss. They would tackle a job and then bring it to me. Sometimes I would "Monday morning quarterback" them, which would really tick them off. They let it be known that I was either to lay out specifically what I wanted and send them off to do it, *or* I was to give them a bare outline and let them create—but I was not to mix the two. It was a good lesson to learn so that I would not get in the way of their creativity lest I kill it.

Finding a Research Home

Brooks provided us with a set of rooms in the basement of the hospital, which we quickly painted a pale aqua blue to offset the dreariness. Later Brooks set us up with offices near his in the main administration building up on the second and third floors. Originally these offices had been part of the living quarters of early superintendents, and there was a hidden back stairway between my office and those of the two interviewers upstairs in the attic. The guys would periodically pop down with questions. During grant-writing season, I would put a single red flag made of construction paper on their side of the door indicating "Only bother me if you are unable to continue without the answer." If the impending grant application was due, there were two crossed red flags on that door. They designated, "I don't care if the building is burning down, please don't bother me!" Any grant writer will understand.

Putting the Instrument Battery Together

We set about piecing the instrument batteries together, which took about 18 months. Robert Shapiro from Mass Mental Health had provided us with 15 structured interview scales and schedules across a wide area of functioning and psychopathology. Questions about areas of function included data on the quantity and quality of work, finances, residence, interpersonal relationships, activities of daily living (e.g., who cooked, cleaned, paid the bills, went to the market, did the laundry?), life events, community involvement, personal resources, strengths, and liabilities. Additional data were collected on struggles with symptoms (both positive and negative), treatment, medications, side effects, hospitalizations, mental status, environmental stressors, and global functioning (a score combining level of overall functioning and psychological status).

We wanted to capture a whole person living in his or her own environment, and we did not want to reinvent the wheel. Some instruments we left intact, and others we blended. Many investigators had made up instruments focusing on a particular domain and asked only those questions (e.g., work and social supports, residence and social supports, leisure time and social supports). We took the ones on work from all the instruments, for example, and found that if we combined all the questions on work that did not overlap, we could then have a complete set of questions on the topic without constantly repeating ourselves and annoying interviewees.

This strategy led to a tradeoff. Tradeoffs are always present in making decisions about research. On one hand, an intact instrument allows comparison with its use in other studies. On the other hand, changing the context of the surrounding questions in which the question is asked may change the way a person answers the question, and so the instrument becomes less comparable to other studies, even though we could reconstitute the original instrument electronically. But we chose to cluster all the questions about work in one place and all the ones on other areas of functioning together. This positioning allowed us to have a sensible flow and ease in the interview. It made sense and promoted the comfort of both the interviewee and the interviewer. This sense of ease was critical to both the quality of the answers and toleration of the process.

The Final Instrument Batteries

We ended up with two interviews, one cross-sectional and the other longitudinal. The first interview focused on how the person was doing now and over the past month. Known as the Vermont Community Questionnaire (VCQ-C),[4] it included 135 interview questions and 98 additional items to be answered by the rater based on observational information gleaned from the interviewees or from their environment. It took approximately 1 hour and 15 minutes to administer, although people seemed so pleased to be our consultants that they spent a great deal of time with us, often as many as 5 hours. Our interviewers were "blind" to what was in the subjects' records, including their diagnoses, so that they could see people with fresh eyes. This strategy was very important and is one seldom followed by other research studies. Consalvo and Landerl also tended to have to watch for weight gain because people kept feeding them as they sat in their kitchens talking to-gether. The interviews were generally taped with participant permission for the purpose of supervision. After erasing a couple of tapes to save money, we decided that the tapes provided valuable information in and of themselves. So we swallowed the financial cost and kept as many as possible thereafter.

The interviewers sat under trees by streams on pleasant days in beautiful Vermont after their interviews. They hand-wrote diary notes about their own subjective experiences while questioning the person of the day. Since interviews are a two-way process, it seemed important that the interviewer have his viewpoint about the quality of interaction as well. This follow-up is rarely done but made sense to us. Social worker Janet Mikkelsen, MSW, also helped us put this large instrument together. We found that the interviewers had written dozens of notes in the side margins of observations and more information—a gold mine in and of itself but often missed by just using the coded answers.

The second interview (VCQ-L)[5] was designed to capture the longi-tudinal information that documented status and events over the previous 20–25 years. There was an interview section of 156 questions including a Life Chart with a rater section. It was administered approximately a week after the first interview and included questions on current psychopath-ology (including both prodromal, the very early symptoms, and residual symptoms), substance use, prescribed drug use, and side effects. We waited for week 2 to ask these more difficult questions, after some trust had been established with our interviewees. The VCQ-L took about 75 minutes and also documented past years in a year-by-year follow-back procedure driven by the modified Meyer/Leighton Life Chart. We found that if subjects filled in the current year's activities first, then it was much easier to remember last year's happenings and so forth.

Thomas McGlashan, MD, then working at Chestnut Lodge and later a professor at Yale, helped us with suggestions for our rediagnostic work. That effort was piloted for us by professor and psychiatrist William Woodruff of the University of Vermont (UVM). Eventually John Strauss and Alan Breier at Yale conducted the entire rediagnostic substudy to see if these patients, who were originally diagnosed according to criteria from the Diagnostic and Statistical Manual of Mental Disorders (DSM-I and -II), would have been diagnosed similarly by the new and more stringent criteria of the DSM-III.[6] A later chapter describes this mammoth effort.

The Life Chart

As described in the previous chapter, the Life Chart had an illustrious lineage, from Adolf Meyer (1919)[7] to the Leightons (1949)[8] to the Vermont Project (1980).[9] Vaillant (1980) also found Meyer's Life Chart useful for research in tracing the life patterns of persons with a variety of psychiatric disorders.[10] The chart provided a graphic overview of each person's life and was completed with a set of structured probes, codes, and protocols created for this project. We also added new questions to elicit information on the subjective view of significant shifts or turning points as well as the best and the worst years in the person's life to date. And we included an extra column to record spontaneous additional comments made during that part of the interview.

Our Life Chart was a large, lined sheet, vertically separated from the then current year of 1981 at the top to 1955 at the bottom. It was horizontally separated by 10 outcome domains:

Life Chart Outcome Domains (VCQ-L)

Residence
Hospitalization
Work
Source of income
Significant others
Deaths of significant others
Other life events
Use of community support systems
Health
Medications

I pilfered my children's Monopoly[11] boards and put the codes in place of Boardwalk, Park Place, etc. The boards were carried in car trunks and fresh new sheets were placed in the middle as needed. Each Chart became as individualized as the life it reflected. Eventually the field interviewers were able to detect which Chart belonged to which person without looking at the case number at the bottom. Barry Nurcombe, MD, at UVM before moving to Brisbane, Australia, and H. Peter Laqueur, MD, both psychiatrists, helped us learn more sophisticated mechanics of the interview process.

We ended up with 2,600 bytes of information across the battery on each person. The next questions to be broached were "How can we tell if we are asking the right questions?" and "Can the interviewees be rated the same way by different raters?"

The Validity Studies

Validity seeks to measure the real thing in the real world. Consalvo and Landerl hired a group of individuals from a senior housing complex in Burlington to serve as consultants to test the validity of the interviews. These people were the same age as most members of the study cohort, whose average age was 59, ranging up to 83 years of age. The consultants were very helpful in smoothing the process. These test cases led to the addition of questions about a sense of powerlessness, disability income, and general medication adherence. They also told us to take deaths of significant others out of the life events category and make them a separate category. These seniors said that we would see more clearly the growing impact of losing one's friends and family members as one aged. We were all too young to have realized this fact of life and were grateful to them for pointing it out.

Another valuable addition to the Life Chart was made one day by an elderly man in the general hospital cafeteria connected to the medical school. Unknown to us, he was listening to our excited conversation about our new version of the Life Chart. He asked if he could become a volunteer tester of the Chart. We were delighted because he was a retired professor of romance languages who could provide detailed feedback, as well as being in the same age bracket as our future study participants. He followed us back to our offices, and we conducted our first full-fledged Life Chart interview. He was a wonderful consultant, and we could see his life emerge across the paper. We were all startled by how the patterns and trends jumped out at us as the paper became filled. In fact, he saw immediately that every time he lost a significant person in his life he would engage in an alcoholic binge. At age 82, he announced that he had decided to find a clinician to explore reasons for this pattern. We knew then that we had a very powerful instrument for collecting a life's worth of data.

The Life Chart ended up not just reliable but people also really enjoyed doing it. We discovered that if you provided a structured template with common probe questions, even people who had lived difficult lives were able to give accurate accounts. Ironically, the one area that they were unable to recall reliably was the beginning and end dates for hospitalizations. Of course, we had those hard data from the records.

We also cross-checked answers with designated family and friends and found that these participants had volunteered information (e.g., illegitimate children, etc.) that their families were certain they would not. We developed a structured interview (the Verinform) to verify the history provided us with not only family members but also with other designated people, such as general practitioners, aftercare workers, vocational rehabilitation specialists, and friends—whoever the participants thought knew them the best and had provided permission. At this time in science, investigators and clinicians were convinced that people who had been diagnosed with psychiatric problems (especially schizophrenia) were mostly unable to provide much accurate information about anything. We found that assumption was generally not true and that they were quite capable.

We chose colors for each component of the interview and record review batteries, and, to this day, we can tell from across the room which instrument is which. It also helped the data people and maintained consistency and reliability. In Washington, DC, the study became known as The Rainbow Project because everything else in their file cabinets was otherwise white.

Abstracting Records From Across Decades Was Also a Real Challenge

I next hired William Deane, PhD, the sociologist who had worked at the hospital for years. He participated in the original project for its first 10 years, ran the 5-year follow-up, and therefore knew the hospital records forward and backward. I also hired Janet Forgays, PhD, a psychologist, and she and Deane conducted the interrater trials together. These two record abstractors worked with UVM psychology Professor Jon Rolf, who had taught me that graduate course on schizophrenia research while I was an undergraduate. Rolf converted the World Health Organization (WHO)'s interview instrument, called the Psychiatric and Personal History Schedule (PHHS), into a structured and systematic record review.

This schedule was part of the interview battery used in the WHO's Collaborative Project on Determinants of Outcome of Severe Mental Disorders.[12] In addition, the Record Review had to be applied to multiple time periods, which turned out to be a real challenge. The WHO format and coded answers were maintained but assigned to repeatedly document five different time periods: (1) first admission, (2) episodes between first and index, (3) index admission, (4) a topical life history, and (5) episodes during the years post release. The record reviewers were blind to outcome and interview data.

Index admission was that admission preceding entry into the rehabilitation program set up in 1955. This time period was the only common denominator across all subjects because they all had different dates of onset, hospitalizations, and episodes. Sometimes the first and index hospitalizations were the same (e.g., a person could have had one admission and stayed in hospital for 20 years and then entered the rehabilitation program). We also had to capture critical information from intervening episodes between first and index admissions, as well as any which occurred after discharge from the program. This review turned out to be a major enterprise. We also ran interrater trials between the two record abstractors so that we would know if they rated the same data in the same way.

The records were truly amazing. The people we were now studying had originally been in Brooks's Thorazine study in the early to mid-1950s. There were occupational, social, and family histories, as well as the expected medical, drug, and side-effect notations, all systematically collected. Unfortunately, much of social and occupational information is missing from today's recordkeeping. In addition, there were whole conversations between clinicians and patients recorded for posterity. In addition, Susan Childers, ACSW, from Smith College Graduate School of Social Work, put together the case books which provided an overall narrative history and an appreciation of each person. Thus, by translating personal histories into cohesive stories, we were eventually able to better understand the magnitude of what we found and not solely rely on data points.

In addition, I had Edgar Forsberg of Underhill Center, Vermont, translate from the German to English many of the other long-term studies completed just before ours so that I could see how these studies were conducted. At the time, American psychiatry was pretty ethnocentric and rarely gave a glance at work not done in the United States. I later brought this work home to American audiences who were only vaguely aware of it. Fortunately, times have changed.

Our Unexpected Treasure Trove of Other Data

As mentioned earlier, Bob Lagor, the Department of Vocational Rehabilitation (VR) counselor who had participated in the original study, told us of a secret cache of VR records which he had saved from the paper shredder back when he was higher up in the system. An order had come down from the state to purge records, and he had taken all the records from the VR side of things on the early *Vermont Story* studies and stashed them away in the hospital basement in cardboard boxes, then moved them into the attic. He said he thought that someday someone might be interested in seeing them. Admittedly this hoarding could have been considered, 20 years later, as ethically inappropriate. The records were full of mildew and smelled awful, but we could still read them. We all copied and copied and copied, put the copies under lock and key, and shredded the originals.

The state government had also recently ordered that, if the hospital record room wanted more file cabinets, it had to send old records to Montpelier, the capital, to be microfilmed. This order included our own clinical research records. Brooks let us copy them, and it was a mad rush by Andrea Pierce, the project's stalwart secretary, to get this done before they were sent off and stripped of valuable information before being microfilmed. Afterward, the government threw away all social and occupational data, as well as clinical notes. They kept only the diagnoses, medical illnesses, and medication records.

Finding the Remaining Missing People

I hired Patricia Reid and Joan Jarvis, who had returned to college to complete their BSW degrees at Trinity College nearby. I was able to wangle credit for them to spend the summer tracking down the last 35 members of the sample (plus 87% already found of total 269). Because Vermonters either never moved, or, if they did, it was usually inside Vermont, these detectives were able to find all but 7 of the original 269-person cohort at an average of 32 years after first admission. Their hard work gave us a *97% found rate*, which is nothing short of spectacular. Most studies of less than 5 years usually find about 30% at 5-year follow-up. The Vermont success rate lent much stronger validity to the findings. Northern New England turns out to have been an excellent place to conduct longitudinal studies.

These intrepid detectives searched hospital records for addresses of family members who had visited the person in the hospital, as well as for hints of places previously lived. They looked at Vermont and New Hampshire telephone books, talked with Departments of Motor Vehicles, and spoke to postmistresses in very small towns, as well as the owners of country stores. They received intel such as, "Oh John, well, he moved to East Corinth and lives up the hill in a cabin." To protect the privacy of our subjects, again, we used the guise of researchers from the University of Vermont studying older Vermonters. The Vermont office of the Social Security Administration even allowed us to provide a few sealed letters without addresses for them to address and send out for us. Each letter explained the study and included a return envelope for a reply if the recipient wished to speak with us. This strategy allowed contact without telling us where the person was living. Most of these approaches probably would not be open to investigators today because internet search engines as resources may have replaced them.

Searching for Other Hidden Biases

The biggest bias, in the opposite direction, was one that took us a very long time to figure out. The key question was: "Who was still missing from this sample?" One day, quite out of the blue, it dawned on me that other studies had shown that about 10% of young males with schizophrenia complete suicide. Thus, there was a very high probability that the hopeless and impulsive ones never lived long enough to make it into our cohort (see Mary Ann Test and colleagues' 1990 discussion of her group in Madison, Wisconsin).[13]

A large team was assembled to accomplish this study, and an incredible amount of thought and effort went into the work before we saw a single subject in the field. This investment was worth every minute. Furthermore, we had a wonderful time being so creative.

The Impact of Psychology Training

Studying design, methodology, and statistics forces the mind to be disciplined and analytic, states of being unaccustomed to me! I had struggled through Professor Larry Gordon's classes, thinking with relief that it was required just for graduation, and that, in the end, it would not be useful for me in nursing. Was I ever mistaken! Later, in working with Professor Maher at Harvard on the design and methodology for the Vermont Longitudinal Study, suddenly everything Gordon had tried to teach me made sense for nursing, too. In the end, design, methodology, and analysis were the bedrock of Phase III of the Vermont Longitudinal Study. Left to my own devices, and without the participation, generosity, and creativity of my many collaborators, the study would have gone down in flames.

9

Tough Questions From the Chief of Medical Biostatistics

A Cross-Cultural Experience Solving Puzzles

Once we were funded, I called our grant application statistician, Dr. Joseph Fleiss, in New York. He was preparing to become Dean of the Columbia School of Public Health, and he suggested that we contact Dr. Takamaru Ashikaga, Chief of Medical Biostatistics at the University of Vermont School of Medicine (UVM). Fleiss said something complimentary like, "Dr. Ashikaga knows all the stuff that I have forgotten!"

I contacted Ashikaga, and we have been working together ever since. He is related to the famous Shogunate family in Kyoto. In fact, most of his family heirlooms are in museums. Fortunately for me, he is also a very patient and kind person, and he taught me to read printouts repeatedly to evaluate what our findings meant. Even though I eventually passed three classes in graduate statistics myself, the science is so complicated that I was relieved to have guidance from someone who spent his entire career keeping up with this ever-changing field. My advice to researchers: always consider working with a statistician as soon as possible on a clinical research project. Today, most journals and the National Institute of Mental Health (NIMH) seek statisticians to review submitted papers and grant proposals. Ashikaga also sat on several review committees at the NIMH.

Ashikaga began by asking tough questions about our study and study participants. He used language that I was acquainted with such as: "What are your main questions? Which variables of interest are independent or dependent? Which ones are categorical, ordinal, or interval?" However, I had never applied these queries to the 2,600 items that we would be asking our

Recovery from Schizophrenia. Courtenay M. Harding, Oxford University Press. © Courtenay M. Harding 2024.
DOI: 10.1093/oso/9780195380095.003.0009

subjects and abstracting from their records. Ashikaga's analyses depended on these specific levels of measurement as well as on whether or not the distribution of the sample means was expected to be normal or not. On the face of it, they seemed to be simple, direct, and understandable questions, but I was blown away by their complexity as perceived by Ashikaga. Here was the direct application of some of what l had learned in freshman statistics.

Statisticians and Psychologists Have Languages All Their Own

Among the many things that statisticians talk about are the chi-square goodness of fit, Kruskal Wallis, Wilcoxon-Mann Whitney tests, factorial logistic regressions, analysis of co-variance, ANOVAs, McNemar, and two independent sample t-tests.[1] Each of these tests has been designed to suit the specific nature of the variables under investigation. These are orderly and logical processes (but not to a disorderly mind like mine).

Psychologists often talk about intricacies such as therapy, behavioral models, observable fact, and neuropsychological test results. Because Ashikaga worked in the medical school, where he collaborated with investigators across many fields, he understood me better than I understood how to apply statistics to such a large dataset. Fortunately for him I was not trying to measure phenomena like double binds, sensorimotor attachments, presymbolic learning, or psychosexual development.[2] Our collaboration was, in the end, however, a cross-cultural experience—meaning that psychology and biostatistics had two different cultures, especially for me. Slowly and surely, we began to understand one another better.

Dealing With Potential Biases in the Sample Selection

Learning about the early days and how the Vermont participants had originally been selected for the rehab program was an important task. Ashikaga asked about this one day, and so we turned our attention accordingly. We first found out that 22 participants had concurrent and significant intellectual disabilities in addition to psychiatric diagnoses, such as schizophrenia or major affective disorders. We decided to interview the entire cohort but deleted those 22 people from our Diagnostic and Statistical Manual (DSM III)-qualified schizophrenia group because they represented a substantially different subsample.

We also interviewed members of the original clinical team (all but one was alive at that point). They told us that all staff, including aides from the back wards of the hospital, were encouraged to recommend people for the new rehabilitation program back in the mid-1950s. One of the staff said, "I just happened to notice Joe. He was pushing a cart up and down in the tunnel. I discovered that he has been doing this for five years."[3]

It should be noted that after a conversation with George Brooks, Thomas McGlashan, MD, inaccurately reported in his famous paper on recent North American follow-up studies, published a year after our findings, that the participants in our study were the same people who had essentially been running the hospital for years, doing the electrical, plumbing, and custodial work; managing the hospital farm; and so on, and who were just "sitting around without a place to go in the community."[4] In actuality, those who worked in the hospital were from the back wards and who had responded to the Thorazine trials ($N = 178$) and were discharged *before* Brooks's rehab program. McGlashan later admitted to me that he wrote up the draft of his important review of North American Follow-up Studies while working on another project in Copenhagen. He said that he had forgotten to call me when he returned home to double-check on the inclusions in our cohort; he had also thought that their average age of onset was 30, which was later than our group. He apologized and told me that he had corrected these errors the following year in a publication in a small journal for private hospitals. I considered him to be a friend and colleague who, because he was highly respected, so many more colleagues read his article and thought less of ours. This unfortunately and accidentally made it tougher for readers to understand what we had really done.

Our study actually contained only those remaining people ($N = 269$) who had only a modest response to the drug regimen. Remember that they were considered to be "very slow, concentrated poorly, seemed confused and frequently had some impairment or distortion of recent or remote memory. They were touchy, suspicious, temperamental, unpredictable, and overdependent on others to make minor day-to-day decisions for them."[5]

Before the study, our cohort members were without a doubt considered to be some of the worst cases ever studied in the world literature. Thus, they were expected to have some of the worst outcomes. To prove that they were the worst cases, we had conducted the substudy of the entire group of hospital residents before the selection was made, as described later. I think that many psychiatrists had a difficult time imagining that significant improvement and even recovery might be possible for such a profoundly disabled group, but, fortunately, many investigators kept searching for answers.

What Did the Other Patients in the Hospital Look Like?

We decided that it was essential to find out who occupied the remaining beds in the hospital. In 1954, the hospital population was as high as 1,300 beds for a general state population of only 377,000.[6] Vermont had only one state hospital and no community mental health centers caring for severely disabled outpatients—only families and children then, so those who were struggling ended up at the state hospital, brought in by the local sheriff, the state police, or the family. We wanted to know if the Vermont cohort was really the most ill and disabled in the hospital. This substudy was called the Parametric Study of the Hospital Population in 1954.

Irene Bergman, Lynn Forrest, and Mary Herzog ended up conducting this important substudy. Items studied were diagnosis, age, sex, and length of hospitalization. They pulled a 10% random sample of the entire hospital population and found that the members of our cohort had much more schizophrenia, much longer length of stays, and were more often males with the most severe cases.

The Children-at-Risk Substudy

Given the advanced age of the cohort (average age of 61 ranging up to 83 years), we decided that we should also study their children and grandchildren. We had the distinct advantage of working with Thomas Achenbach, PhD at UVM, who had developed many well-used instruments such as the Child Behavior Checklist.[7] Lucinda Cummings and Lisa Nurcombe worked on the preparation of this new proposal. Even though we had already found 98 of these second- and third-generation subjects and had secured permissions to interview them from their parents and grandparents, a later NIMH site visit team refused to fund the study because it was not a "genetic study." This decision was enormously frustrating to all of us because, at that time, geneticists were still arguing about one of their algorithms, known as the *LOD score*, which stood for a "logarithm of the odds"; it concerned the probability of whether two specific genes might be located together on the 48 chromosomes.[8] Eventually computers predicted that the numbers of families needed for linkage studies had to be exponentially larger. And so it turned out that the genetic algorithms of that early time, especially for schizophrenia, were not very helpful after all. Again, this episode reveals how myopic science can be. Assessing these children and grandchildren might have been helpful in advancing our understanding about the impact of schizophrenia on one's personal life and family because it appeared that most of these relatives were leading healthy lives. I am still cross about this narrow-mindedness and even 40-plus years later, the field of genetics has not produced any definitive usable data for schizophrenia. Professor Jane Murphy and I were once listening to a group of NIMH-sponsored genetic investigators at the Society of Research in Psychopathology apologize one after another for their lack of findings. The director of the NIMH Genetics Section, Elliot Gershon, started the discussion following the presentations by quipping that he was glad that he had not given all these investigators his checkbook!

What Did We Do About the People Who Moved Out of State?

Most people in Vermont simply do not move out of state, but there were 17 in our cohort who did, and we needed to find out if they were somehow different from those who stayed. I gave my two interviewers a "See America" ticket from a major airline, and they had a wonderful time interviewing people in California, Arizona, Oregon, Texas, Florida, and Canada. I wasn't at all sure they would want to return to the snow and ice of a New England winter. They found that some people had recovered, some had definitely improved, and some had not—just like the group that had stayed in Vermont.

What About the People Who Had Died?

The group of deceased cohort members comprised 26% of the original sample, not surprising in a three-decade follow-up. In most studies, a comparison of the demographics (e.g., age, sex, etc.) and the illness characteristics (e.g., diagnosis, etc.) between the live group and those deceased, using statistical means, would be made and that would be that. We expanded the process because we were curious and we did things differently. The information we had on these people, while quite complete and accurate, was not of the first-hand, observable kind we had secured from the live people interviewed in our study, and so we reported the data on the deceased separately.

Stanley Miller, MD, a medical student at the time, piloted this expanded protocol to find out just how those who had died were functioning beforehand. We decided that not only would we conduct the usual comparison of demographics and illness characteristics presented in most studies, but we would also gather together the families and friends of those who had died and use another structured protocol. To interview those who had known the deceased person well, we used key comparison questions from the longitudinal protocol (VCQ-L) already employed for the living and interviewed participants and described in detail in the previous chapter. This strategy turned out to be very important to our understanding of the findings.

After consulting with Professor Paula Clayton (Chair of Psychiatry at the University of Minnesota) who was working in the area of death and families,[9] we decided to trace the activities and status of the deceased subjects up until the last 6 months of life. The last 6 months prior to death hold the possibility of all systems going awry (called by the British, in their own inimitable style, as "terminal drop"). The data for the deceased were kept separate from those for the living subjects. Often investigators mix the two, but our way was much more stringent.

This systematic assessment of the deceased persons in our cohort turned out to be an important strategy because the field expected that those who had died would of course have been the most disabled by schizophrenia and that they would die early. We found something quite different. Their outcome trajectories demonstrated the same proportion of recovered, significantly improved, or unimproved as the live group.

How to Deal With the Impact of Federal, State and Local Policies and Program Changes

When a study covers more than 30 years, of course many changes in policies and programs will have occurred that affect the outcome of participants. Unless we understood these changes and overlaid the longitudinal data with their timing, we were at risk for misinterpretation of movement. For example, official board-and-care homes did not come to Vermont until around 1968. If we saw a mass shift into such care that year, we might have misinterpreted it as a sudden change in cohort functioning instead of simply a new system opportunity.

As described in a later chapter on the Maine-Vermont Comparison Study, Michael DeSisto, the Maine Project Director, used the Vermont Longitudinal Study Life Chart history format to graph both state policy and program changes from 1777 to the 1990s. His work with both state historians is described in more detail in the literature.[10] DeSisto and his policy historians produced two remarkable documents using the format from the 1940s onward and were also extremely helpful in our state-to-state comparisons.

The Joy of Mixed-Methods Design

Each person's history was derived from multiple sources: structured personal interviews, prospectively written records (meaning written at the time they occurred in research terms), third-party interviews (e.g., family, friends, and clinicians), life histories, audiotapes, and interviewer diary notes describing the interview process and their subjective experience in working with each person. The difference between a single structured cross-sectional interview, typical of most research protocols, and the in-depth data acquired through both quantitative and qualitative approaches allowed us to learn a great deal more. The analogy of a single snapshot versus a play in a theatre-in-the-round allowed the investigators to recognize the richness of the mixed-methods and longitudinal strategies.[11]

How a Picnic in the Lauterbrunnen Valley Helped Me Understand the Beauty of Cross-Sectional Data

At the outset, I was extremely frustrated with colleagues who studied such things as eye blink reflex and the like. It seemed as if they did not really know or care who owned the eye, nor any of the particulars about its owner other than standard demographics and illness characteristics. Furthermore, government entities were beginning to push for a 6-month turnaround time for data so that it could be used to inform significant service system decisions. These approaches just did not make sense to me. They were reductionistic and splitting hairs while I considered myself to be a holistic and integrative type of person. To me it was important to find out how people got to where they were currently and, perhaps even more important, what happened to them later.

Then, one day in May, I had a wonderful opportunity to sit in a field full of flowers at the foot of the Jungfrau Mountain in Switzerland, with its lofty waterfalls of melting snow, for a picnic with a friend. I thought to myself, "I do not care what the history of this place is nor what each of these flowers is named. This is one of those peak moments and a cross-sectional one at that." I began to appreciate my colleagues' efforts, and indeed how important their work was in solving some of the puzzles. We are complementary and essential. This was yet another learning experience, uncovering my own biases and assumptions.

How We Dealt With the Days of Punch Cards

The reader needs to know that during my undergraduate years in the mid-1970s, we were assigned to computer "Gandalf" boxes.[12] (It seems that many statisticians have a keen sense of humor.) These boxes allowed us to visit, with an appointment, the university's mainframe computer, housed somewhere else, to find out where our school projects were in the work queue of the entire university. We also had the "advance" of IBM punch cards[13] on which all collected data were punched. Professor Rolf told me a nightmarish story featuring a student who had punched in all his dissertation data without specific critical identifiers, and then dropped all the cards on the floor. To avoid such horrifying accidents, we used a 20-item field on every card that included the identifying information of the subject number, which instrument, which section, what date of interview, and so forth. It made for a good night's sleep but a mammoth job for Ashikaga's team. Over the years, we converted data to 5¼-inch floppy disks and then to 3½-inch disks as time and computers progressed. We backed up everything, with copies locked and stored in different file cabinets in different buildings in case of fire or other disaster. The risk of catastrophic data loss continues to haunt investigators, especially graduate students.

The Beauty of Direct Coding, Double Coding, Code Books, and Master Categorical Clumping of Variables Across the Instrument Batteries

Many studies even today have code sheets that are then separated from the original instrument, but we decided to have the scoring done directly onto the interview or record review instrument itself. Since every subject had a personal unidentifiable study code, this approach did not break confidentiality but reduced most coding errors. Such a plan also allowed the rater to add a variety of sidebar comments to the margin, which could help us better understand the actual recorded code. Mary Ellen Fortini, PhD, and Lori Witham poured over the final instruments for data cleaning, making sure that they were complete and entered correctly.

Ashikaga insisted on his team double-coding each battery for comparison, looking for errors in key punching—another good idea. His staff (Sue Ledeux, Sandi Tower, Dorothy Myer, Mary Noonan, and Joanne Gobrecht) also developed comprehensive code books detailing all of the instruments with their ratings. Each item was assigned a unique and identifiable study instrument number from across the huge dataset so that we could look at a question and know exactly from where it was derived.

Furthermore, one of the most helpful and creative strategies was designed by interviewers Landerl and Consalvo. They took giant poster boards and titled each one with a category, such as symptoms, family, or work. They then proceeded to list all variables having to do with each category from across the entire dataset. This catalogue was then typed up on regular sheets of paper by our hardworking administrative assistant, Andrea Pierce. This compendium was a life-saver whenever we wanted to design data analyses to answer specific questions with specific variables using specific time periods. In studies this large, reliance on memory is less dependable than this strategy.

Tracking Data Across Institutions

Our main offices were at the state hospital in Waterbury, about 27 miles from the medical school. Our hard-won data were precious to us, and I wanted to track them very carefully. I devised a system whereby anyone who handled the data had to sign off on receiving them and indicate when and where, using triplicate sheets and carbon paper so that everyone would have a copy. The sheets went from the raters to me to the Biometry Division at UVM, where they were coded, and then back to our locked file cabinets. This tracking felt very bureaucratic but we never lost anything.

Reliability Studies

Each of the component instrument batteries had to be tested for reliability, which asked the question, "Do these raters assign the same answers to the same questions?" Many of the individual instruments had been put through this process earlier by their creators and others using them in research projects. Because we had new raters and also had integrated questions from a wide variety of existing instruments, as described earlier, new trials were warranted as well.

Each battery was subjected to two sets of interrater trials under test-retest conditions, 6 months apart. Both raters attended, together, a cross-sectional and longitudinal interview for 21 subjects and then another 18. Each rater scored the interview independently, and then the pairs of ratings were compared. The statistical method that we used was Cohen's kappa coefficients from the first and second set of trials. Instead of just looking at the percentage of agreement on each question, Cohen's kappas were specifically designed for just a pair of raters, and they introduced a modifier that would also adjust for the possibility of a random answer and be more stringent.[14] Our trials found statistically significant findings, indicating that the degree of agreement was generally reasonable at p < .01 and p < .001 levels.[15]

The Life Chart was scored separately because it was considered highly experimental, but it turned out to be very reliable as well, with kappa coefficients of .98 and .78. All these figures have been reported in the academic literature as well.

Landerl and Consalvo went out together to interview participants. The biggest difficulty appeared to be the reliability ratings for cleanliness of the home place. I looked at their desks at work and could understand why because one was neat and one was not. They solved the problem by developing a rating scale of all the greasy spoon restaurants in which they met after the interviews. We thought we ought to publish a guide to such restaurants in Vermont as an additional money-generating project.

The Abnormal Involuntary Movement Scale (AIMS) had a history of variable reliability at that point but now has been widely used in the assessment and degree of tardive dyskinesia.[16] This instrument was also scored separately from the rest of the VCQ-L. Even though we had Professor Alan Gelenberg, the author of the instrument, to train us, the reliability was considered now only modest at .55 and .57 (p < .01). This may have been also due to two non-physicians conducting the assessments and who were not used to performing neurological tests.

The Hospital Record Review Form (HRRF) with its 1,800 items was also subjected to interrater trials. Kappa coefficients ranged from .41* to .95** depending on the section, but all were considered moderate to highly significant except the two at .41, which would now be considered poor.[17] (The score had to do with one rater very familiar with the records and one who was less so.) In the end, however, we resolved the matter and only had one rater review those records.

Our conclusion was that rating these instruments was indeed reliable. Furthermore, these tests pointed to the utility of the VCQ-C, VCQ-L, and HRRF for research conducted by other investigators measuring the adjustment and functioning of people with prolonged and episodic histories of serious psychiatric problems now living in the community.

Time to Go Talk With Everyone

The interrater trials were completed successfully, and we could be sure that all the raters would rate questions consistently. Landerl and Consalvo finally went out the door to visit people. Remembering that they had become discouraged during their years of outpatient clinical work, they were about to be quite amazed—as we all were. People's lives were as individual as they were, and many were faring much better than expected.

PART THREE

Surprise Discoveries

I0

Surprise Discoveries Out in
the Field

How Many People Did We Find?

Due to the strong relationships that he built in the 1950s, George Brooks received replies to 87% of his initial letters 20 years later. Essentially, his letter went, "Hi! How are you? Where are you? What are you doing?" In the end, we were able to locate and/or account for 97% of the original cohort (or 261 out of 269).

This group had an average of 32 years after first admission, with the range between 22 and 62 years, making this study one of the longest in the world literature, much to even my own surprise.[1] As a group they also constituted the longest study of deinstitutionalized state hospital patients in the United States, interviewed an average of 25 years after the initial rehab program.[2]

All of our participants taught us many important things about the recovery process and also why it is so important to interview people who have left the system of care. Many other shorter studies interview only those who are *convenient*, meaning that they are still in the system. That approach significantly skews findings and perpetuates myths.

Phase III of the Vermont Story: Initial Findings an Average of 32 Years After First Admission

We indeed had found that "one-half to two-thirds of our sample had achieved significant improvement or recovery."[3] Their achievement was even more remarkable given their original levels of chronicity.[4]

Recovery from Schizophrenia. Courtenay M. Harding, Oxford University Press. © Courtenay M. Harding 2024.
DOI: 10.1093/oso/9780195380095.003.0010

As noted, the follow-along period ranged from 22 to 62 years, for an average of 32 years after first admission. This stretch of time provided new perspectives on what might be possible for once severely impaired and disabled persons. In Europe, this kind of study was called a "catamnestic study" or one that studies the course of an illness after diagnosis and treatment. However, we started at first admission and stretched all the way through time until the last interview, and, given the length of time following this sample, we were certainly closing in on our cohort's final prognoses.

Who Was Interviewed for Our First Glimpse of Long-Term Outcome?

As discussed, we removed 22 people from the original sample of 269—those who had been diagnosed with significant intellectual disabilities—because they were considerably different from the rest of the sample. They would have been excluded in a similar research protocol today and subject to their own study. We did interview many of these individuals because we wanted to know how they were, but we withheld their data from the final analyses. That left 247 people in the cohort, with 168 (68%) to be interviewed, 7 (3%) lost to follow-up, and 61 (25%) deceased.[5] Again, as noted, 11 people (4%) participated in interviews but became wary about how their data might be used and subsequently refused to release it. Unbelievably, only 7 people of 269 (3%) were never found or accounted for, even though we checked death records and conducted a wide search. This low figure is unusual because investigators have often found it difficult to find even 30% for a 5-year follow-up study and we had accounted for 97%! This high percentage helped to smooth out most of the potential biases embedded within earlier long-term studies. The high percentage is one of the reasons New England is a great place to conduct research.

Demographics of the Interviewed Group

Members of this cohort were born between 1897 and 1942. The age range of interviewees was 38 to 83 years with a mean of 59 years. Two-thirds of the group were older than 55 years. There were 81 men and 87 women. Fifty-one percent of the live group had not finished high school. This was expected because tuitions were very expensive for those who went to high school outside of a rural community without one. Up until about 1940, completion of eighth grade (early on in the century) and tenth grade (later) was all that the state required.[6] This explains why Brooks's parents had to send him away to Montpelier for high school at age 13.

Overall Combined Psychological and Psychosocial Functioning

The predecessor to the current Global Assessment of Functioning (GAF)[7] was the Global Assessment Scale (GAS).[8] Both scales were designed to capture a comprehensive score (with one number from 1 to 100) which represented, as a composite proxy measure, a person's combined psychological and functional health. The later GAF separated psychological health and functional health.

Our team felt that a score of 90 to 100 would be nearly impossible for most mortals to achieve ("no symptoms, superior functioning in a wide range of activities, life's problems never seem to get out of hand, is sought by others because of his [or her] warmth and integrity").[9] I once teased one of the scale's creators (Robert Spitzer) that he and his collaborators might be the only people who could score in that category.

The common cutoff for significantly improved was 61 and above. At this level, people were described as having "some mild symptoms (e.g., depressive mood and mild insomnia) OR some difficulty in several areas of functioning, but generally functioning pretty well, has some meaningful interpersonal relations and most untrained people would not consider him [or her] 'sick'").[10] Sixty-eight percent of the entire sample (114 of 168) scored above the cutoff of 61, and most were over 71. A score of 71 meant that "minimal symptoms may be present, but no more than slight impairment in functioning; varying degrees of 'everyday' worries that only occasionally get out of hand."[11] Scores of 81 to 90 were described as "transient symptoms may occur, but good functioning in all areas; interested and involved in a wide range of activities, socially effective, generally satisfied with life; worries may occasionally get out of hand."[12] All these descriptions get to those fuzzy borders of what could be considered perfectly "normal" functioning.

Sex Differences in GAS Scores

Looking at sex differences, there were many more men (68%) in the 31–70 age ranges and many more women in the 61–90 range (62%), as expected. Although when a comparison was made between the sexes on this scale the apparently strong differences washed out to a trend level because most were clustered between 60 and 80.[13] This means that the original impression of differences became statistically less significant. In general, men tended to have an earlier onset of serious problems, which left them with a less sturdy platform on which to pull themselves up and out of the avalanche of serious psychiatric issues, so it seemed to take longer for them to get their lives back. Women, on the other hand, generally had a later onset, often leaving them time to finish school, have work experience, and develop more relationships before succumbing to the avalanche. Therefore, they often seemed to get better faster, benefiting from a stronger foundation on which to build their recovery.[14]

Achievement in Levels of Functioning at Follow-Up With Slight or No Impairment in Overall Functioning

Using the components of the Strauss and Carpenter's Levels of Function (LOF) scale, which included more variables than the GAS score, 92 people (55%) fell into the category of "No impairment was rated for subjects [sic] who were asymptomatic and living independently, had close relationships, were employed or were otherwise productive citizens, were able to care for themselves and led full lives in general."[15]

This scale also revealed that a large push to reclaim lives had continued long after the original clinical team had left, a little discouraged that these improvements hadn't occurred for a third of the group still struggling in 1965. Across the board, so many people were so much better than we had expected. In fact, a quick perusal of most of the existing literature (with the exception of some long-term studies and a few shorter ones) would have indicated that all such people were supposed to achieve only marginal levels of functioning at best. The LOF total score turned out to be highly correlated with that of the GAS described earlier.[16]

When examining the individual items on the LOF, one-half to four-fifths of people had restored their functioning and got much if not all their "normal" lives back.[17]

- One hundred and forty people (83%) were not in the hospital in the past year;
- One hundred and eleven people (66%) met with friends every week or two;
- One hundred and twenty-eight people (76%) had moderately close to very close friends;
- Seventy-nine people (47%) were employed in past year;
- One hundred and twenty-one people (72%) displayed slight or no symptoms;
- One hundred and thirty-three people (79%) met their own basic needs;
- One hundred and twenty-eight people (76%) led moderate to very full lives; and
- Ninety-two people (55%) had slight or no impairment in overall function.[18]

Averaging all these scores means that 69.3% were doing quite well. Our own very stringent research criteria for "fully recovered" were no further symptoms, no odd behaviors, no more medications, living in the community, working, and relating well to others. In addition, we found about 30% fully recovered, with 40% significantly improved, having retrieved or developed all but one area of functioning. An additional 30% of this group did not seem to flourish at all. Remember, too, that this lowest subgroup was 30% of the bottom 19% of the lowest functioning people of 1,300 patients residing at the only public hospital in the state. We have certainly been underestimating people.

The Significantly Improved Group

The significantly improved group revealed continued heterogeneity in functioning and taught us many important things. For example, we found that people had invented ingenious ways to cope with residual symptoms and still could work, relate well with others, and live in the community. As an example, some interviewees told us that they learned not to tell anyone about their symptoms because, as one person put it, "It seemed to upset other people." Others, who appeared asymptomatic, revealed that they had developed coping skills to deal with any residual symptoms.

Many other people were working, living in the community, had no symptoms, and appeared to be relating well to others. However, on closer assessment, some members of this group had learned to carefully regulate their social relationships. These varied groups of people gave us many crucial insights into human ingenuity and persistence. (We looked around at some of our colleagues in the field and saw that some of them had also adopted the same strategies.)

As discussed earlier, while 47% were still working, with an age range in the sample up to 83, other people had fallen victim to the disincentives of the entitlement system. They had been working, lost their jobs, and needed their entitlement payments to bridge the gap before they could start working again. But these had chosen not to work again for fear of having to go through the very lengthy Supplemental Security Income/Social Security Disability Income (SSI/SSDI) process (during the 1970s and 1980s this usually took 2 years or more) to retrieve their monthly payments. And this with the possibility of losing yet another job and having to go through the system still again.

Even though we rated them as "not fully recovered" but "significantly improved," from a research point of view, each one had achieved a much higher level of function than they, themselves, had originally expected, and they had indeed gotten their lives back.

Hospital Use and Symptom Reductions

Eighty-three percent of the sample ($n = 140$) had not been in the hospital during the year of the follow-up assessment. These were the very people who were "supposed" to grow old and die in the hospital.

Seventy-two percent ($n = 121$) displayed slight or no symptoms.[19] This finding alone is a significant challenge to those clinicians who assume diagnosis to be a lifetime label. As I pointed out earlier, the second set of National

Institute of Mental Health (NIMH) site visitors had declined to pay for rediagnosis from *Diagnostic and Statistical Manual* (DSM-II)[20] criteria to the new DSM-III criteria.[21] Because of their training, those reviewers believed that "these patients were just a bunch of old chronic schizophrenics [sic]." We fixed the problem later when Strauss and Alan Breier carefully rediagnosed them all according to the DSM-III. More will be said about this important process in a later chapter, with more surprises revealed.

Places of Residence

One hundred forty-eight (88%) lived in rural and residential settings, as expected for Vermont, and not in industrial or commercial areas. Eighty-one people lived in independent housing, described as a house, an apartment, a mobile home, or a rooming house.[22]

Of the group living in board-and-care facilities (called "dependent housing"), seven could have been living independently and often managed the house. Twenty-three others were "actively involved in activities within the house, at the local community mental health center, or in the community and were self-motivated."[23]

Meeting Basic Needs

Readers must remember that this was a group that had become so institutionalized and disabled that they had had trouble telling time, using a fork, combing their hair, and brushing their teeth.

Our interviewers went to their homes and neighborhoods. They sat at kitchen tables and observed, first-hand, the condition of the homes, the safeness, and "the degree of ghetto-ness" of the neighborhood (meaning were these people living only with others who had once been patients at the state hospital). Instead, most people were living next to typical Vermont neighbors, not on the margins of society.

We asked such questions as, "Who does the laundry? Who does the grocery shopping? Who pays the bills, and who does the cooking and the cleaning?" Much to our surprise, 79% (or 133) were able to do those important tasks, though these people were on the elderly side.[24] (Now that

I am over 80, I realize what a set of assumptions I myself had then about aging.)

Hospital and Nursing Home Care

Five single middle-aged men were in the hospital at the time of the study. In fact, the longitudinal picture of hospital use was amazing. We found that, contrary to expectations, men were often released much earlier than their female counterparts before the rehab program in the 1950s. They were temporarily released due to requests by families who needed help with planting or harvesting crops, but the families then returned them to the hospital after the season had ended. This strategy often happened across the country in rural farming communities.

There was an average of only two readmissions, mostly early on, for a third of the sample after the rehab program and their initial release from the hospital, when some people were not quite sure that they belonged in the community. Since Brooks had a strategy of meeting returning people in the admissions office with their discharge planning papers in his hand, they got the point and eventually stayed out. As described earlier, they received substantial supports in the community as they were reclaiming their lives. In addition, seven people were found in Level II nursing homes because, while they did not need 24-hour care, they did need some supervision.[25]

Many Still Working After All These Years

Today, across the United States, statistics for persons coping with serious and persistent problems report only about a 12–20% employment rate.[26] Work had been the hallmark of the early rehabilitation program because there was little financial support to be had and vocational rehabilitation was a key component of getting people back into the community.

Forty-seven percent ($n = 79$) were still employed at follow-up even though so many people were retired and were elderly.[27] Half of those jobs were listed as unskilled, which was also predictable given the original low level of education. These jobs included farm laborer, construction worker, grocery and other store clerk, dishwasher, seamstress, and painter. Fourteen more people contributed many hours of volunteer work to their communities, while eight women were housewives. Forty-four people were considered in the elderly, retired, and widowed group, leaving only 23 people unemployed.[28]

Level of Work Depends Mostly on Education

As an important side note, I was interviewed on National Public Radio's "Morning Edition" about this study in 1987. After the program aired, I received many calls from all over the North American continent. Callers said, "Thank you for telling our story." "I am a physician . . . an engineer . . . a college professor . . . a nurse . . . a high school teacher." "I once had schizophrenia. I just don't tell anyone because of the discrimination and stigma."

What a person does with his or her life seems to depend more on the level of education acquired along the way, not necessarily on psychopathology. Such information is vitally important to our understanding of mental disorders, but it is often unknown or unacknowledged. Programs that prioritize helping people to finish their educations are critically important, but this goal is also often forgotten by overloaded clinicians busy simply trying to put out fires (crises) and by those academics and administrators in higher education who ironically have succumbed to lack of knowledge about the potential of this group of future students.

Income and Quality of Life

In 1982, Vermont was listed as the 36th state in the nation in per capita income, with an average of $9,979 annually (equivalent to the purchasing power of $31,516 in 2023).[29] Eighty-five percent of our group had a gross income of less than $10,000. We employed the Community Care Schedule (CCS)[30] and budget sheets which were filled out with each person. We found that 77% (or 199 people) had adequate income, which was defined by the CCS as "the amount of money received will cover the subject's [sic] basic needs comfortably."[31] In fact, as I discussed in an earlier chapter, Vermonters often end up with a better quality of life than their income suggests, typically by using bartering (such as exchanging dental work for fixing a roof).

Interpersonal Relationships

Thirty-two people were married; another 11 were widowed. That finding left 39 people who were divorced as well as 86 who were still single.[32] Serious problems with relationships are often an underlying precipitating factor or sequelae when coping with serious and persistent disorders. We had a large number of measurements of social functioning in the instrument battery. Our findings revealed that 111 people (66%) actually met with friends every week or two, and 128 (76%) enjoyed one or more moderately to very close friends. This capacity had reconstituted and even developed further in more than two-thirds of the people being interviewed.[33]

Fullness of Life

Based on a very large number of observations and assessments, the interviewers rated 128 people (76%) as having achieved a moderate to very full life.[34] Our initial finding of significant improvement and even full recoveries was a major challenge to the centuries-old assumption that people living in the back wards of state hospitals are chronically deteriorating patients for whom there is no hope.

Challenges to the Rule of Thirds and to Kraepelin's 90/10

Across many disciplines there is a rule of thumb that "one-third get better, one-third stay the same (marginal functioning), and one-third become worse" in the entire population of people diagnosed with medical problems. Because 30% of our participants were fully recovered and another 40% were significantly improved from the most severely disabled and chronically hospitalized, we definitely challenged that old saw. In our assessments, the middle 40% were definitely no longer marginal but fully recovered, with the exception of one area. However, readers may forget that our sample already represents the most impaired 19% of the hospital population, which I knowingly reiterate here, because many people seem to have difficulty imagining that such once profoundly disabled people might possibly retrieve their lives, especially those who were running around with no clothes on, speaking animal gibberish, and smearing feces on the walls!

Resistance seems to come from training, adherence to the early work of Emil Kraepelin, day-to-day clinical work in impoverished traditional settings, and lack of feedback about or from former clients. According to our work, Emil Kraepelin, who still influences psychiatric training and diagnostic systems today, got the percentages significantly backward. As such, repeating his pronouncements perpetuates a cycle of pessimistic expectations. Kraepelin wrote that, in his opinion, only 10% or fewer might improve, while 90% of patients would deteriorate over time.[35] What the field of psychiatry also seems to forget is the fact that Kraepelin was somewhat unaware of the composition of his caseloads. Many patients did not have what he called dementia praecox but advanced syphilis, while others had undiagnosed encephalitis, such as those patients portrayed in the film "Awakenings."[36] Put those facts together with hospital administrative policies at the time to discharge no one after 2 years of inpatient stay, and I can see why Kraepelin thought what he thought. But he was wrong.

How Difficult Was It to Accept the Vermont Data?

The field was incredulous in its disbelief. "Those people, who succeeded, must have been misdiagnosed and had affective disorders instead." Or, "But what was the very long-term outcome just for 'core' schizophrenia?" "Did some members of the group really truly have what we consider today as schizophrenia?" "What about the new DSM-III criteria?" "Did they really have 'real' schizophrenia?" "Did they do less well than other people diagnosed with schizoaffective and major affective disorders?" "They must have had a very expensive program." "Vermont is so beautiful; it must have helped them get better." Vermont Community Mental Health Centers were indeed threatened by some of the centers in nearby states that proposed using "Greyhound therapy," bussing out-of-state patients up to Vermont for care. These questions and many others are discussed in the next chapters.

Joe Zubin, former head of the Biometrics Research Department at the New York State Psychiatric Institute at Columbia, had an answer for these inquisitors.

> Where in the world would you go get the natural history of schizophrenia if not under the best circumstances? You wouldn't want to go to the ghetto, where people are suffering from a lot of other sources of distress, to see whether the outcome is good there. You would want to go to the best place, where the triggering mechanisms are at a minimum.[37]

What's Next?

So now we had all the data in the house, double coded, and we were looking for errors. Brooks kept running the hospital and Deane re-retired. Consalvo went back to school to get his doctorate, studying the importance of humor. Landerl went back to Howard Mental Health Center with an entirely new appreciation for what was possible. I raced off to Yale to show off what we had found to John Strauss, the renowned schizophrenia investigator and one of our original NIMH site reviewers. He had been a believer in this outrageous proposal from the start.

I I

A Whole Bunch of People
Got Better

Getting Out of the Trees to See the Forest

When the entire study was completed in 1982, I headed off to Yale. After all,
Professor Strauss had moved to New Haven from Rochester, and Professor
Bowers was Vice Chair of Psychiatry there as well. They were two of the
four people (including Loren Mosher and Jack Maser) who had faith in
us from the time of the first National Institute of Mental Health (NIMH)
site visit.

Strauss said to me, "Well, Courtenay, what did you find?"

With great enthusiasm, I started bubbling in my excitement, "This percentage did this and this percentage did that. . . ."

"No," he said, "what did you find?"

Puzzled, I said, "Well, this other percentage did this and that other percentage did that!"

With a slight tinge of irritation in his voice, Strauss said once more, "No,
Courtenay, what did you find?"

I still didn't understand what he was after, and I persisted with more
percentages.

Finally, and with consummate patience but tinged with a little more irritation, he asked for the fourth time, "What did you find?"

I was feeling stupid and confused, and I simply blurted out, "Well, a
whole bunch of people got better!"

"That is what you found," he said quietly. And, sure enough, that is what
we had found.[1]

Recovery from Schizophrenia. Courtenay M. Harding, Oxford University Press. © Courtenay M. Harding 2024.
DOI: 10.1093/oso/9780195380095.003.0011

I had gotten lost in the trees, and Strauss, using his standard operating strategy, was up on the hill overlooking the forest.[2] He understood, much better than I, how important the main message would be to the field. We were challenging over a century's worth of pessimistic thinking about the long-term outcome of people diagnosed with schizophrenia.

Strauss and I outlined four major questions that the study might be able to answer. They were, "Who got better? When did they get better? In what ways did they get better? And were there any predictors of who got better?" I had to embroider those four questions onto a piece of fabric, frame it, and put it over my desk to keep my focus on them because the requirements of academia can pull one away at any given moment. It has taken the rest of my career to try to provide some answers and acknowledge that some are still out of reach.

The remainder of this chapter will provide more clarity into the human side of all those percentages. Stories such as these are not usually published along with study statistics.

From Chambermaid to Manager

My first glimpse of "Helene" was a surprise during the pilot study. She was a tall woman with curious green eyes peering out from under a cloud of white hair. When I reminded her that she was my consultant, her remembering smile brought out the laugh lines around those green eyes. She invited me into her small home with starched white curtains fluttering in the breeze from the slightly opened window. After all, this was Vermont, which even in the height of summer, was apt to be chilly. As I looked around at the photographs clustered on a nearby table, I could see that Helene had indeed reclaimed her life.

She had snatched it back from the misery of a long stay in Vermont State Hospital (VSH), from howling in despair, from forgetting how to comb her hair, use a fork, or tell time. She had come back from a death sentence; she was supposed to grow old and die in that hospital. When the staff saw that she had ripped off her clothes and spoke unintelligible nonsense, they had despaired themselves, and relegated her to a back ward. The staff had saved Helene's life several times, but why, she did not know or care.

Then, one day in the mid-1950s, an earnest young psychiatrist at VSH named George Brooks came onto the unit and began to ask questions of even the most profoundly disabled people. He asked astonishing questions, such as "What do you need to get out of here, because I don't know?" He expected to get a reasonable answer. Together, a group of patients, this psychiatrist, a nurse, a psychologist, a sociologist, and a vocational rehabilitation counselor developed many of the concepts used today in modern psychiatric rehabilitation and a new form of community psychiatry.[3] All have been described in earlier chapters.

Slowly but surely, Helene saw that this team retrained by Brooks truly believed that she and the others, the so-called hopeless cases, could live worthwhile lives outside the hospital and in the community. She began to comb her hair and brush her teeth. After all, there were now men on the unit. Until this point, men and women had always been segregated. Men, too, began to spruce themselves up. Staff started to ask Helene what kind of work she would like to do outside. Work? This seemed an amazing question to be asked of someone who had not worked in years. Slowly she began to hang on to little threads of hope. Every once and awhile Helene would test the staff to double check that they still meant what they said. Miracle of miracles, they kept persisting. They taught her the skills associated with being a chambermaid, which was her choice. They taught her how to talk with guests who happened to wander back into their rooms. But Helene was very shy and would just give a somewhat frightened little smile.

One day at a ski inn, Helene's first job, she met a new supervisor who was very demanding and berated her for not making the corners of the bed in the best military style. She broke down in tears and decided that the person speaking on the TV in the room where she was working was actually speaking to her. The supervisor became frightened and immediately called the vocational rehabilitation professional on the hospital team. This counselor, Robert Lagor, drove out to the inn, calmed Helene and the supervisor, and gave them both a new set of coping skills to try. After several false starts, the lessons took hold for both parties.

When I found Helene for pilot research interviews before the third follow-up wave so many years after her first admission, she had become the assistant manager of the inn. This challenging role required excellent social skills. She had found both her niche and herself and had obviously flourished. Helene, and so many other people living in the back wards at VSH, had found their way back from the brink of oblivion and reclaimed life. Together, and in collaboration with a remarkable staff, friends, and often family members, they pioneered new pathways to healing and recovery from persistent extreme emotional and cognitive distress.

Some More Assumptions Ambushed

One of the first participants in the formal field interviews was a man I'll call "Geoffrey." Consalvo found him in the city of Rutland, the second largest Vermont town, with a population in 1980 of 18,486.[4] He greeted Consalvo with a hearty handshake and settled them both in rocking chairs on the front porch of a neatly kept Cape Cod style house.

Geoffrey was tall, well-built, and 62 years old. He had a little bit of silver on his sideburns and a warm smile. He had just been married for the first time. He had taken care of his mother for many years, and, when she died, he had decided that it was time to marry his long-time girlfriend. He had a brother and sister nearby and spent time with them now and then when he wasn't working. They had all tried, with support and money, to be helpful when their mother was ill. Geoff had been the last caretaker. He also had work friends and those of his wife as well as a village priest.

He had become a licensed plumber and made a decent living. He made some wry comments about other patients who were "on the dole" and weren't working. He was very proud that he had been working ever since the rehab program in the 1950s.

He stated that "Back in the day, if you wanted to get out of the hospital you had to go to work. If you got out and didn't work, back you went to the hospital."

He also pointed out that the local community mental health center did serve a purpose and had helped him. He made a comment, however, that some patients who were using the center thought that their clinicians would and could solve all the problems that they brought to them. Consalvo noted that Geoff's hand trembled a little and wondered if that was a neurological problem or the side effect of years of early medications. He would conduct the AIMS Plus EPS Test a week later during the longitudinal interview to find out. It turned out to be possibly the result of some undiagnosed condition. At their first meeting, however, Consalvo was using the cross-sectional ("How are you today and in the past month?") interview. Geoff invited Consalvo for a meal, as many people did during ensuing interviews.

Consalvo met Geoff's wife and her son and watched the family positively interact.

Back a week later, Consalvo conducted the longitudinal interview which covered all the years since discharge from the rehab program in the mid-1950s. Geoff felt that all of his early hospitalizations were due to life events. These life events had to do with family, finances, and work stress. He said that he only stayed a couple of months to get his equilibrium back. After the first three episodes early in his life, there were 13 years before the next and last. He tried medications but gave them up after a few months. When back for an admission, he was put on medications again and again he stopped as soon as he got out.

Interestingly, Geoffrey had gone to work with his father in order to get to know him. His parents had been divorced when Geoff was a boy, and he hadn't seen him very much. They conducted surveys together. But Geoff found it tiring, decided to become a licensed plumber, and had been doing that job ever since. Consalvo reported that Geoff demonstrated an excellent memory and was very personable. He had no psychiatric symptoms but smoked a lot and drank three beers every day.

In looking at his psychiatric record, Dr. Deane, the record reviewer, found that Geoff had been hospitalized at age 20 as a new recruit in the Army. The Army hospital did not agree to release his first admission record of his 7-month stay. After his release, he worked as a helper in construction and for truck drivers. It was noted in the Vermont records that he consistently maintained a good work history. In his second admission at age 28, in Vermont, Geoff had been disruptive during a church service. He described having a gun under his pillow the night before but that was to do with "deer hunting." He was confused and evasive. Geoff wandered around all night when in the hospital and woke others trying to sleep. He had demonstrated being suspicious about ordinary things and would sit down on the floor and start talking to himself. He told the staff that "No, I am not sick." He was thought to have auditory hallucinations and was given a substantial amount of Thorazine. His brother gave permission to provide electroshock but there was no evidence that he had participated—probably a good thing.

Another episode at age 33 occurred with similar behaviors. On this admission, he received imipramine (Tofranil), trifluoperazine (Stelazine), and procyclidine (Kemadrin; a drug for involuntary movements caused by the other two). He was vague, disorganized, and mildly belligerent. He said he had no idea why he was there in the hospital but that he had lit a small fire in the church which had burned holes in the rug.

But when he showed up at the hospital again 13 years later, the admission description was of an unkempt, fidgety, tense, restless person. He seemed confused again, but he did remember what events made him seek help. It was noted that he seemed to have some insight and was competent at providing general information. Although his hospital diagnoses across time were listed as schizophrenia, his symptoms appear to have crossed other categories as well. This situation has been increasingly observed by the field of psychiatry.[5] Since then, it seemed that his relationship with his community mental health counselor has helped him settle down and stay out of the hospital with no further problems and a full life being lived.

Great Success but Followed Around by a Little Black Cloud

The interviewers kept finding astonishing stories. "Tom" was so well known that I am unable to say what state Tom lived in or what his company does in retelling his story. Many years earlier, Tom was hospitalized three times for a total of 7 years with a diagnosis of schizoaffective disorder. During his last admission, his mother had become ill. She asked her son to sign out of the rehabilitation program (before the staff felt he was ready) and come home to help her. He was 45 years old. She eventually died 2 years later, and he then plowed the equity in her house into a new company. Over time, he became a multimillionaire, making more money than all of the clinicians who had worked with him. He later married, and, because it was too late to have children, he and his wife mentored the younger people in the business.

At some point in the long interview process, Tom quietly asked Landerl if he was still on "conditional release"? It turned out that, back in the 1950s, instead of being discharged, people were released on the condition that if they became ill again or did not behave correctly, the hospital could immediately readmit them. Imagine living with that little black cloud following you around! Tom was reassured that the law had been changed. We realized that probably most of the members of our sample needed to be told this as well, and we worked this information into our protocol, assuming that many other worried people might not have asked.

Helene, Geoff, Tom, and many other people found their way back from the brink and reclaimed their lives. Together, and in collaboration with friends, family members, rehab workers, and some clinicians, they pioneered new pathways to healing and recovery from serious and disabling sets of severe psychiatric problems.

The Mute Person Who Wasn't

During the interrater trials, Landerl and Consalvo went off to interview a person named "Albert" who had been reported to be mute. They entered a farmhouse that was full of shrieking women who layered on stress as thick as a bank of heavy fog rolling into San Francisco. Fortunately, the two interviewers quickly hustled the participant off for a walk around the "South Forty" (referring to a portion of a Vermont farm's acreage). During the stroll, this so-called mute person said that he didn't speak in the house because he could not get a word in edgewise, and it was a way to cope. For the record, the community mental health center record said he was mute, and staff there had never investigated further or considered the environment in which he lived.

The "Niche" People

Helene, now the ski inn assistant manager, had been a shy young person as a chambermaid but had clearly found a niche in which she could grow and flourish. In another instance, an older woman, "Myrtle," had become a boarder in one family's home. Over time, she had become the esteemed grandmother. These niches allowed people "to function at a higher level of productivity, intimacy, and independence than might have been expected given their history."[6]

The Self-Regulators

Another group of people were more active in selecting their environments and shaping their interactions with people around them. One of

the self-regulators was a woman in her 70s. "Martha" had put together a
jazz trio of others in her age bracket. The trio played concerts for a wide
range of audiences, and she was the master of ceremonies as well. She was
vivacious and charming, and we all wanted to adopt her as another grandmother. However, during our interviews, we found that she very carefully managed her social relationships and had no close friends. She was
rated as "significantly improved" but not fully recovered. We had already
observed that some of our clinical colleagues also carefully regulated their
social interactions.

Who Struggled Mightily but Didn't Make It Out?

Most of our publications and presentations focused on the exciting findings
of significant improvement and recovery because this was an era in which
the field of psychiatry had continually emphasized doom and gloom. After
all, one-half to two-thirds of the so-called "worst cases," the back-ward
"hopeless cases" with severe forms of what was labeled as schizophrenia and
chronic versions of affective disorders, made it out of the avalanche and reclaimed their lives. "Recovery," in terms of our research criteria, meant that
a person had no enduring symptoms, no odd behaviors, received no further
medication, and was living in the community, working, and relating well
to others. "Significantly improved" research criteria meant that a person
was recovered in all areas but one. In the late 1980s, these results were reported in the front pages of the esteemed *American Journal of Psychiatry*.[7,8]
The results were a surprise and a joy, to me anyway, but mostly disbelieved
by the field no matter how many times I wrote or spoke about these data
or pointed out that there were also nine other two- and three-decade-long
studies of schizophrenia from across the world reporting some similar findings.[9] We completed an additional three-decade study later in the state of
Maine, which found even more evidence of improvement. All these studies
will be discussed in Chapters 15 through 18.

   That said, it is important to look also at the third of this group that did
not make it very far shoveling themselves out of the blizzard of mental
health problems, even with help. Remember that this struggling group represents not one-third of the population of people diagnosed with schizophrenia at the hospital, but one-third *of the bottom third* of the only hospital

in the state for public patients (or about the bottom 10% of the overall hospitalized population).

Those who did not significantly improve or recover had the classic profile of slightly being comprised of more male patients (but only by 10%), mostly single, with lower educational status, longer hospitalizations prior and post rehab program, and living still in sheltered care. They had decent levels of system support, but only one-third had good levels of social companionship with family and friends. Eighty-four percent were not employed. Fifty-one percent still had definite or probable signs of schizophrenia, 55% with severe levels of functioning (meaning not able to take care of themselves).[10] These are classic and expected findings *for everyone with schizophrenia*. These are some of the people that Bill Deane had worried about at the 5-year follow-up, written up earlier in Chapter 5.

Helpful Clinical Information

These people have much to teach us as well. They did not pull themselves out despite the innovative programming, the optimism of the staff, and the possible opportunities presented to them. They remained stuck under the avalanche. That highly caring and pioneering rehab program run by George Brooks did not reach them. Neither diagnosis, symptoms, length of stay, medications, demographics, nor a wide variety of other variables collected predicted who would be completely recovered, significantly improved, or not improved. Many who looked just like these individuals became significantly improved, some fully recovered. Manfred Bleuler had a patient with schizophrenia completely recover after 40 years of illness.[11] Implications of this discovery are astounding. *We should never triage, lower our expectations, or give up on people who are still struggling because we simply cannot predict yet whether they may still recover.*

Stories of the Group Stuck in the Avalanche

We found a variety of possible reasons in re-reviewing the records and talking with this group. "Edith" had been imprisoned in her family's attic for 15 years before coming to the hospital. She seemed to have simply lost her spirit, her reason for being, and clinicians were unable to break through. Several other people, such as "Albert," "Harry," "Earl," "Clara," and "Velma," after many attempts at community living, decided that they did not belong outside of the hospital because they felt that they were too old to adjust to a whole new way of life. Then there were five men, "Phillip," "Alvin," "Herman," "Maurice," and "Vernon," who were found to be living in individual single rooms over hardware stores or in similar situations in different villages of Vermont. When asked why they weren't working, a common reply was, "Well, my family gave up on me, so I gave up on me." Because these middle-aged men seemed to be employable, we speculated that their comments might indicate a loss of resilience under significant rejection, a personality style, or a desire simply to strive no further. But, after all, they did feel that getting out of the hospital was a major accomplishment.

A person in New York City, "John," who was a brilliant mathematician, was still trying to find the exact formula for a problem he was going to solve. A couple of decades earlier, Brooks had sent his scribbles to a professor of mathematics at a prestigious university, and, indeed, the patient was deemed brilliant. But he couldn't let go of this focus, even for a minute, trying instead for perfection.

Several others were still living in Vermont board-and-care homes and functioning at fairly low levels. A few of these people, mostly elderly women, such as "Constance," "Adeline," "Annie," and "Gertrude," as well as "Clarence" and "Rufus," were all suffering from tardive dyskinesia (TD), a side effect of psychotropic medication which can become permanent over time.[12] The uncontrollable facial grimaces and other movements of arms, torso, and hands with rapid twitches were quite disfiguring and made it difficult for some to eat, walk, or even talk. They were socially unacceptable to others who did not understand their condition. Imagine recovering from psychosis and still having TD.

Then there was "Herman," who met the interviewer with a shotgun on the front porch of his remote cabin in the woods. Even though they had an agreed upon appointment, his persistent paranoia got the better of him.

"Willie" was reported to be living in an isolated fishing shack on the outskirts of town. Our original assumption was that he was probably not functioning at all well and was a loner, too. However, when the interviewers found him, they discovered that he had made a sort of life for himself. Every morning he made the rounds of certain businesses, which provided him with coffee and doughnuts. He was well known and had been taken under the town's wing. We also found that he had a bunch of drinking buddies with whom he hung out in the summer, and so he had something of a social life. But still he was living on Supplemental Security Income (SSI) and on the fringe of society. We discovered that small towns were often accepting of people whom they didn't quite understand, but would tolerate only a couple of them.

During a trip out West to interview the people who had "escaped" from Vermont, the interviewers had found wide heterogeneity of outcome. One person, "Charlotte," who was living in Portland, Oregon was quite recovered and was putting on one-woman art shows in galleries. One study participant, "Mack," was homeless in Houston, Texas. Of interest, he had carved a niche for himself in a specific alley and had his clothes hung up neatly on hangers stuck to nails in the wall, with shoes neatly lined up underneath.

We also found two people, "Warren" and "Francis," who had figured out the system and would routinely get themselves hospitalized in Florida for the winter, returning to New England and the VSH every summer.

We found a few couples who had married one another after meeting in the rehabilitation program. This group included a female patient, "Beatrice," who had married a male aide, "James," from the rehab unit. Some couples had managed to achieve decent relationships, while others had made poor relationships, with their residual psychopathologies eating away at the bond.

In looking at more records, we found that some study participants, such as "Angus," "Peter," "Jenny," and "Mabel," were still diagnosed with schizophrenia and had family members who had suffered from neurological problems such as epilepsy, brain tumors, and strokes. We wondered about those connections to our participants. Perhaps there was a subgroup whose genetic heritage included problematic neurological functioning, which showed up in different ways and indicated possible pathway vulnerabilities?

Possible Cohort Biases

We had been reassured by the original research team that the only people who were *not* selected from the back wards for the original Vermont Study were the 178 responders to Thorazine. These responders were able to get out of the hospital *before* the rehab program was initiated. In the 1950s, the rehab program was funded by the Office of Vocational Rehabilitation (OVR) in Washington, DC. The OVR wanted people to work. It excluded people older than 65 with the assumption that people at that age could not and did not work. (My still-working-at-80 grandmother would have said, "Oh, fiddledeedee" to this assumption!) In addition, we excluded people in the hospital on legal mandates who, of course, were unable to be discharged.

The Issue of Suicide

We also began to consider why there had been only two suicides since index hospitalization for the rehabilitation program because the literature often indicated an approximate 5–13% young male suicide rate in serious mental illness.[13] It suddenly struck us that the biggest bias in the study, other than being skewed toward the most disabled and profoundly ill participants, was the fact that we did not have the young males in the cohort who had committed suicide before the cohort was assembled in the 1950s, and we had had only two suicides once it was put together. Although two was too many, it was several years into the study before we recognized that fact. In 1980, it was hard to see who was possibly missing in the cohort selection way back in 1955.

The Jump in the River

"Ernest" killed himself early on after the rehab program began in the 1950s, and "Elmer" took his life by jumping in the Winooski River running by the hospital. It happened several weeks after we had interviewed him with our Life Chart, which reviewed a life lived to that point. We were stunned and saddened. We had no idea whether the review was the direct cause or whether it had to do with intervening events or both. But we looked at Elmer's record and saw that he had had many periods of major depression, which had occurred in the past, and other suicide attempts had been made. But we still felt that we might have contributed to this sad event. Unfortunately, maintaining blindness of the field interviewers to the records and of the record reviewer as to who was being interviewed out in the field prevented us from being able to issue any advance alerts.

Recognizing the Power of the Process

We decided that this kind of research, particularly as a longitudinal study, is a clinical intervention of sorts. Investigators build relationships and review what is going on in a person's life. Using the mutual participation method described earlier, the Life Chart divides, before a person's eyes, his or her sequential years of life into 10 areas such as work, residence, and significant others while revealing patterns of events.[14] It is like the proverbial "life flashing in front of you." As clinical investigators, we made the determination, after Elmer's suicide, that we would add to the closing section of the protocol a strong positive finish to a life lived by identifying whatever we could in the Chart to demonstrate that the person had lived a life of meaning. This included having had a beloved big dog, sticking by a friend over time, or being a volunteer in the town library. Whatever could be found, we pointed it out. This approach would be considered a breach of protocol if there was to be another follow-up, but we knew this would be the final one.

Overall, we were struck with the ingenuity and persistence of this part of the sample to gain a toehold on existence even though they were still coping with ongoing symptoms, problems, personality quirks, loss of opportunities, medication side effects or long-term use, the effect of stigma and discrimination from society, a sense of hopelessness, or a lack of perceived meaning and purpose of their lives.[15]

Life Chart Now a Clinical Instrument Called The Lifeline

Since the project, the Life Chart has been molded into a clinical interview called the Lifeline,[16] and it includes the same joint process, concluding with the positive ending protocol. Instead of being used at the end of a research interview, it is used at the beginning of an early clinical encounter to start building a therapeutic relationship focused on a whole life, and it is updated across time. It provides an instant snapshot and captures the context in which the person grew up instead of focusing only on current distress. This instrument has been given in training workshops across the world, including in Beijing when I interviewed another mentor, Professor Byron Good of Harvard Global Health, Social Psychiatry, and Medical Anthropology, in front of a large group of excited Chinese psychiatrists.

Powerful Faces

During the first week of the follow-up, Paul Landerl, who was a semi-professional photographer on the side, came back very excited by the wonderful faces he had found and asked permission to photograph people who were willing. We went back to our Harvard Law professor, Stan Herr, and he helped draft a new permission form. About 150 people allowed one or the other interviewer to take their pictures. The faces were amazing. They were strong, dignified, and proud. They revealed determination and resilience. They looked like every other Vermonter, our friends and neighbors.

Some of Landerl's stories that went with taking the photos included one of a person well known in one town. "Peter" had lived in people's barns in the winter and had a shack in the summer. He did handyman's work around town. We found him now in a nursing home as an elderly man who had his eyes closed in the first picture and wide open in the next one. If we had only one picture (the one with the eyes closed), the photo would have conveyed a completely different impression. In fact, there were several cases in which one picture would not have been enough. These "before-and-after" pictures revealed much more about each person.

One man, "Richard," grabbed his guitar to show us one of his talents. Another person, "Lorenzo" was unshaven and insisted that he be allowed to shave and "clean up" and have a second photograph taken. It made all the difference in our impression of him. Another was a woman, "Alice," who was somber and serious during the interview. She suddenly brightened up for the camera and announced "I am really '*quite*' a woman, you know!"

Another older gentleman, "William," took considerable interest in the camera and told Landerl that he had also been a photographer in his younger days. Landerl later noted that this skill was something which this man's clinicians did not know about and could have been used to further his re-entry into the community.

For the few people suffering from residual TD's disfiguring movements, both Landerl and Consalvo figured out ways to take photos which enhanced the real person underneath this drug side effect. One woman, known as "Marilee," stuck out her tongue, even though she did not have TD according to her assessment in the protocol. Viewing this single picture, an immediate assumption would be made that she did have the side effect, but later ones reveal her incredibly playful sense of humor.

Other Uses of the Photos

We made sure each person received a copy of their photo with the project's thank you letters. We heard tales of people going around their villages showing them off. Many participants said that they had never had a picture of themselves except for the admissions photo taken at the hospital. Imagine!

In some ways, these photos say more than our data do about hard-won recovery. Because many people gave us permission to show these photos at scientific meetings, we did in the early days, before our audiences included nonprofessionals who were not included in the permissions. The response to these photos was overwhelming. Suddenly the data came alive: most listeners remembered the faces more than the statistical displays and, many years later at other conferences, will often talk to me about their experience of seeing the faces. I have often wished I could just show all the pictures and tell each life history instead of the "scientific data." I remember how, at one annual American Psychiatric Association meeting, Professor Martin Harrow, who had just begun investigating his sample in the new Chicago Study, said to me: "You have the happy faces and I have the unhappy faces" (Martin Harrow, personal communication, May 6, 1992). Now that 20 years have passed, many of his faces have become happy ones too.[17]

Independent and Dependent Housing Were Not Necessarily So

Another discovery made by our two interviewers was about more of the usual assumptions made in the field and thus were reflected in common instrument ratings about "independent versus dependent" housing. Much to their surprise, instead of just finding very disabled people in board-and-care "dependent" housing, the raters found at least five levels of functioning ranging from sitting in a rocking chair on the porch to actually running the house as the manager. We had to change the instrument battery to register this new discovery. Landerl and Consalvo also found one person, "Lyle," who had been working for the state of Vermont at a semi-professional level. He replied to our surprise that he still lived there, pointing out that "Well, it is the cheapest housing around!"

Low Income Level Did Not Necessarily Mean Poor Quality of Life

In a very interesting discussion with Joe Fleiss, our original statistician at Columbia University Mailman School of Public Health mentioned earlier, we began talking about using the measurement of the Hollingshead and Redlich's ratings.[18] These scores were based on income and profession of parents to quantify the socioeconomic levels of our participants. Although Vermont was one of America's poorest states, the quality of life seemed so appealing that scores of "Flatlanders" from New York and Massachusetts were buying up homes there. What happened in Vermont was bartering. People might barter for dental work, gasoline for their car, groceries for the family in exchange for a new roof for a shed, or deer meat for a freezer, or even some land with sugarbush on it, such as the Brooks family had done all those years before. Bartering enabled a higher quality of life than would have been possible based just on income, and it also indicated the level of our participants' integration into their communities.

12

"I Don't Believe a Word She Just Said!"

Learning to Present These Exciting Data

In June of 1982, just as we were completing our initial data analysis of the Vermont Longitudinal Study, I received an invitation to present some of our brand-new findings at a big meeting being held at the National Institute of Mental Health (NIMH), the International Conference on Schizophrenia, Paranoia, and Schizophreniform Disorders in Later Life.

Because we had the newest data, our study was given two 10-minute presentation slots, while other investigators were given just one. I was never a teaching assistant as a graduate student because I was grant-funded, and therefore I had no real idea of how to provide a 10-minute overview (or any length presentation for that matter), especially about such a massive dataset. What I didn't realize was that a short, 10-minute presentation is the hardest to pull off. Someone told me later that President Woodrow Wilson had responded to a question from one of his Cabinet members about to how he learned to give very precise speeches by replying, "It depends. If I am to speak ten minutes, I need a week for preparation; if 15 minutes, three days; if half an hour, two days; if an hour, I am ready now."[1]

I was very pleased to be asked to speak but still totally ignorant about how to actually do so. Everyone around me assumed I knew, and I thought 10 minutes would be easy, so I did not ask. I decided that the first 10 minutes would focus on: "What Happens to Chronic Psychiatric Patients as They Grow Older? The Vermont Story" and the second 10 minutes would discuss "Social Functioning in Chronic Patients 22–62 Years After First Admission."

Recovery from Schizophrenia. Courtenay M. Harding, Oxford University Press. © Courtenay M. Harding 2024.
DOI: 10.1093/oso/9780195380095.003.0012

I sat bravely between John Strauss, such a major force in the research world on schizophrenia (with his colleague Professor William T. Carpenter, Jr. and many others) and Professor Dr. Med. Luc Ciompi, of Switzerland. With his colleague, Professor Dr. Med. Christian Müller, Ciompi had completed the longest catamnestic study of schizophrenia, known as the Lausanne Investigations.[2] One of the features of a catamnestic study is that it follows the course of people's lives often from their first admission. This study had an average length of 36.9 years and ranged up to 64 years after first admission. (A later chapter provides information on the Swiss study as well as on other contemporary two- and three-decade-long studies.) In fact, nearly every investigator that I had ever read about in schizophrenia research was there in the auditorium that day. To make matters even tougher, my NIMH program chiefs were sitting in the front row, with the refunding decision to be made the following week for continuation of our project. Gulp!

All I had were 3× 5-inch cards clutched nervously in my hand, a few slides, and no practice nor any mentoring on how to give a formal presentation. In those days, slides were physical objects edged in cardboard to be ready for a large carousel. They were made by each med school's Audio/ Video Department.

What happened next was my worst nightmare. The microphone went out and my soft voice was revealed. Professor Joseph Zubin yelled out from the second row, "I can't hear you!" He had been the developer and chief of psychiatric research at the Biometric Department in the New York State Psychiatric Institute at Columbia University. He was now in his 80s. I struggled on. Then the slide projector and podium light also went out. I finished as best as I could and slunk back to my seat, wishing I could disappear.

To top things off, during a panel following the morning's presentations, Professor George Winokur, an esteemed clinical researcher and one of the investigators on the other long-term US follow-up study at the time, the Iowa 500, said, "I don't believe a word she just said."[3] I wanted to crawl under the chair by then but I was sitting on the dais with the other speakers for the discussion session. I wasn't allowed to get a word in edgewise. I just smiled because I knew what we had found was real. Little did I know that this was just the first of many instances of people yelling at me in disbelief in our findings over the next four decades.

While the conference participants and I were at lunch in the cafeteria, up sauntered another famous researcher from the University of Pittsburgh.

Professor Gerard (Jerry) Hogarty, MSW, had been our outside reviewer from the second site visit. It was he who had encouraged me to apply for graduate school, and he had described how challenging it would be in the research arena. Was he ever right! With his hallmark Boston Irish cheery demeanor, he took me back to the auditorium to fix all that recalcitrant machinery. As he was making certain that all the repair work was done, he taught me how to make clearer slides. He told me to only put a few key words on each slide to underscore important points, and not to put lots of tables and figures on them. He made me laugh so much that by the time the afternoon session started I felt much better. In fact, my mood was so improved that I was able to tell my audience that "speakers usually do not get a reprieve," and I proceeded to do at least an adequate job on the next presentation. The Vermont Longitudinal Study was refunded the next week. It was my baptism by fire.

Ever since that day, I have passed Hogarty's advice and my story on to as many scared students as possible. He saved the day for me and indubitably for many others. In fact, organizers of conferences often made him "the clean-up batter." This baseball analogy refers to the person who could bring all the players on base back home in order to score multiple times by hitting a home run. Thus, at the end of a long sequence of speakers, some of whom were interesting and some of whom were unbelievably boring, Hogarty would re-enliven the audience. He would send them all off for the break refreshed and anxious to return for the afternoon sessions. (Not all of us have a background of putting ourselves through college as a stand-up comic though—but Hogarty was another wonderful mentor to have.)[4]

The Second Fiasco

Shortly after I learned to talk off my slides as Hogarty had taught me, I had the honor of presenting at the 1983 annual meeting of the American Psychiatric Association during a session chaired by its president, John Talbott. Talbott had spent years devoted to the care of public patients and mental health systems.[5] Just as I was going up to the microphone, the man who was managing the presenters' slide carousels removed the retaining ring on the top and dumped all of mine to the ground. I did not even have my 3 × 5 cards to guide me, so it was not a good presentation. I was chagrinned yet again because I had a hard time talking off the cuff and still do. From that day forward, I have carried hard copies of my slides, just in case, and it does pay off every once in a while. As I began to receive invitations to meetings across the United States and Europe, I became better at presenting our data. Practice really helped most of the time.

How People Yelling at You Can Be Actually Be Enlightening

What I did not expect was how fierce people would be during the discussions. Members of the audience were often skeptical, defensive, and dismissive. For a while I did not understand how directly I was challenging years of assumptions that persons diagnosed with schizophrenia spectrum could achieve only marginal levels of functioning at best. In my naïveté, I had thought the field would do a jig in the hallway after receiving the good news that many people diagnosed with schizophrenia could and did get their lives back. It was a shock to hear things like, "Are you from a different planet?", "Your patients must be all affective disorders in disguise", "My patients are much sicker", and "I can't decide if you are a revolutionary or just a romantic." Eventually I ended up putting all of these comments on a slide to preempt them popping up at the end of presentations.

Although I had heard that schizophrenia patients were expected always to go downhill, I was so new in the field that when I saw that so many people had gotten their lives back I was delighted and surprised, and I wanted to share our findings with the world. When I heard that Professor Dr. Med. Manfred Bleuler, one of the "grand old men of European psychiatry," received the same kind of negative reception to similar findings from his long-term study,[6] I began to appreciate that we had on a different set of glasses through which to look at the world.

How Can an Adversarial Audience Teach the Speaker?

It took me a while to understand that these challenges could be helpful. They showed me what would eventually concern those who read our papers. I learned to listen better, and thus my discussion sections in papers were also much improved and better attuned to the real concerns underlying those questions. I also learned three more essential lessons about being challenged. First, challenges allowed me to think more deeply about things; second, when someone yelled vehemently or was really derogatory, my audiences would stick with me if I kept my cool and refrained from crying or being angry at the podium (even though I felt like it sometimes): and third, these challenges pushed me to sneak in more information to bolster my case.

Another Important Lesson About Belief Systems

Another lesson to be learned was not only how impermeable the belief system about schizophrenia was, but also that I was challenging the very core of my audiences' clinical practices. The more my audiences questioned everything I said, the more data I provided. More data did not often make a difference, with a couple of exceptions. I recall one clinician who asked question after question until I thought I would burst. Afterward, he said, "I just had to make sure before I change from private to public practice." I have followed his career, and, indeed, he did make the change. Another clinician said, "I have read the original German monographs of Eugen Bleuler [the doctor who had renamed "dementia praecox" as a group of schizophrenias], and he was optimistic about improvement." Although doubtful, I thanked him and went off to check it out. Sure enough, Professor E. Bleuler had once been optimistic and had discharged 60% of his patients from Burghözli Hospital in Zurich in his early days there. However, over the years, his son Manfred, who had taken over the hospital, wrote about how his father had succumbed to prevailing notions of pessimism about outcome from schizophrenia. As the story went, every summer E. Bleuler went back to Rheinau, a village which was his old stomping grounds. He had lived there during his early days before he became the first Swiss psychiatrist to take over the famous Burghölzli Hospital in Zürich. Burghölzli is now known as the Psychiatrische Universitätsklinik Zürich, a research hospital associated with the University of Zürich. However, Rheinau was a small clinic, and, while there visiting, year after year he saw a few of his old patients. It discouraged him enough to write that it seemed to him that these patients, suffering from the "group of schizophrenias," never did return to their original selves, or "*non resitutio ad integrum*."[7]

Acknowledging Where the Doubters Were Coming From Made Them Listen Better

In the mid-1980s, I collaborated with Strauss and Zubin on a paper eventually titled "Chronicity in Schizophrenia: Fact, Partial Fact, or Artifact?"[8] In this paper, we pointed out that we recognized not only the training that clinicians receive based on the pessimism of both Kraepelin and later E. Bleuler, but also the everyday realities of their working lives. Such clinical positions were almost all in the public sector, with overloaded caseloads, severely disabled people, and underfunded services. These challenges perpetuated a treatment model of stabilization, maintenance, medications, and entitlements—not recovery.

These beleaguered clinicians were also significantly deprived of follow-up information about their very own clients. If they had time to think of them at all, the conclusion would most likely be that they had found their way into someone else's caseload across town. It was no wonder they thought I was from a different planet! In a way, the other long-term study investigators and I were indeed seeing things from an entirely different angle. We had the *fun* job. We went to talk to people after years of treatment and living in the community to find out what their lives were like. As we learned to appreciate the doubters perspective, and after the publication of both the short[9] and long[10] versions of our paper, clinicians began to hear us better.

When Yale Calls, You Go!

Finally I had met all the on-campus requirements for my doctorate because most of my coursework was completed and the data collection period ended. John Strauss invited me to work with him at the Yale Department of Psychiatry in one of its five sections, the Connecticut Mental Health Center. I was able to transfer to Yale to work with him. At Yale, I was to complete my last two general courses in psychology.

Strauss had been a schizophrenia investigator for many years by then, and he had just started a new NIMH grant, "The Role of Work in Recovery from Serious Mental Illness." I began work with his lively team, Alan Breier, MD; Hisham Hafez, MD; and Paul Lieberman, MD (three young psychiatrists), and with clinical social worker and a professor at a local university, Jaak Rakfeldt, PhD. We were all learning more about schizophrenia.

First, I discovered that the diagnosis of schizophrenia—or whatever it was—could not be established as fact. There were many theoretical models under discussion and problems galore with definitions and scanty biological evidence. Because of this uncertainty, I learned that *a diagnosis, per se, was only a cross-sectional working hypothesis and not something graven in granite.* I also learned that the field was woefully ignorant about etiology, the impact of psychotropic medications, and how systems of care were making people more chronic. Meanwhile, angry ex-patients were acquainting us with the mistreatment, stigma, and discrimination they had experienced throughout their lives.

The pendulum had swung 180 degrees again, this time from psychoanalysis and the "schizophrenogenic mother"[11] to biology. The field of psychiatry was rushing headlong into studying the medical underpinnings of disorder, "the broken brain,"[12] genetics,[13] neurodevelopmental theories,[14] and drugs, drugs, and more drugs.[15] But so far nothing had paid off with any certainty.

The Argyle Sock Model of Iterative Research

I found that Strauss opted for acknowledging his lack of knowledge, as George Brooks had done earlier. He earnestly approached all of his study participants as "consultants" who could teach us what it actually felt like to have a psychosis and how the recovery process evolved for each individual.[16]

I, on the other hand, kept pushing for structured scales as I had been taught and as I had used in the Vermont protocol. I allowed that we could interlace all those questions from scales and schedules with open-ended ones, especially at the beginning, the middle, and the end. The most important ones, which we had used in Vermont as well, were (1) "How are things going?"; (2) "Now that we have gotten half-way through the protocol, are there any things that you might want to add?"; and last, my all-time favorite (3) "Is there anything, about which I didn't know enough to ask, that you might want to tell me?"

To have a structured instrument, we needed to better understand how the processes and components of work helped or hindered recovery from psychosis, as well as other factors. Since very few people had investigated these questions, Strauss wanted to pioneer the research. The usual approach was to review the literature, create a questionnaire, use it with a class of psychology undergraduate students, and publish "a large N, significant p study." That meant a study with a large group of interviewees, with significant results would be published—assuming one was asking the right questions.

Strauss was a "closet psychologist." During his senior year in medical school, he opted to study with Piaget, the Swiss observer of how children think. These crucial studies were learned from watching Piaget's own three children.[17] Given that example, Strauss endeavored to discover some of the component parts of recovery from psychosis by taking this bright idea and a few questions to interview a small subset of patients. These participants added some new ideas and could tell us we were off kilter on others. Then we would go back later and ask again: "Are we getting closer?" So, again and again, the battery grew, the validity grew, and we learned a lot through this iterative process. I affectionately called it "The Argyle Sock Model of Iterative Research."

Some Important Things We Found Out About the Recovery Process

Our sample consisted of 28 people who had been hospitalized for functional psychiatric disorders at Yale-New Haven Hospital located next door. This was an intensive follow-along study with interviews shortly after hospitalization, bimonthly, and at 1 year and 2 years after hospital discharge. We learned many important things about recovery during this process.

We found out about the differential use of social supports right after a psychosis through Breier, an original team member. For example, early in the recovery process, patients said they wanted "reassurance that they were 'still loveable'" and only later did they want "help with problem-solving."[18] These findings were important because clinicians often rush in to help and don't worry so much about reassuring the person that he or she was still "loveable," meaning still acceptable as a human being after such an alienating experience as a psychosis.

Later, when Rakfeldt worked with us, he wrote about "low turning points" when people had had enough of the struggle, hit bottom, and decided to go forward again[19]—something learned by Brooks as well decades earlier.[20] Strauss wrote papers with us focused on ways people learn to cope with symptoms as another explanation of negative symptoms (e.g., withdrawal from social situations, loss of interest in things, passivity) and another on how people continued on with adult development.[21,22]

Ann Holstein and I, while she was getting her master's degree in nursing, wrote about the unrecognized multiple stressors that the ill women in our sample experienced, in contrast to the males in the Yale Study. These women were faced not only with conquering severe psychiatric distress but often also with the challenges of home and child-rearing responsibilities, as well as of earning a living. Researchers need to take these factors into consideration when trying to understand ratings of symptom severity and appreciate these women as being functional but more stressed.[23]

The team also identified many different phases of the recovery process, and the resulting paper won an award from the American Psychiatric Association.[24] The paper outlined eight longitudinal principles, which included

1. Nonlinear course,
2. Identifiable phases (e.g., moratoriums, change points, ceilings),
3. Mountain climbing,
4. Time decay of vulnerability or reduced reactivity,
5. Phases in environmental response (e.g., convalescence, backlash, perhaps moratoriums, and change points, too),
6. Identifiable sequences of individual–environment interaction (e.g., exaggerating feedback, corrective feedback, and cumulative effect),
7. The active role of the patient, and lastly,
8. The meaning of environmental events and personal behaviors (e.g., loss of a job can be interpreted as awful or an opportunity to try something else).

Embedded within one of the phases was "woodshedding," as suggested by Paul Lieberman. He had worked as a college radio announcer and told us about a habit among jazz musicians. Apparently, when working on new material or styles of playing, they head for the proverbial woodshed to work on things alone before appearing in public.[25] We found one person in our study who was mute and who had stayed in bed ever since her psychosis. One day she got out of bed and simply said "hello" to the postman and proceeded to do so daily. When we asked her about those encounters later, she said something like, "I was beginning to perhaps, maybe, start again." We were asked how many existing protocols would capture this important stage of "practicing to re-enter the world" in the recovery process. The answer was none that we knew of at the time.

Some of the papers focused on one person or three people (especially those studies led by Lieberman and Hafez). They employed qualitative research methods only but were not considered "publishable" in the 1980s, during the push for "real science" and quantitative data. This situation seemed slightly ludicrous to us since biological investigators would often publish 10 papers on different measures taken on 10 patients. (Maybe we can dig these papers out of our dusty file cabinets and publish them as a book now that qualitative research is in vogue again.)

Paying Attention to Social Policy Implications

Strauss, in New Haven, and George Albee, in Vermont, both suggested that I introduce myself to Professor Edward Zigler in the psychology department on the main Yale campus. He had conducted many studies of schizophrenia,[26] so I trotted over and met with him to talk about my last two courses. Zigler was one of the founders of the well-known program for pre-kindergarten children, Head Start.[27] He also had served at least six or seven US presidents by then. In 1977, he started a program, the Bush Center for Child Development and Social Policy, funded by the Archibald Bush Foundation in Minnesota. (In 2005, the Bush Center became the Edward Zigler Center.[28]) He listened to my wild story of receiving a NIMH grant with a bachelor's degree, hiring experienced professional-level people to collect and analyze our data, and our initial findings.

Without a pause, he said: "Courtenay, your findings have significant public policy implications. How about becoming a Bush Fellow?"

I replied, "Sure. What is a Bush Fellow?"

He said, "Well, it will pay for the remainder of your Yale education, and you will learn about social policy."

Although the Yale Admissions Office must have swallowed hard upon seeing my low math Graduate Record Examination (GRE) score (reported recently but based on long-ago high school math), Zigler called a former student of his, Thomas Achenbach, PhD, one of my professors at the University of Vermont (UVM)'s psychology department, and discovered that I had already passed three grad courses in statistics. None of those math questions was on my GRE. That news apparently relieved Yale, and the university accepted me as a Fellow because Zigler backed me. So, every Friday thereafter for 2 years, I took a brown bag lunch across campus and went to a lecture on social policy. In the course of things, I also went to my last two additional general classes in psychology (one of which was child psychology taught by Zigler) and finished my graduate school course requirements.

Zigler taught me many other things. One of the first was that Congress and legislatures prefer "one-handed psychologists." Lawmakers want to be told what works. Apparently, they do *not* want to hear about all sorts of possible options, and I later used this information in my work with a few legislatures to up the ante for recovery programs.

Second, he expressed to me that I had to break the rules, taught to all psychology students, about being aloof and impartial about findings in the discussion sections of papers. Although researchers always strive to be objective and unbiased about their projects, Zigler told me that, in his experience, many investigators would translate findings in any way they saw fit to back up their own thinking. Sure enough, he was right. As an example, some authors found support for the lifetime use of drugs while others reported support for family therapy. Several other areas were declared effective as well, but I had data on none, nor had I written about them. He strongly suggested that I break with tradition and write exactly what I really thought about the social policy implications of my work. I did so and was criticized for it, but never regretted it. He also taught me how to play poker, which was very helpful in dealing with audiences. site reviewers, and funders.

Being at Yale taught me so many critical lessons, but it also gave me a national podium (e.g., a National Public Radio "Morning Edition" interview and opportunities to do many international presentations). I knew it was the same me presenting the same data as I had at the UVM, but I was grateful for all opportunities to talk about our findings.

Doing a Career Backward and Finally Learning to Be a Clinician

After graduation from the UVM, the psychology division in the department of psychiatry at Yale also allowed me to complete clinical training with an internship and postdoctoral fellowship with three very sharp supervisors. The patients with whom I worked kept giving me a new appreciation for human resilience and persistence. I continued to work at the Connecticut Mental Health Center, which at the time in the early 1980s was providing training for residents on the classic "50-minute hour" in psychodynamic and psychoanalytic psychotherapy and, of course, medications for its public patients coping with serious problems. I found that questions such as "Where are you living now?" and "Are you getting enough to eat?" were never asked. When I asked them, the answer was often, "Sleeping in my car and eating every other day!" I learned to help people find jobs and homes, as well as friends and a new sense of self. It just made sense. It had taken me an average of 32 hours a week just to work with eight complex people. One even asked me, "Are you practicing on me?" Since psychologists are not taught about such things, I was indeed learning, and I admitted it. She and I had a good laugh. In some way, I think that the knowledge that she was giving me provided a pathway for her own rehabilitation and improvement. We were "walking the path together," as George Brooks had described to me earlier. She gave me her wisdom, and I tried to share what little I had accumulated.

Changing the System of Care

I spoke with the commissioner of mental health in Connecticut, Michael Hogan, PhD, about funding for case management. Hogan asked me to document a month's worth of efforts and then declared he would fund such efforts. Recognizing a source of new funding, Yale suddenly reorganized the Center, already under Boris Astrachan, into teams and hired actual case managers and vocational counselors, all who had the training that I did not have. They were a wonderful resource, and people were much better served from my standpoint as well. However, starting in the 1990s, consumers of services began informing clinicians that they were neither "cases" nor did they want to be "managed." So we keep learning. I think that partnerships are the way to go.

Thus, I continued to do things backward, as usual, but these experiences also helped me gain a better "seat of the pants" understanding about whatever schizophrenia was, as well as other serious and persistent disorders. I found that these experiences also allowed me to ask even more clinically relevant questions in future research. And Hogan went on to become commissioner of mental health of Ohio and then for New York state, where he kept innovating new programs. He also played a key leadership role in the 2003 President's New Freedom Commission on Mental Health Report during the George W. Bush years.[29]

Our Vermont Sample Rediagnosed: The New DSM- III Versus the Old DSM-II

During all this learning and growing, I kept presenting, defending my dissertation, and drafting out more of our Vermont findings. It became very clear that many of the public challenges to our data had to do with the diagnostic question, "Could these significantly improved or fully recovered patients in the Vermont Longitudinal Study really meet the new diagnostic criteria for schizophrenia?" There was great excitement about the new diagnostic system, the *Diagnostic and Statistical Manual of Mental Disorders*, third edition (the DSM-III), which offered more precision and reliability, although George Vaillant had already challenged its validity.[30] Audiences kept pushing for answers in their disbelief. Surely the new DSM-III must show that our original findings were wrong. The questions went on and on. Some of the answers are discussed in the next chapters.

Remember that our second NIMH site review team had declared that "We all know that they are just a bunch of old chronic schizophrenics [sic]," and they refused funding to apply the new criteria. The DSM-III,[31] published in 1980, was being used by the field then, and would be through the rest of the decade. Now, at this writing in 2024, the DSM has gone through five iterations (DSM-III-R, DSM-IV, DSM-IV-TR, DSM-5, and the DSM-5 TR).[32,33,34,35,36] The schizophrenia section has not changed all that much except in the DSM-5, which removed the subtypes because the symptoms of many patients seemed to switch from one subtype to another.[37] But, in the 1980s, all of our audiences wished to know the cohort's DSM-III status at selection and current diagnostic state, and to then have that factored into the outcome of our study participants. We desperately had to figure out what to do next, but we had no funding for it.

13

Did Rediagnosis for Contemporary Schizophrenia Make a Difference in the Rates of Improvement and Recovery?

The Critical Decision to Rediagnose Our Sample

Strauss and I huddled over the problem of rediagnosing our participants in the Vermont Longitudinal Study. I had no money left to hire psychiatrists to review the records and try to determine whether members of the study sample would qualify for the brand-new criteria of the *Diagnostic and Statistical Manual*, third edition (DSM-III),[1] These criteria had been published by the American Psychiatric Association (APA) in 1980—just as we were going out into the field. The deal was to see if our study participants would actually qualify, particularly for schizophrenia, as they were at index hospitalization in the late 1950s, under the now ancient DSM-I and -II.[2,3] The DSM had not been updated since version II in 1968, and version III was now considered to be the gold standard for the profession.

Audiences at our presentations were as frustrated as we were that we did not have modern diagnostic labels for our cohort. In the early 1970s, an important study had been conducted between London and New York by John Cooper and Barry Gurland, among many others.[4] They found that the levels of diagnosis of schizophrenia in the United States were much higher than in London. Their findings indicated that psychiatrists in New York

Recovery from Schizophrenia. Courtenay M. Harding, Oxford University Press. © Courtenay M. Harding 2024.
DOI: 10.1093/oso/9780195380095.003.0013

were much too liberal and that many people had probably been misdiagnosed over the years. Conversely, I have also been told that many American psychiatrists secretly thought the British were too fond of affective disorders. However, doubters thought that members of our cohort who got better had affective disorders instead of schizophrenia. The expectation was that if they truly had schizophrenia, then their prognoses would have been only marginal improvement or a downhill course. We had to try to address these doubts and find out.

A Brief History of the Diagnostic Classification Systems Used in the United States, Especially for Schizophrenia

The DSMs have evolved over time to reflect the prevailing thinking, observations, research, training, and politics within psychiatry. In the late 1920s, the Armed Forces, the Veterans Administration, various medical schools, and the international community all had different ways of diagnosing patients, which led to significant confusion.[5] The original *Diagnostic and Statistical Manual of Mental Disorders* marked the first edition of what has been referred to ever since by shorthand as the DSMs. The first edition was finally produced in 1952 by a committee that had formed to discuss the problem in 1932. People in the field told me that the work was done in smoke-filled rooms. These meetings were full of men with strong opinions, perhaps similar to that of political caucuses.

Adolf Meyer, director of the Phipps Clinic at Johns Hopkins and later its chair, was highly influential in American psychiatry.[6] In describing Meyer's approach to diagnosis, a more recent chair, Raymond DePaulo, Jr., stated that Meyer "would pick the one [a diagnosis] that seemed to suit the patient best but be prepared to use another if that failed. It wasn't about doing this kind of psychotherapy or giving that kind of drug. It was figuring out how best to help and continuing to learn."[6,7]

Later, as described by Robert Spitzer in the Foreword of the DSM-III, Meyer felt that "mental disorders represented reactions of the personality to psychological, social, and biological factors."[8] However, Meyer was known more for his "psychobiological" theories, and it was actually his student Alexander Leighton, then at Harvard, who had emphasized a stronger social component to mental disorder in the quest for equilibrium in 1949.[9] Thus, the biopsychosocial theories and approaches of today essentially evolved more than 70 to 100 years ago. But from the DSM-II committees onward, most groups have considered "reaction" to social interaction as only a "theory" of causality and have removed it as a criterion.[10] This is perhaps much the same as the way that "brain disease" is the new theory of causality today. "Even if it had tried, the DSM-III committee could not establish agreement about what this disorder [schizophrenia] is; it could only agree on what to call it."[11]

The DSM-I Published in 1952

The skinny gray pamphlet of the DSM-I manual contained only of 130 small pages, most of which were devoted to how to document with correct numerical codes in order to be more congruent with international classifications and keep proper statistical records. Of the 31 pages describing different disorders, only two and a half were devoted to "Schizophrenic Reactions" (a la Meyer); these included simple type, hebephrenic type, catatonic type, paranoid type, acute and chronic undifferentiated types, schizoaffective type, childhood type, and residual type.[12]

The only prognosis for long-term outcome presented in the manual was for Schizophrenic Reaction, residual type, with the DSM declaring that "This term is to be applied to those patients who, after a definite psychotic schizophrenic reaction, have improved sufficiently to be able to get along in the community, but who continue to show recognizable residual disturbances of thinking, affectivity, and/or behaviors."[13]

The DSM-II Published in 1968

The mustard-colored spiral bound DSM-II came along 16 years later, after a long effort to work internationally for classifications that everyone could use and agree upon.[14] It was based upon the World Health Organization's International Classification of Diseases- (ICD-8), which had worked with APA committee members.[15] The DSM-II contained 134 pages with 39 devoted to descriptions of disorders. Three pages were devoted to "The

Schizophrenias." An effort was made to be atheoretical, and the manual dropped the term "reaction."[16]

The DSM-II manual had only two prognostic statements: "For Catatonic Type: In time, some cases deteriorate to a vegetative state."[17] For Acute Episode: "In many cases the person recovers within weeks but sometimes his disorganization becomes progressive. More frequently, remission is followed by recurrence."[18]

The designers had hoped that the new classification would "facilitate maximum consistency within the profession and reduce confusion and ambiguity to a minimum."[19] However, they went on to admit that "No list of diagnostic terms could be completely adequate for use in all those situations [every clinical setting] and in every country and for all time."[20] Ernest Gruenberg, Chairman of the Committee on Nomenclature and Statistics, added that "Psychiatrists know full well that irrational factors belie its validity and that labels of themselves condition our perceptions."[21]

The DSM-III Published in 1980

Professor Robert Spitzer was then the new Chief of Biometrics Research at the New York State Psychiatric Institute (NYSPI). Spitzer had participated in the creation of the DSM-II as a consultant[22] and now was the chair of the APA task force and a major contributor to lists of criteria in the making of the DSM-III. Published in 1980, just as the Vermont Longitudinal Study was collecting its data, the new hard-bound green book now had 493 pages, with 300 pages devoted to disorders. Twelve and a half pages were on "Schizophrenic Disorders."[23] This book was a huge enterprise, consisting of 18 subgroups which worked for many years with advisory groups, consultants, other disciplines, and councils. Spitzer circulated drafts and admitted that reactions to them included "alarm, despair, excitement, and joy."[24] As I stated in an earlier chapter, when he asked US psychiatrists to tell him just what his or her primary theoretical framework was, only one doctor wrote back: "I am omnivorous!" That responder was George Brooks of Vermont. No surprise there. Brooks read everything he could get his hands on.

Among the goals of the DSM-III task force were to make the classification system (1) clinically useful for designing treatment, (2) compatible with ICD-9,[25] (3) use familiar language, (4) reflect research data, and (5) help to pick similar patients for research studies.[26]

Because Spitzer was from the field of biometrics, he naturally initiated an unusual set of field trials before publication to check on reliability. The field trials were funded by the National Institute of Mental Health (NIMH) and deployed 550 clinicians from 474 institutions to rate 12,667 patients. There were 137 clinician pairs who rated 331 patients with psychosis.[27] This effort averaged only four cases per pair. In the end, they recognized that there were gray areas between disorders and health. Therefore. they looked for a picture of symptoms that caused pain and significant behavioral problems that disrupted lives. Symptoms included a list of delusions and hallucinations, incoherence, illogical thinking, little emotion shown (flat affect), grossly disorganized behavior (e.g., catatonia), deterioration from previous status, and a duration of 6 months.[28]

In general, disorders were now detected by what was unfortunately declared to be a "Chinese restaurant menu" system. For a possible schizophrenia diagnosis, the clinician could select at least one symptom from a list of six symptoms from criterion A. Then the clinician must check if there is deterioration from "previous levels of functioning in such areas as work, social relations, and self-care as criterion B." Clinicians must then check to see if the illness had a duration of at least 6 months as criterion C. Next, for criterion D, the clinician must check to see if any affective symptoms had developed before, during, or after the psychosis. Criterion E was onset before age 45, and F not due to any organic mental disorder or retardation.[29] The checklist was made more complicated. Overall, the forest-green DSM-III was declared by Spitzer to be descriptive in nature because of the lack of knowledge about etiological factors, and thus it had no "sharp boundaries."[30] Five subtypes of schizophrenia were still listed: disorganized, catatonic, paranoid, undifferentiated, and residual. In general, and across time, schizophrenia and other diagnoses were considered by many clinicians and investigators to be more categorial before there was enough evidence for this.[31]

As far as the prediction of outcome went, the same pessimistic prognostications were assumed, but, for the first time, the rare possibility of a better outcome was mentioned, probably due to the publication of so many European two- and three-decade-long follow-up studies translated into English. The DSM-III declared that

> A complete return to premorbid functioning is unusual—so rare, in fact, that some clinicians would question the diagnosis. However, there is always the

possibility of full remission or recovery, although the frequency is unknown. The most common course is one of acute exacerbations with increasing residual impairment between episodes.[32]

The big question for us was, "Is this prognosis true for the Vermont cohort?"

Sharing the First Results for Readers Now

Colleagues have suggested that some readers might like to skip the design and methodological discussions in this book, plus the actual data that shore up the evidence, and skip right to the findings, while others might like to look into the process. Therefore, I will provide a brief summary of the findings first and the details of how we did this important study later.

To answer the question posed by the title of this chapter, "Did rediagnosis for contemporary schizophrenia make a difference in the rates of improvement and recovery?" The answer is emphatically, "No!" It did not make any difference in the findings whether we used DSM-I, DSM-II, or DSM-III diagnostic criteria. In our paper published in the *American Journal of Psychiatry* and rigorously reviewed, we wrote the following:

> For one-half to two-thirds of those subjects, who retrospectively met the DSM-III criteria for schizophrenia, long-term outcome was neither downward nor marginal but an evolution into various degrees of productivity, social involvement, wellness, and competent functioning.[33]

More Overview of Results First

The most stringent DSM-III diagnostic criteria failed to produce the expected downward course for what was considered to be hard-core schizophrenia. In the entire original cohort of 269 people, 118 (44%) met the new DSM-III criteria for schizophrenia. Furthermore, 31 (12%) met the category of schizoaffective disorder, 47 (17%) of affective disorders, 18 (7%) of atypical psychosis, 22 (8%) of organic disorders (always known), and 32 (12%) people were assigned to the "other" category.[34]

Of the 82 people in this substudy with just schizophrenia who were still alive and interviewed (our hardest data), 68% had *neither* positive nor negative symptoms of schizophrenia. Eight people still displayed definite signs of schizophrenia while another 14 still had probable signs. Nine people had shifted to probable affective or organic disorders and one to alcohol abuse.[35]

Only 25% were using their antipsychotic medications as prescribed. Fifty percent were no longer using their medications, plus the other 25% were using drugs only when they felt "shaky," then taking themselves off in a self-management approach.[36]

Forty percent were still employed, in addition to all those who were retired, elderly, or widowed. The expectation in the field was that perhaps the number would be closer to 10–15% working.

Vaillant has written about more than 16 attempts to decide what to do with "remitting schizophrenics" [sic]. In 1984, he declared that "diagnosis and prognosis should be considered to be different dimensions of psychosis."[37] Yet the field of psychiatry continues to proclaim the 125-year-old slogan: "Once a schizophrenic, [sic] always a schizophrenic [sic]." This continuing mindset sets up programming as custodial, expecting crisis intervention, stabilization, maintenance, medication, and entitlements as primary treatments, with rehab efforts considered ancillary.

These clinical approaches may be helpful for a small subset of patients for whom we have not been able to figure out what is actually going on and for whom we have minimal ways to intervene and help. For the majority of people with the lived experience of profound emotional and cognitive distress, many rehabilitation strategies continue to help them escape the avalanche of mental disorders and emerge into a meaningful life. Examples of rehab client–clinician collaborations can be found in early and later chapters of this book.

How We Accomplished This Study

Now that we had the new diagnostic system in place, Strauss and Alan Breier, our chief resident and member of our research team at Yale, decided that the task was urgent enough to try to rediagnose all 269 members of the Vermont sample, without funding, on their own time. Because the DSM-III had specific criteria, we were able to conduct interrater trials to establish decent reliability between the two investigators. The chronicity criterion was taken care of because people had already been selected back in 1955 with a requirement of being ill and impaired for at least 1 year. Most people were hospitalized for more than 6 years, and some had been hospitalized up to 25 years. "Impairment" implied not being able to function in several areas of routine daily living such as work, social relations, and self-care or "the inability to function in one's ordinary day-to-day capabilities."[38]

All of us recognized that clinicians who were on the spot interviewing a patient in those early years probably saw and heard things which were not always recorded to help them make a diagnosis. In fact, in reviewing many records across the country, I have seen some clinicians simply write the diagnosis of schizophrenia without any justification. We also acknowledged that criteria for schizophrenia would continue to change, so we decided to use a standardized collection of raw data. We had already chosen the Strauss Case Record Review (a signs and symptoms checklist)[39] and the World Health Organization's Psychiatric and Personal History Schedule.[40] These two instruments were used in the International Pilot Study of Schizophrenia (IPSS) to pick up not only symptoms but also behavioral indicators.[41] Furthermore, the Research Diagnostic Criteria (RDC) Screening Interview,[42] the Brief Psychiatric Rating Scale,[43] and a reduced version of the Mini-Mental State Examination[44] plus the Global Assessment Scale[45] were all included to assess psychiatric symptoms. In their earlier work, Strauss and Harder had found that a structured review was helpful in overcoming the pitfalls of "narrative formats, under-reporting, or ambiguous observations."[46] Remember that Vermont State Hospital records were remarkably complete, having been part of the first Thorazine trials with full social, occupational, family, medical, psychopharmacological, and other treatments and patient–physician conversations documented.

The raters worked independently, and, in the first set of 21 records, did not achieve as good a level of success as we had hoped due to the newness of the DSM-III process. Therefore, they independently reviewed 19 more records. All in all, they evaluated 40 records, or 15% of the sample. In the first trial, they agreed 57% of the time. When they didn't agree, we found that the second diagnosis of one rater often agreed with the first of the other rater. The second trial netted a kappa level of .78 which was highly significant and equivalent to that of the DSM field trials themselves of .79 for schizophrenia, and therefore we felt good about proceeding.[47] The kappa coefficient statistic strips out the possibility of sheer luck between scoring parties and is thus more rigorous.[48] Spitzer had made sure with his checklist strategy that there was more reliability between clinicians, and that was good. But as George Vaillant reminded us in a famous debate at the 1984 APA Annual Meeting, with the introduction of the DSM-III, "Validity has been sacrificed on the altar of reliability."[49] This meant that although raters could agree on the checklist, it did not mean that the diagnosis was correct or real.

In the original sample, the DSM-I had determined that 79% or 213 of 269 study participants were considered to have schizophrenia, primarily paranoid and catatonic subtypes, with clusters of symptoms shown in Table 13.1. The remaining 21% (34 of 269) were considered to have affective disorders, and 8% (22 of 269) had severe developmental delays.[50] The data from latter group, which we inherited from the original Vermont Study, was removed from the analyses as being inappropriate in this type of study.

Using the DSM-III criteria, the 213 people originally diagnosed with DSM-I schizophrenia were reduced to 118 with DSM-III schizophrenia.[51,52] It was of great interest to us that the remaining 95 patients who had once been given a diagnosis of schizophrenia did not shift, as expected by the field, to major affective disorders but to atypical psychosis (not otherwise specified) or schizoaffective disorder. In the DSM-III, there were no actual criteria for schizoaffective disorder. However, the common feeling was that if there were affective symptoms along with schizophrenia symptoms, then that is where they belonged.[53] Schizoaffective disorder has always lurked in the middle ground between the two major diagnoses, and people diagnosed

Table 13.1 Symptoms and behaviors found in Vermont cohort

Hallucinations: Mostly auditory, and some visual, olfactory, gustatory, and tactile	Depression
	Distractibility
	Grandiosity
Bizarre delusions	Flight of ideas
Negative symptoms	Pressured speech
Affective flattening	Hyper- or hypoactivity
Poverty of speech/ content	Impaired role functioning
Apathy	Markedly peculiar behaviors (e.g., talking to self in public settings, hoarding food, poor hygiene, expressing odd beliefs, or magical thinking)
Anhedonia	
Problems with attention	
Neurovegetative signs (disturbances of sleep and appetite, loss of energy, excessive guilt, psychomotor retardation)	Expressing self with over-elaborations or vague digressions
	Catatonic Excitability[48]
Catatonic waxy flexibility	

as such were expected to have a slightly better outcome than those people diagnosed with schizophrenia. Schizoaffective disorder generally remained close to the schizophrenia category up until the release of DSM-5.[54] However if we were to look at only the "core schizophrenia" group, we would be deleting people assigned to the schizoaffective category *and* atypical psychoses for this set of analyses. Those clinicians involved in the committees working on the future DSM-5 wrote that "Characterization of patients with both psychotic and mood symptoms, either concurrently or at different points during their illness, has always posed a nosological challenge and this is reflected in the poor reliability, low diagnostic stability, and questionable validity of the DSM-IV schizoaffective disorder."[55]

The field expected the shift to affective disorders because of the more than 125-year dictum by Kraepelin, who wrote that people with such disorders were expected to have much better outcomes. Therefore, anyone who became better with a diagnosis of schizophrenia was always considered to have been misdiagnosed. But Brooks suggested that when clinicians spent time with patients and got to know them well, symptoms and behaviors sorted themselves out more clearly. His statement sounds like Adolf Meyer's caveats mentioned earlier. Consequently, it was no surprise to him that the rediagnostic effort kept almost everyone within the schizophrenia spectrum and not in the affective disorders.

A Formal Challenge to the Assumptions Embedded in the DSM-III

The hypotheses that we used in the evaluation of outcome for the new schizophrenia subsample were taken from two assumptions stated explicitly in the DSM-III. Therefore, we used the DSM-III to challenge itself. These hypotheses were the following:

Hypothesis 1

Members of this cohort diagnosed as having met the DSM-III criteria for schizophrenia at index hospitalization would still have signs and symptoms of schizophrenia at follow-up.

Hypothesis 2

Members of this cohort diagnosed as having met the DSM-III criteria for schizophrenia at index hospitalization would have uniformly poor outcomes in critical areas of functioning such as work, social relations, and self-care at follow-up.[56]

Confirmation of these hypotheses would lend support to the validity of the statements about the long-term course and outcome of schizophrenia that are made in the DSM-III.[57]

And, as I have said before, it should be noted that these assumptions have been made by psychiatry for more than a century.

The Methodological Improvements Over Earlier Follow-Up Studies in the Field

As a review, our improvements consisted of the following ingredients:

1. The reliable application of operationalized current diagnostic criteria, both at follow-up and retrospectively, for the index hospitalization;

2. The application of standardized assessments of psychopathology at the time of follow-up and retrospectively at the time of index hospitalization using DSM-III criteria[58] as well as the other five instruments rating psychopathology and function listed earlier.

3. The assessment of outcome according to a wide variety of course and outcome measures, including both psychopathological and psychosocial measures;

4. The documentation of intervening variables (such as life events and social support systems);

5. The development of a longitudinal picture of what happened to the person, with permission from the person him- or herself, through the use of a number of sources for information. This included detailed medical records, interviews with the person, and interviews with general practitioners, vocational rehabilitation workers, after-care workers, families, friends, clergymen, and other important informants, particularly clinicians (who have known the person throughout the entire follow-up period);

6. The reconstruction, as accurately as possible from various records, of the types of treatment the person received, including drugs and interpersonal forms of treatment; and

7. The record reviewers were blind to what was being found in the field; the field interviewers were blind to what was in the records; and the re-diagnosticians were blind to previous diagnosis because I personally redacted all previous diagnoses given in copies of the records.[59]

A Description of the Core Schizophrenia Subsample

Of the core group of 118, 28 people had died, 4 had refused after completing the interviews, and 4 were lost to follow-up. Our most meaningful data then would be those 82 people whom we had interviewed face to face. With a set of classical scales and schedules used by the field, studying both psychological and levels of functioning, we had assessed their outcome 20–25 years after the rehab program in the 1950s. Time since their first onset of illness at follow-up in Phase III ranged from 22 to 62 years, with an average of 32 years.[60] This length of time makes the Vermont Longitudinal Study one of the longest in the world literature.

Almost half of this group had been hospitalized for more than 6 years before the rehab program. Ironically, they were split half and half between males and females. (Investigators are always grateful for such a balance.) This subset ranged in age from 41 to 79 years with an average age of 61 at follow-up, with most people being single, divorced, or widowed. Ninety-three percent were still living in Vermont. This stability makes Northern New England a good place to conduct longitudinal research. The two interviewers flew to wherever the other 7% ended up. They assessed them to see if, some how, they were different from those people who had stayed in Vermont. They weren't. The same protocol described earlier was provided, and all the interrater trials between field interviewers, between record reviewers, and between diagnosticians were accomplished with highly significant scores, as reported.[61]

Family Involvement

As with the cohort at large, we had also conducted a structured interview with families, friends, and clinicians of the 28 deceased members of the cohort to document the lives and functional levels of each deceased member until 6 months before they died. We chose to end the assessments of the deceased at that point because research had shown that often there is a continuous decrement in function during that time. And, as we had done with the larger sample, the analyses for the deceased patients were accomplished separately in case those results would skew that of the live sample. *It turned out to be the same proportions of recovered, significantly improved, or unimproved as in the live sample; many clinicians would assume that the worst cases died.*[62]

Life Histories

Narrative life histories were constructed for each participant, and these provided a glimpse of the ways psychopathology, personality characteristics, life events, environmental supports, treatment, and just plan luck interacted to produce specific outcome patterns that would have been lost in group statistics.

More Findings for the Newly Rediagnosed DSM-III Core Schizophrenia Subset

Two major surprises were published as part of our pair of lead articles in the *American Journal of Psychiatry*, in 1987. As revealed earlier and bears repeating,

> For one half to two thirds of these people, who had retrospectively met the DSM III criteria for Schizophrenia, long-term outcome was neither downward nor marginal but an evolution into various degrees of productivity, social involvement, wellness, and competent functioning.[63]

The results rocked us back on our heels! We were sure that the more stringent criteria of the DSM-III would result in a more pessimistic picture and validate what psychiatry had said all along.

Yet all the structured questions and ratings, the clinical observations, and the interviews of others who knew these people well kept verifying over and over what we had found. Sixty-eight percent of those participants no longer displayed any signs or symptoms (either positive or negative) of schizophrenia at follow-up.[64] *In fact, 45% displayed no symptoms whatsoever— all in the fully recovered group (29%) plus the remainder in the significantly improved group.* Eight people still displayed definite signs of schizophrenia,

while another 14 still had probable signs. Nine people had shifted to affective disorders, and one person to alcoholism. This was definitely a different picture from what had been expected.

The Role Medication Played in Outcome

The second major surprise had to do with the use of medication. All of
these people had been on Thorazine in the mid-1950s, and, after 2 ½ years
of trials, they had not responded well enough to get out of the hospital, as
178 others in the back wards had done. They and the staff created that innovative rehabilitation program, described at the beginning of this book,
and that helped to get them out into the community. When we asked them
about medication use, lo those many years later, 16% had no prescriptions
and 84% first reported using their prescriptions.[65] However, after learning to
trust us during an average 5 hours of interviews across 2 days, many sheepishly admitted that they picked up their prescriptions but had put them
away "in case they needed them again." They showed us bedroom drawers
and pantries full of these medications prescribed over time. It turned out
that once they had revered their physician, Dr. Brooks, and had taken medications as willing participants. During rehabilitation, they had learned to
take an active role in their own treatment, and, after discharge, they began
to rethink their own care with the new physicians whom they did not
know as well. They realized that community physicians had not seen them
come through their worst days into some of their best, and they found that
significantly unsettling. In the end, we found that, along with 16% who had
no prescriptions, 34% had simply stored away their medications. These figures meant that *50% were no longer using medications*.[66] Of those who were
still using prescriptions, 25% had invented their own targeted medication
strategies, long before Marvin Herz[67] and William Carpenter[68] came up
with the idea in the 1980s. For instance, when this group felt "shaky," they
would medicate themselves a little, and, when they felt better, they would
take themselves off. It has been suggested that "targeted strategies" may not
be particularly good for the brain.[69] However, since then, many discussions
about careful tapering strategies have been conducted.[70] In any event, only
25% took their medications carefully and exactly as prescribed. When we
asked the non-users why, their answer was generally that, somewhere along

the way, their community mental health psychiatrist had yelled at them and threatened them with life-long psychosis if they did not take their meds. All of the fully recovered people (29%) were no longer on medications. Of the significantly improved people (39%), some were off completely, some were using targeted strategies, and some were compliant with their psychiatrist's wishes. The remaining unimproved group members all followed their doctor's orders to the letter.

Remember that our stringent criteria for recovery was no further medication use, no symptoms, no odd behaviors, living in the community, working, and relating well to others. Also remember that these patients were considered the most ill and most chronic cases ever studied. The significantly improved group had achieved all but one of those recovery criteria. That included some use of medication in a few cases; or all of the above criteria, but with distant social relationships; or everything except employment, et cetera.

Diagnosis of Schizophrenia Appears to Have Little Predictive Value Especially Over the Long Term

We compared the differences between scores for those people who had been diagnosed as meeting DSM-I criteria for schizophrenia in the first pass-through and those who now also met DSM-I and DSM-III criteria for schizophrenia. And we looked at those people who had met DSM-I but not DSM-III criteria.[71] Once again, there was wide heterogeneity of functioning and nothing significant stood out. *These findings meant that the diagnostic systems had little predictive power about outcome across time.*[72]

The Word "Recovery" Might Finally Enter Into the Language of Psychiatry?

Both of our hypotheses, based on the expectations of clinicians for more than a century, did not hold up to intense scrutiny. Our study had the best design, the toughest methodology, the most comprehensive measures assessing the most chronic cases, and still people managed to get better. Now we found that a person could have had a bona fide diagnosis of schizophrenia (whatever that is) and nonetheless begin to function well over time, lose the diagnosis, even change the diagnosis, and then get their lives back. This was a bombshell (so we thought), and we were grateful to the *American Journal of Psychiatry* in 1987 for publishing our findings as two back-to-back lead articles, with an unusual introductory editorial by Ronald Manderscheid describing a possible impact on service systems.[73]

Walking Into the Lion's Den

On October 3, 1986, I was invited to provide the grand rounds lecture at the New York Psychiatric Institute and the Department of Psychiatry at the College of Physicians and Surgeons at Columbia University. I decided to go because (1) I was honored to do so and (2) October 3 was my birthday and I wanted to be in Manhattan to see friends and colleagues.

They warned me, in advance, that a faculty member of the Institute, Robert Spitzer, who had spent so much of his time orchestrating the publication of the DSM-III, was also tough on speakers. He was known to sit in the front row, right next to the podium, one foot away, with his co-researcher and wife, Janet Williams, beside him. Both would be in heavily starched white coats with names etched on their pockets and, at the end of each presentation, would immediately pop up to ask difficult and challenging questions.

When I was backstage before the presentation, Spitzer came behind the curtain and welcomed me to Columbia.

I said cheerfully. "Oh Bob, I was hoping you were on vacation this week!" I told him that I heard that he was tough on speakers but that I was delighted to be there.

He said "Who me?" and made a mock surprise gesture with his face and hands.

I was indeed grateful for the warning, that I had my street creds from Yale, and that I finally had accumulated more practice speaking—with 33 international and national presentations under my belt by then as well as 48 others with academic institutions and service system providers. I was up for the challenge. I spoke more comfortably off my slides, as Hogarty had taught me to do, and I had hard copies of them hidden on the podium, just in case the projector went down again. When I was through, and just as predicted, up pops Spitzer.

He said, "We all know that John Strauss believes that people can get better. Was it possible that he unconsciously let some cases, that really had affective disorders, slide into the schizophrenia category?"

With a broad smile, I said: "Well, I brought a slide just for you. It reveals the raw data interrater trial results for the rediagnostic part of the Vermont Study. In it, you will see that, of the two raters, it was Strauss who changed people out of the old DSM-I and -II schizophrenia categories to something else. By and large, the something else was atypical psychoses, schizoaffective disorders, and psychosis NOS [meaning not otherwise specified]." There was a faint chuckle in the audience.

Spitzer popped up again: "Well, I bet your two interviewers unknowingly shifted people to the recovered categories because they were so optimistic?"

I leaned on the podium and laughed. I said, "Those two guys had been so burned out and discouraged working in a community mental health system that they had fled to research. They think differently now, and one is back trying to change things at his agency and the other went back to school to get his doctorate." After my two previous major disasters speaking in important lectures, I am happy to report that experience and coaching can make a big difference.

Then I brought up the work that Professor Patricia Cohen, in the Psychiatry Department, had done with her husband, Professor Jacob Cohen at NYU down the street. They were premier statisticians, and Jacob had written the well-used textbook *Statistical Power Analysis for the Behavioral Sciences*.[74] I explained that their 1984 study found that physicians from many specialties, including psychiatry, found in their caseloads that *2% of the worst cases (those with the most severe forms of illnesses) were seen 64 more times in their caseloads than 40% of people with the least severe version*. That experience changed their outlook about what outcome was possible for certain diagnoses. The phenomenon was called the *clinician's illusion* (hence the title of their paper).[75] Pat seemed pleased that I had brought it up. And I think it is important to think about.

I myself had succumbed to the same problem when I was working at Boston Children's Hospital many years before. It appeared that in our Neurosurgical intensive care unit, an international referral center, every third child had a brain tumor of one sort or another. It seemed to me that the world must be full of them. I even wrote a note to my family's Vermont pediatrician, David Ellerson, and asked him about it. He wrote back that he had the same number of patients as three pediatricians and that he had seen one kid with a brain tumor in 10 years. I knew that he was an expert diagnostician so that I, too, had fallen under the misperception of the clinician's illusion. Unfortunately, it is easy to do, without the clinician realizing it.

Shortly after my presentation, in the hallway, Spitzer asked what I would like to see written under prognosis for schizophrenia in the revised DSM-III-R. When I told him that at least 50–68% might significantly improve or some might even recover, his comment was, "You've got to be kidding!" (Robert Spitzer, personal communication, October 3, 1986).

The DSM-III-R Was Published in 1987

The same year our research was published, the sailor-blue DSM-III-R (R for "revised"), with 567 pages, was released.[76] It referred to such diagnostic dilemmas as, "Criteria were not entirely clear, were inconsistent across categories, or were even contradictory."[77] The writers, including Spitzer, who was now head of the work group to revise DSM-III, also acknowledged that most etiologies were still unknown and that the borders between disorders were gray and poorly defined.[78] In the 12 pages on schizophrenia, outcome had reverted to an earlier skepticism but there was an admission that symptoms might diminish over time.[79] (pg. 191)

> A return to full premorbid functioning in this disorder is not common. Full remissions do occur, but their frequency is currently a subject of controversy. The most common course is probably one of acute exacerbations with residual impairment between episodes. Residual impairment often increases between episodes during the initial years of the disorder. There is some evidence, however, that in many people with the disorder, the residual symptoms become attenuated in the later phases of the illness.[80]

Believe it or not, I thought that this statement actually showed some forward movement, but it was perhaps wistful thinking on my part.

The Umpire

This story reminds me of one that a colleague, Joe Zubin, told me. He was asked to provide a testimonial at a party celebrating Spitzer's retirement because Zubin had been the original chief and founder of psychiatric research in biometrics at the Institute for many years before Spitzer. He told this baseball analogy in a great New York accent.

"When a new baseball umpire is asked how he makes his calls of strikes and balls, he says: 'I calls [sic] them by the book.'" "When you ask a middle-level umpire, he says: 'I calls [sic] them as I sees [sic] them.'" "When you ask the senior level umpire, he says: 'They ain't balls until I say they are balls, and they ain't strikes until I say they are strikes!'"

The implication was that Spitzer had pushed the field to accept the DSM criteria for a bunch of disorders which were not necessarily written in stone—but as he himself saw them.

Zubin said, in mock puzzlement, that, "*For some reason*, Spitzer asked me not to accept any further testimonial invitations if someone asked" (Joseph Zubin, personal communication, Bern, Switzerland, September 11, 1987).

14

Vermont Data Supported the DSM-5 Deletion of Subtypes in Schizophrenia

An excellent review of the schizophrenia literature was written by Assen Jablensky in 2010.[1] Jablensky was at the World Health Organization for many years and then was a professor at the University of Western Australia in Perth. He outlined the struggles psychiatry has had in defining and understanding schizophrenia. The long-standing subtypes in the Western world have been paranoid, disorganized, catatonic, undifferentiated, and residual.

Caveat to Readers

For those readers less interested in statistics, know that the remainder of this chapter explores how psychiatry has changed its ideas, especially about the diagnosis of two subtypes of schizophrenia in particular (catatonia and paranoid) over time. The situation has reached the point of omitting all of the subtypes of schizophrenia in the next-to-newest diagnostic manual, the fifth edition of the *Diagnostic and Statistical Manual of Mental Disorders* (DSM-5)[2] because patients so often slide around from one category to another. The findings from the Vermont Longitudinal Study provide more evidence about why this happened 125 years after schizophrenia was first so subdivided.[3,4]

If you are skipping ahead, the next chapter focuses on the Maine–Vermont Comparison Study, with an average follow-up of 36 years, using the exact same design, methodology, and instrumentation in a state without any or miniscule rehabilitation in the 1950s especially for patients diagnosed

Recovery from Schizophrenia. Courtenay M. Harding, Oxford University Press. © Courtenay M. Harding 2024.
DOI: 10.1093/oso/9780195380095.003.0014

as having schizophrenia. This study asked the question, "Did that rehabilitation program in Vermont make a significant difference in long-term outcomes of schizophrenia?"[5,6]

Catatonia and Paranoid Subtypes: Diagnostic Enigmas in the Vermont Cohort

The National Institute of Mental Health (NIMH) often has shifting priorities. It spent a large amount of money to collect 2,600 data points on each person in the Vermont Longitudinal Study but then, like a fickle lover, turned its attention elsewhere, leaving hapless investigators such as myself to analyze all that data by ourselves with little or no funding to finish the job. Today, there are drawers and drawers full of unfinished analyses sitting in professors' desks all over the country, much to all of our chagrin. Unfortunately, it takes money and collaboration to analyze and report data. Newer professors have figured out sneaky ways to continue old data analyses under the cover of new grants, but we did our best to secure more funding just for more analyses and were very grateful to the Robert Wood Johnson Foundation (grant number 19300) for providing a year's worth of extra support.

The findings I describe next were among those presented at an annual American Psychiatric Association (APA) meeting in San Francisco in 1993[7] and were on Vermont participants diagnosed with catatonia and paranoid subtypes of schizophrenia.

Changes in the Diagnosis of Catatonia Across Time: A Dramatic Behavioral Phenomenon

Professor and Vice Chair of Yale Psychiatry Malcolm Bowers and I worked on this analysis with statisticians Takamaru Ashikaga and Shiva Gautam at the University of Vermont (UVM) for quite a while before Dr. Bowers unfortunately died.[8] We were fascinated with the disappearance of the catatonia subtype of schizophrenia in our sample, depending on which version of the APA DSM was applied. These data provide more evidence about why the DSM-5 committee was smart to drop these subtypes for the first time in over a century.[9]

The neuropsychiatric syndrome of catatonia was described in 1874, by the German physician Karl Kahlbaum (1834–1973).[10,11] He did not know what caused this set of problems but nevertheless categorized them by the symptom picture. He felt that these behaviors emerged as a set of phases, with a person sitting absolutely still, often with an arm raised for hours on end; in some other contorted position; or in a melancholic stupor. Other behaviors included hyperactive manic behaviors, such as walking back and forth or flitting about the ward. Kahlbaum noticed that catatonia was more apt to accompany affective disorders and was a separate problem.

As a nurse assigned to Med-Surg and Geriatrics at Vermont State Hospital in the mid-1970s, I actually saw and cared for such patients. These are not happy states, and I often wondered how people could participate in these behaviors and not collapse from sheer exhaustion.

Another German physician, Emil Kraepelin, followed Kahlbaum and decided that this "disease" belonged as a subtype of his own loosely defined disorder, dementia praecox.[12] Kraepelin also described a lethal form of catatonia which included, in a later description of the excited form, such symptoms as high fevers, altered consciousness, autonomic instability, anorexia, and electrolyte imbalances, among others.[13]

Since the term "dementia praecox" was replaced by the Swiss physician Eugen Bleuler with a "group of schizophrenias,"[14] it has included the subtypes known as catatonia, hebephrenia, paranoid, and disorganized. These subtypes lingered in the diagnostic manuals amid many arguments between psychiatrists in Europe and the United States, which dragged on for over a century until the publication of the DSM-5 in 2013.[15,16] Catatonia had long been connected with schizophrenia, though with many experts dissenting, arguing instead that catatonia should be its own syndrome and applicable across many disorders, both psychiatric and medical.[17]

The Changes in the Vermont Catatonia Group Correlating to Changes in the DSM Across Time

Our catatonic subsample was composed of people given the diagnosis prior to the advent of the diagnostic manuals, or just as the first DSM was published.[18] We could trace them across successive manuals, reflecting the newest thinking of psychiatry at the time, to see how these persons would be recategorized.

The DSM-I was published in 1952, by the APA Committee on Nomenclature and Statistics. Catatonia in the DSM-I was characterized at that point by "conspicuous motor behavior, exhibiting either marked generalized inhibition (stupor, mutism, negativism, and waxy flexibility) or excessive motor activity and excitement. The individual may regress to a state of vegetation."[19] In the Vermont sample, 52 people had this diagnosis. They were tracked all the way through our last evaluation of them in the 1980s. Table 14.1 shows how the understanding of this syndrome has changed over the succeeding years and continues to change.

In the DSM-II,[20] published in 1968, the category of schizophrenia, catatonic subtype, was differentiated into two sub-subtypes: excited and

Table 14.1 Changes in catatonia diagnosis as designated across the First Three Diagnostic and Statistical Manuals (DSMs)

First admission Pre-DSM or DSM-I (1952 or earlier)	Index admission DSM-II (1968) (n = 52)	Rediagnosis by John Strauss and Alan Breier with DSM-III of live participants (n = 49) (3 deceased)
Schizophrenic reaction, Catatonic type 000.20 (N-52) Today's coding = 295.20	Schizophrenia, catatonic type (excited or withdrawn) 295.20 (n = 46)	Schizophrenia, catatonic type 295.20 (n = 14)
	Schizophrenia, paranoid type 295.30 (n = 2)	Schizophrenia, paranoid type 295.30 (n = 11)
	Schizophrenia, hebephrenic type 295.10 (n = 1)	Schizophrenia, hebephrenic type 295.10 (n = 3)
	Manic depressive illness, manic type 296.10 (n = 2)	Schizophrenia, chronic Undifferentiated type 295.90 (n = 9)
	Hysterical neurosis, dissociative type 300.14 (n = 1)	Schizoaffective disorder 295.70 (n = 8)
		Bipolar disorder, manic type 296.40 (n = 1)
		Paranoid disorders, atypical 298.90 (n = 1)
		Atypical anxiety 300.00 (n = 1)
		Intermittent explosive disorder 312.34 (n = 1)

withdrawn. The DSM-I had noted this distinction but did not assign two different diagnostic codes to it. In the DSM-II, the excited subtype was "marked by excessive and sometimes violent motor activity and excitement." The withdrawn type was described as "generalized inhibition manifested by stupor, mutism, negativism, or waxy flexibility."[21]

The following categories were given as alternatives to the diagnostic code 295.20 for catatonia. Category 295.10 was called "schizophrenia, hebephrenic type," which was "characterized as disorganized thinking, shallow and inappropriate affect, unpredictable giggling, silly and regressive behavior and mannerisms, and frequent hypochondriacal complaints."[22] Category 295.30 was designated as "schizophrenia, paranoid subtype" and was "characterized by the presence of persecutory or grandiose delusions" and "attitude is frequently hostile and aggressive."[23] Category 296.10 was now considered to be manic-depressive illness, manic type, and was described as exhibiting "excessive elation, irritability, talkativeness, flight of ideas, and accelerated speech and motor activity."[24] Category 300.14 was considered to be a hysterical neurosis, dissociative type, in which "alterations may occur in the person's state of consciousness or in his identity to produce symptoms of amnesia, somnambulism, fugue, and multiple personality."[25] At this point, the majority of our sample (46 of the 52 [or 88%]) were considered to still meet the criteria for catatonia, but there were inklings of many more changes to come.

The DSM-III was published in 1980.[26] The number of people diagnosed with catatonia subtype who were still alive and who were interviewed (n = 49) in the Vermont sample had dropped dramatically to 14. Thus, cases of catatonia had gone from 52 to 46 to 14. The others had all been reassigned to other categories, in light of newer understandings in psychiatry. The category of catatonia was in the DSM-III defined as a "marked decrease in reaction to the environment . . . a motiveless resistance to instructions, maintaining a rigid posture, excited motor activity, purposelessness, and not influenced by external stimuli."[27]

The third phase of our longitudinal study was our follow-up study, which began in 1980 and was fortunate to coincide with the publication of the DSM-III. By this time most of those same 52 patients had been rediagnosed, leaving only 14/49 (or 29%) of the original group still considered to have catatonia. However, one Vermont person was rediagnosed (category 298.90) as atypical psychosis, a category in which there are psychotic symptoms ("delusions, hallucinations, incoherence, loosening of associations, markedly illogical thinking or behavior that is grossly disorganized or catatonic").[28] The number of hebephrenic patients had gone from 1 to 3; the paranoid subtype had jumped from 2 to 11. All sorts of other categories began to pop up. Eight people had been given a diagnosis of schizoaffective disorder. Nine people were considered to have undifferentiated subtype of schizophrenia, and one was given a diagnosis of bipolar disorder, manic subtype. One person was given a diagnosis of intermittent explosive disorder, and yet another had atypical anxiety disorder. Clearly, the field was struggling in 1980 to classify the same behaviors within the different phases described more than 147 years ago by Kahlbaum.[29] Or symptoms and behaviors had changed, or this was a medical disorder all by itself, as suggested by many investigators, including Gelenberg in 1976.[30]

In our paper presented at the annual APA meeting in San Francisco, we reported many different aspects of the group that we were studying.[31] Two of them had to do with possible sex differences, as well as the main factors which correlated with being diagnosed as having catatonia.

Sex Differences in Catatonia

The original DSM-I group was 60% (31 of 52) female versus 40% (21 of 52) male. We found that the average age of onset for both sexes was very similar (males = 26 years of age vs. 29 years for females) although the range was 16–45 years, with an average for the group of 28. None of the statistics revealed significant differences between men and women.

As reported, we looked at three periods of time: pre-Index status, Index (time of rehabilitation program) hospitalization, and at long-term follow-up (an average of 32 years after first admission). The Strauss-Carpenter Prognostic Scale[32] revealed that 60% had no pre-Index employment, and 69% had few or no social relationships. Twenty percent had onset before age 25, and 50% had serious disability prior to hospitalization (flat affect, psychotic signs and symptoms for at least 5 years, signs of depression or hypomania). Eighty percent had no known precipitating events before this admission although questions about verbal, physical, and sexual abuse trauma were not routine. Utilizing the retrospective DSM-III diagnosis for status at initial hospitalization, the data revealed that there were no sex differences except that nine females had shifted to the schizophrenia, undifferentiated type, which was only slightly significant. That subtype in DSM-III for schizophrenia was described as "prominent delusions, hallucinations, incoherence, or grossly disorganized behavior" and "doesn't reach the criteria for any of the other types *or* meets the criteria for more than one."[33]

Catatonic subtype criteria also included the following: "marked decrease in reactivity to the environment and/or reduction of spontaneous movements and activity or mutism; negativism (an apparently motiveless resistance to all instructions or attempts to be moved); rigidity (maintenance of a rigid posture against all efforts to be moved); excitement (excited motor activity apparently purposeless and not influenced by external stimuli); and finally, posturing (voluntary assumption of inappropriate or bizarre postures)."[34] There was a note in the DSM-III: "Although this type was very common several decades ago, it is now rare in Europe and North America."[35] Brooks once mentioned to me that he saw overwhelming and profound fear in many of his catatonic patients. I found that this observation was also noticed by Moskowitz and others in 2004, positing that perhaps some form of catatonia was an "evolutionary extreme fear response."[36]

Correlations of Signs and Symptoms of Catatonia at Index Admission

Withdrawal, slowed and reduced movements, slow and reduced amount of speech, or mutism were correlated highly and partially verified the observations embedded in the original description of catatonia. *What we did not have was any correlation of the excitement variables at Index.*

Earlier Symptoms and Long-Term Outcome

In these analyses, many outcome measures were used. They include the Strauss-Carpenter Outcome Scale,[37] the Do-for-Self Scale,[38] demographics, work, the Community Adjustment or Care Schedule Scale,[39] and symptoms from the Brief Psychiatric Rating Scale (BPRS).[40] The symptoms of catatonia at Index did correlate with those from the BPRS (e.g., slowed movements then, with disorganized symptoms now; slowed movements then, with mannerisms and withdrawal very significant all these years later;

reduced movements with mannerisms; slowed speech with grandiosity and withdrawal; disorganized with grandiosity; irritable with disorganized symptoms, hallucinations and excitement). The Global Assessment Scale (GAS)[41] scored positively at Index release later correlated with the functioning variables of the Strauss-Carpenter Outcome Scale[42] (e.g., useful work, lower symptom level, fullness of life, level of functioning) and with the GAS at follow-up.

Caveats include the fact that the Vermont Longitudinal Study investigated the most chronic end of the spectrum. We had to conduct a retrospective rediagnostic process to equilibrate the cohort to today's patients, but this was accomplished in the most rigorous manner (see review in the previous chapter).[43] We recognize that 52 people is a small sample,; nevertheless, we found some interesting trends which add to the consideration of this complex syndrome.

Wither Goest Catatonia?

The DSM-III-R revision was published in 1987.[44] It kept the earlier catatonia subtype descriptors. The DSM-IV was published in 1994, and it only added echolalia ("senseless repetition of a word or phrase just spoken by another person") or echopraxia ("repetitive imitation of the movements of another person") to the symptom criteria.[45] Exclusion criteria included neuroleptic-induced parkinsonism or a manic or major depressive episode. Also in this manual, catatonia was considered for affective disorders as well. It also noted that acute observation should be continued for "potential risks from malnutrition, exhaustion, increased temperature, or self-harm" or injury to others, as mentioned in earlier reiterations as well.[46]

The DSM-IV-TR, published in 2000,[47] had the same description for this schizophrenia subtype but also added one for both a general medical disorder (due to infectious, metabolic, and neurological conditions) and as a side effect of medications (e.g., the possibility of the neuroleptic malignant syndrome and as a "specifier" for mood disorders, which are the same as those for schizophrenia).[48]

Depending on the study design, the rate of catatonia reported seemed to be between 7% and 17% in 2004. It was considered to have multiple etiologies[49] and was increasingly associated with the mania of bipolar disorder.[50] However, Philbrick and Rummans (1994) have listed 84 possible causes of catatonia and 31 possible medical complications associated with catatonia.[51] In addition, a scale has been developed which appears to successfully identify such a person no matter the etiology. This instrument is known as the Modified Bush-Francis Catatonia Rating Scale and was developed in 1996.[52] Several scales have since been created as well.

Diagnostic strategies were outlined by Fricchione et al (1983), which included the use of scales, observations, and neurological and other physical examinations.[53] Philbrick and Rummans (1994) also suggested that early recognition was crucial, along with supportive care, discontinuation of drugs, restarting dopamine agonists, and remaining alert for more medical complications.[54]

The DSM-5 (Published in 2013)

In getting the DSM-5 manual ready to be published, the APA committees picked up the challenge once again as the field evolved. The DSM-5, covered in dark blue, ushered in a new era for schizophrenia, comprised of 35 pages out of a total of 991 pages in the volume on disorders and coding. The schizophrenia committee, led by Professor William Carpenter, renamed the many serious and persistent problems under its umbrella as "schizophrenia spectrum and other psychotic disorders."[55] This retitling was meant to include the range of presentations and degrees of severity encountered and to boost the reliability of the diagnostic process.

The second biggest change was that the DSM-5 dropped subtypes of schizophrenia used over the previous 120 years, such as paranoid, catatonic, disorganized (known earlier as hebephrenia), undifferentiated, and residual. It seems too many patients slid between categories over time, and the subtypes were no longer as helpful as hoped.[56]

The third major change was prognosis. Up until 2013, as illustrated in this chapter, prognosis was expected to be either marginal or downward for nearly everyone. In this version, "symptoms were expected to diminish across the life course" but not disappear.[57] Prognosis was seen as primarily affected by one's gender (females doing better), by genes (no schizophrenia in the family doing better), or by culture (stability and low levels of discrimination doing better). However, there was a discussion about less education and work life attained that never mentioned the fact that systems of care are primarily funded and managed to provide stabilization, maintenance, medication, and entitlements—although these are often mislabeled as rehabilitation. Perhaps the lack of comprehensive rehabilitation programs described in the final two chapters of this book contributes to reduced opportunities to complete one's education and obtain better job opportunities?

The DSM-5-TR (Published in 2022)

No updates have been made to the schizophrenia spectrum disorders category, with the exception of coding to match the International Classification of Disease (ICD-10) for catatonia due to another medical condition.[58]

Our Conclusions on the Understanding of Catatonia in Vermont

At Index hospitalization in Vermont, there was a tight correlation between the withdrawn type of symptoms and the expectations of the syndrome, but this correlation was not seen for the excited version. Things changed across time, either with patients or diagnostic systems. Later, catatonia ended up more in the affective disorder realm and not so much the schizophrenia group. Those cases, rediagnosed with affective symptoms, had much better outcomes at long-term follow-up, as expected. Catatonia appeared to be a fairly uniform motor behavioral syndrome at first admission in Vermont but displayed wide variation at follow-up, all of which spoke to a hidden underlying heterogeneity due to multiple etiologies. The death rate was surprisingly lower than that of other subtypes of schizophrenia, which was entirely unexpected. Other samples have found this, too. Early detection and intervention appear to reduce the remaining lethality of versions of this syndrome.[59,60]

What Did the DSM-5 Do With Catatonia?

As stated earlier and given increasing evidence, the DSM-5 removed catatonia as a subtype of the new schizophrenia spectrum and other psychotic disorders categories.[61] The text added that, "It may be diagnosed as a specifier for depressive, bipolar, and psychotic disorders; as a separate diagnosis in the context of another medical condition; or as another specified diagnosis."[62] It includes three subtypes of catatonia (stuporous, excited, and malignant) caused by at least 18 medical and neuropsychiatric risk factors and has 27 medical complications including death.

There are now five steps suggested by some investigators that could be implemented to provide treatment: IV lorazepam, electroconvulsive therapy, a glutamate antagonist, an antiepileptic drug, and, finally, an atypical antipsychotic medication.[63,64] What this discussion highlights are the huge challenges facing the field of psychiatry and the struggles to solve them. It also displays how important it is to conduct a thorough assessment of other possible medical disorders such a person might have before jumping to the conclusion as a specifier for schizophrenia and other serious psychiatric problems.

The Validity of Paranoid Subtype in Long-Term Outcome

As reported earlier, Alan Breier was one of two investigators, along with John Strauss at Yale, who took it upon themselves, without pay, to rediagnose the Vermont sample using the new criteria of the DSM-III. Before Breier went on to work in the intramural section of the NIMH and then on to Eli Lilly and now as the Raymond E. Houk Professor of Psychiatry at the University of Indiana in Indianapolis, he and the Vermont team had a particular interest in looking at a subsample of people diagnosed as having a paranoid subtype to see if it belonged with schizophrenia or with affective disorders (or all by itself).[65]

The research team first divided the entire sample into four groups: paranoid subtype of schizophrenia ($n = 70$), nonparanoid schizophrenia ($n = 48$), schizoaffective patients ($n = 30$), and affective disorders ($n = 47$). Breier then posed a series of questions to help figure out whether the paranoid subtype belonged to schizophrenia, affective, or schizoaffective disorders.

Using a variety of scales listed earlier, including the Strauss-Carpenter Prognostic Scale,[66] the team compared and contrasted these subgroups on a wide variety of outcome measures. It turned out that social functioning (both quality and quantity) once again was the better predictor of outcome. It distinguished the nonparanoid schizophrenia group from everyone else, whereas work or community adjustment did not differentiate the groups very much at all. The predictors affecting long-term outcome with the least strength were symptoms (both positive and negative), and again this validates Strauss and Carpenter's open-linked systems.[67] The term "open-linked systems" means that past work predicted only work, a past ability to meet basic needs predicted only future ability to meet basic needs, and so on. Past social functioning was the only variable that crossed over to predict not only future social functioning but also the ability to work. It should be noted that symptoms and prior hospitalization did not predict anything.

However, one dividing cluster appeared using a combination of 16 variables. This grouping separated people with schizophrenia (both paranoid and nonparanoid) from people with affective and schizoaffective disorders, thus moving schizoaffective disorder further away from schizophrenia, where it had been vacillating since the time it was invented and closer to the affective disorders. This switch has only recently been appreciated by the field.[68] Some investigators also think that paranoid delusions have a strong affective component to them.[69,70] And, as far as outcome goes, the ranking of best to worst very-long-term outcome for the subgroups remained as long expected: affective disorders, then schizoaffective disorder, then paranoid subtype of schizophrenia, and last, the nonparanoid subtype of schizophrenia. Contradictions persist.

What Else Did the New DSM-5 Declare in 2013?

What did the DSM-5 developers decide to do not only with catatonia but also with paranoid subtype of schizophrenia? It eliminated *all* the primary subtypes. It went on to state that they *"were eliminated due to their limited diagnostic stability, low reliability, and poor validity."*[71]

The manual has designated only one set of diagnostic criteria for catatonia, which will cover the expanded list of possible combination diagnoses for schizophrenia, major affective disorders, other psychoses, schizoaffective disorder, brief psychotic disorder, and substance-induced psychotic disorder, as well as general medical and metabolic conditions.[72]

In addition to the expected categorical method passed on from DSM–III, the DSM–5 suggests a renewed dimensional approach, which might be used to highlight the heterogeneity and severity of symptoms in schizophrenia spectrum disorders among many others. In other words, psychiatry may be in the middle of a significant shift from continuing to accept perspectives primarily developed over a century ago as well as the hidebound categorical approach and go back to the drawing board.

Introduction to Part 4 of This Book

In the following chapters, I shift focus onto one of the most important components of our studies. A good, solid treatment research project should provide a control or comparison group that did not receive whatever intervention is under study. We searched and searched for a group commensurate to the task. There was no one at Vermont State Hospital who could fill the bill because everyone who could be in the rehab treatment was already in it. In Chapter 7, I explained the effort to which we went in order to solve this puzzle. We finally found our match in Augusta State Hospital (AMHI) at the suggestion of Dr. Michael DeSisto, the Maine State Director of the Bureau of Mental Health at the time. In the 1950s, AMHI had little to no rehabilitation available for chronic patients, especially those with schizophrenia, as Vermont did. Two hundred and sixty-nine patients in Maine were matched to the Vermont sample by age, sex, diagnosis, and length of hospitalization.[73]

Chapter 15 describes the work and the findings of this important and unique comparison long-term study of 36 years. The question posed had to do with rehab versus no rehab. Did that rehabilitation program in Vermont make a significant difference in the long-term outcome? The Maine–Vermont Comparison Study also provided much more information than we expected,[74,75] including findings about the relative environments of the two states outlined in Chapter 16. In my experience, the environment always plays a much larger role in people's lives than expected. It is a good idea to study it, but researchers rarely do—and even when they do, it is seldom reported on.[76]

15

The Role of Rehabilitation, Neural Plasticity, and Public Policy in Long-Term Outcome

The Maine–Vermont Comparison Study

The critical question now was "Did Vermont's innovative rehabilitation program make any difference in such positive long-term outcomes?" In the late 1970s, I consulted with Professors Brendan Maher,[1] Jane Murphy,[2] and Bonnie Spring[3] at Harvard University, as well as with Lee Robins[4] at Washington University. The decision was made to identify another state hospital, preferably in New England, with solid record keeping and little to no rehab, from which to draw a matched sample from the 1955–1959 era. This was not an easy task.

The Vermont team began checking out hospitals in other states. Most had little to no rehab in the 1950s, but their records were not as comprehensive as we needed. Then one day in 1985, after presenting a lecture in Maine on the Vermont Longitudinal Study at a large meeting, I met two important people that would help solve the problem. Dr. Michael DeSisto came to speak with me after the presentation. He was the director of the Maine Bureau of Mental Health, and he asked me to check out Augusta Mental Health Institute (AMHI) as a possibility for a comparison group. DeSisto was a psychologist, a former hospital administrator, a researcher, and a professor at the University of Maine. Furthermore, he was passionate about his system of care, his family, and sailing in Maine's Boothbay Harbor. He assured me that the AMHI records were comprehensive, and he was right. We also found that "both states had similar distributions of age, gender, household size, per capita and household incomes, and low numbers of

Recovery from Schizophrenia. Courtenay M. Harding, Oxford University Press. © Courtenay M. Harding 2024.
DOI: 10.1093/oso/9780195380095.003.0015

racial minorities that were found [by comparing both Vermont and Maine] state demographics, from the United States Bureau of the Census, 1950, 1960, 1972, [and] 1982."[5]

The other person from Maine who would help us was Priscilla Ridgway. When she approached me after the presentation, she said that she had been blown away when I spoke about real people in a real mental health system instead of just data. She related one of her own stories from early in her career. At AMHI, formerly known as Augusta State Hospital, she had sat daily as an aide next to a woman who had been mute for a long time. Every day, Ridgway quietly sat nearby and offered the woman something from her lunch bag. One day, she offered the woman an apple and the woman said suddenly, "Yes!" I understood, then and there, that here was someone who already understood some of the principles of rehabilitation. Later, Ridgway received her doctoral degree and has become one of America's best-known writers and consumer advocates for helpful systems of care.[6]

Ridgway was then working at the Bureau of Mental Health (now known as the Maine Office of Substance and Mental Health Services, under the Department of Health and Human Services). I drove over one wintry weekend from Burlington, Vermont, to Augusta, and we met at the state office building to begin writing another National Institute of Mental Health (NIMH) grant application. The state of Maine had decided, in its infinite wisdom, to shut off the heat in all of its buildings every winter weekend in an effort to save money. There Ridgway and I sat, gathering state information and trying to type with our hats, gloves, and parkas on. I do not think that the general public has any idea what researchers go through to get their work done!

If funded, the deal at the NIMH was that the grant funding had to go to the state of Maine even though the project would be an exact replica of Phase III of the NIMH Vermont Longitudinal Research Project in its design, methodology, and questions asked.[7,8] As in that study, the data were to be analyzed by Ashikaga and his team back at the University of Vermont (UVM) College of Medicine. The grant was submitted under the Maine Bureau Director's name as principal investigator (PI), and, when the money came through, DeSisto also became the study's project director. It was tough for me to give up the co-PI job; Yale, at that time, would not allow co-PIs with research teams from other institutions. I am sure it had to do with having to split the indirect costs, something universities have a keen interest in avoiding. Yet, having the funding to complete the matched comparison study was key to those of us in Vermont.

Augusta State Hospital

The August State Hospital had an even longer history than the hospital in Vermont. Opened in 1840, thanks to the efforts of its native daughter, Dorothea Dix, who was busy establishing hospitals across the country,[9,10] the large and imposing hospital in Augusta sat on a promontory right across from the capitol and its legislative buildings on the opposite riverbank. Apparently, this site was deliberately chosen so that lawmakers would "not build it and forget it."[11] Similar to other hospitals in the nation during in the 1950s and 1960s, Augusta eventually began to add services slowly over time, such as dentistry, a pharmacy, departments of social work and psychology, occupational aides for industrial therapy, a night hospital, a vocational counselor who visited one day a week, a sheltered workshop, and a large library.[12]

The focus of any rehabilitation in those early days was on higher-functioning people in the hospital, especially those with affective disorders, and no programs existed in the community. According to DeSisto, in 1947, there were 47 people in our newly selected Maine–Vermont cohort who, early in their years hospitalized, had participated in a brief work placement and/or housing program administered by a single social worker. However, these 47 people ended up back in the hospital, became chronic back ward patients, and were selected as members of our new study sample from the mid-1950s. Of those 47, only 19 were alive at follow-up.

Along the way, the hospital was renamed Augusta Mental Health Institute, and it became overcrowded repeatedly, as did every other state hospital in the nation. By the late 1940s and early 1950s, 1,837 patients were crowded into spaces designed for 1,270, which made the hospital 44% over the planned number of beds.[13] In the early 1970s, a new superintendent insisted that people be actually discharged rather than sent out on "conditional release" as they had been in Vermont. That decision turned out to be a good thing for everyone, as we had found out earlier from members of the Vermont sample.

The hospital in Augusta participated in the national movement toward deinstitutionalization, or, as DeSisto would call it, "depopulation." In

1962, many elderly patients were sent to nursing homes. In the early 1970s, hospitals across the nation put people into new board-and-care homes, a process known as *transinstitutionalization*, or they were sent home to their families. Many states simply dumped people out with few or no supports. The number of AMHI Maine hospital residents dropped from 1,837 to 350 within 5 years, and care was refocused primarily on patients with severe and persistent mental illness.[14] A small replacement hospital with 92 beds was built in 2004 and was labeled "Riverside Psychiatric Center." It was designed to promote "patient comfort, patient self-determination, and re-covery."[15] Maine has a second hospital in Bangor up north.

Matching Mainers to Vermonters

Being a hospital with good records and minimal or no rehabilitation for persons in the back wards in the 1950s, Augusta made it possible for us to match its patients to participating patients in the Vermont sample. It was Ridgway and then two others, Margaret Fuller, MSW, and Millard Howard, MS (from the Department of Social Work), who transferred data from 8,000 3 × 5-inch hospital admission summary cards onto a computer. That amazing feat allowed Ashikaga's group back in Vermont to generate possible matches. Those people with organic disease, primary drug and al-cohol disorders, or on criminal mandates, as well as those admitted later (from 1956 to 1961) were excluded. There turned out to be 1,944 possible matches from those early years with people born from 1900 onward, and so we were able to find 269 very close matches to the Vermont cohort. This achievement was very helpful and reassuring.[16]

Mainers were matched to Vermonters as they were in 1955 on four key indicators (age, sex, diagnosis, and length of hospitalization). In research, matching samples on four critical domains as well as using the same time period is an important approach to studying the impact of exposure to two different treatment strategies. The first approach (Maine) was traditional care (stabilization, maintenance, medications, and little to no rehabilitation); the second (Vermont) was significantly enhanced care, described in great detail in earlier chapters and in our published articles. Matching on those four significant variables imposed controls on the results because such fac-tors would have had a significant confounding effect on the outcome if not held constant. Race is usually included but Northern New England was primarily of Caucasian descent at that time and is still, at 94%.[17]

We were concerned about whether there might be other outcome differences found according to variables on which we did not match. Were those four areas strong enough to withstand partialing out the impact of many other critical factors, such as urban/rural residence, education, year of discharge, policy differences between the states, socioeconomic levels, and acute onset after having been matched?

The Process of Finding People

After the matching process occurred in Vermont, diligent work went into finding addresses in records, talking with families, chatting with the postmistress of a small town, or asking after folks in the local general store. "Oh yeah, I know Old Roy. He lives up around the corner in the yellow house." Most people had stayed close by their original homesteads. An impressive 94% of our 269 Maine matches were accounted for, while Vermont researchers had found 97% of the original 269 members of their study sample.[18] Again, these findings were remarkable and illustrate why Northern New England was and still is a great place to conduct longitudinal research (although younger people are more mobile now than they were in the 1980s and 1990s). Currently, long-term research is typically considered to extend to about 3–5 years, not across three decades (as was the case with our studies), and the expected follow-up number is usually less than one-third at the 5-year point. The significance of our multidecade achievements meant that our findings could provide a more balanced view of possible outcomes for people diagnosed with severe and persistent mental disorders.

Conducting the Maine–Vermont
Comparison Study

DeSisto selected a group of 30 people who brought their skills and talents as multidisciplinary investigators and contributors, similar to those on the Vermont team. Two energetic young clinicians with several years' experience under their belts, Alan McKelvy and Christopher Salamone (both

MSWs), were chosen to scour the landscape and conduct the designated field interviews. It turned out that Mainers interviewing Mainers was as important as Vermonters interviewing Vermonters. This matching process engendered more trust among those being interviewed as well as a greater understanding of the local culture on the part of the investigators.

Paul Landerl of the Vermont team went to Augusta to train the interviewers while Carmine Consalvo, the other Vermont interviewer, consulted on the process. Landerl and the Maine team conducted two sets of interproject and intrarater trials of 48 people to make certain that the interviewers would be asking the same questions and scoring the answers the same way as the Vermont team had.[19] Professor Alan Gelenberg, MD, author of the AIMS+EPS Scale, trained interviewers in both states to assess abnormal movements.

Outcome Areas Assessed by Interview

Using the Vermont Community Questionnaire (VCQ-C) with its 15 established scales, the interviewers assessed such areas of life as work, social functioning, social supports, weekly activities, self-care, use of treatment and social services, environmental stressors, levels of competence, continuing symptoms, and degree of overall satisfaction with one's life.[20]

DeSisto and the team added a new scale called the "Do for Self" instrument, combining areas of self-sufficiency that included summed scores for work, social functioning, and symptoms present.[21] Anyone doing massive data collection is always appreciative of summed scores from the raw data to conduct analyses if they do not mask the underlying data from discovery and accurately reflect the large dataset.

The VCQ-L (the longitudinal interview) and the Meyer-Leighton formatted Life Chart assessed the interim history between index discharge and current status presentation.[22] The Chart included work, source of income, residence, periods of hospitalizations, life events, deaths of significant others, important relationships, health, use of community supports, and medications. The Chart was a large sheet of lined paper indicating years and domains. It was placed in the center of a Monopoly[23] game board with each original square, such as Boardwalk or Park Place, covered with small typed sheets of questions and probes, while others had the scoring protocol. Just as we had found in the Vermont interviews, the Chart turned out to be a powerful clinical assessment tool. The entire cross-sectional battery took about 60–90 minutes, and the longitudinal battery took about 75–90 minutes; the two were completed about a week apart.[24]

Appointments were made and the person's rights were presented and discussed. Interviews took place either at the person's residence away from others or at an isolated spot in a local coffee shop chosen by the interviewee. And again, the interviewers sat down after each interview and wrote about their experiences with each person being interviewed. This important piece of information about the person–interviewer interaction added to our understanding about both parties and the time they spent together, and yet this important aspect of interviewing has been neglected in most studies. Many important pieces of information not asked about but offered by the person being interviewed were jotted down on the margins of the instrument battery and written into the narrative by the interviewers in both studies. Much of this valuable information becomes lost if only computerized data are retained.

Areas Assessed by Record Reviews

Two very senior people mentioned earlier, Margaret Fuller, former head of Social Work at the hospital, and Millard Howard, educated at Harvard and a long-time member of the social work department, conducted the record reviews. They were extremely familiar with the records as well as with these patients and their histories, having worked at AMHI for most of their careers. But they were usually not aware of former patients' current status unless they had landed back in the hospital. This meant that they were not aware of community outcomes, thus keeping this part of the study "blind" unless they happened to stumble on a former patient in town. Janet Wakefield, PhD, one of the Vermont record reviewers, also trained the Maine record abstractors and conducted reliability tests.[25]

The Hospital Record Review was created from a World Health Organization instrument, the Psychiatric and Personal History. It had been used during their large collaborative study known as the Determinants of Outcome of Severe Mental Disorders,[26] done between 1977 and 1979, just before the Vermont Longitudinal Study began its work. This interview was

reconstructed by Professor Jon Rolf at UVM into a structured hospital record review capturing different time periods spent in hospital (first admission, interim admissions, index hospitalization, post index admissions) and
included a section on personal and family history.[27] (All of these strategies
have been described in more detail in Chapters 7, 8, and 9, and in our published papers.)

Further "Blindness" in the Data Collection Process

As in the Vermont Longitudinal Study, the Maine field interviewers did
not know what was in the records nor did they know the interviewees'
original diagnoses, and the record reviewers did not know what outcomes
were being found in the field. In that way, the raters had fresh eyes and
rated without preconceived notions of what ought to have happened, just
as the Vermont team had done. All the data acquired were then sent back to
Ashikaga and his biostatistics team at the UVM College of Medicine (especially Dorothy Meyer, who supervised the data entry and coding of both
studies) for later analysis. Most studies are coded and analyzed by the study
leader, but by having an independent medical school biometry group doing
the work, the findings could be considered even more valid and reliable.

Descriptions of the Maine Sample Versus the Vermont Sample

Thus, 269 Mainers were matched to all 269 Vermonters, with 144 women
and 125 men in each sample. One hundred and seventy-eight surviving
Vermonters (66%) and 119 surviving Mainers (44%) were interviewed. The
discrepancy in live sample count happened because of the 7 years' difference
in follow-up time. Eleven people in Vermont had participated in the interview process but then refused to have their data used (4%), and in Maine,
14 had refused (5%). Again, these are very low refusal rates. These numbers
revealed that the interviewers carefully approached people as consultants
and asked them to teach us what they knew. In addition, Fuller and Howard
had formed previous long-term relationships with people and were critical

to our accessing people, some of whom might ordinarily have been shy about participating. Only 7 people (3%) were never found in Vermont, 16 (6%) in Maine. Identical to the Vermont work, two sets of interviews were conducted within a week of one another.[28] The first interview included questions about current levels of functioning, while the second focused on how people had fared since discharge.

DeSisto et al.'s first paper revealed all the statistics, not only of the matching variables, but also of some important factors (called covariates) mentioned earlier. This strategy was an effort to determine whether any of those factors (such as education, urban/rural origin of both the person and his or her father, economic status, acute onset, and the year of interview) might negate the differences between the two states.[29] Vermonters had more education, came from more rural settings, and suffered more prolonged onsets, but they had been discharged under the rehab program 16 years earlier than their Maine counterparts.

What Happened to Those Who Had Died Earlier?

For those study members who had died before the interview sequence, a special instrument had been devised in Vermont. This instrument mirrored key indicators from those instruments used for the living participants. It was designed to find out, from relatives, friends, and clinicians who had known the deceased person, how he or she had functioned previous to the 6 months before dying.[30] Other studies typically looked only at the demographics and diagnoses of deceased samples, comparing them to the live sample. We took the extra time to collect systematic levels of functioning across time. This is especially important in very long-term studies because otherwise assumptions might have been made that those who were the most psychiatrically ill had died first, leaving the better functioning people to represent the outcome—thus skewing our results.

The study in Maine was conducted 7 years later than in Vermont, and more people had died by then. They were, on average, older, and more had the diagnosis of schizophrenia than the live group.[31] In the literature, people diagnosed with schizophrenia have been found to die almost 25 years earlier than those without the diagnosis, from a wide variety of problems.[32] We thought that perhaps, in this case, the older and more seriously ill had died first, but the statistical analysis revealed no differences between the surviving and deceased groups on any of the matching variables, just expected attrition due to time. Furthermore, no differences were found on two very important indices (the Global Assessment Scale [GAS] rating,[33] combining both health and mental health, and the Community Care Schedule [CCS]),[34] nor on the rates of death between the two states.

The rediagnostic work to move patients' diagnoses from criteria from the *Diagnostic and Statistical Manual of Mental Disorders*, second edition (DSM-II) to DSM-III was completed by two psychiatrists, Owen Buck and Victor Pentlarge, after interrater trials.[35] Of the 119 Maine people still alive out of 269 (44%), 38% carried the diagnostic label of schizophrenia, 13% were schizoaffective, 22% were diagnosed as having affective disorders, and 26% had other diagnoses; all were considered to be long-stay patients. Such percentages were nearly identical to Maine's original cohort of 269.

In looking at other critical indices prior to becoming part of the Maine cohort, the schizophrenia group had 56% men, 68% with useful work, 42% never married, 54% prior hospitalizations, 68% with diminished affect, 62% with severe thought disorders, and 28% had co-occurring severe depression.

Of the affective disorders group 69% were women, 82% had useful work, 10% never married, 34% had prior hospitalizations, diminished affect was seen in 19%, severe thought disorders were present in 32%, and 79% suffered from moderate to severe depression. Everyone had more than 5 years since original onset of symptoms. Almost everything revealed significant differences between the two groups (affective vs. schizophrenia diagnoses), as we had expected.

The project was supported by many people from the state of Maine, including Kevin Concannon, MSW, Robert Glover, PhD, and John LaCasse, Eng. ScD. Linda Clark managed the project's office, and Lois Frost found all the records. The original Maine data ended up back in Augusta, to be stored as privileged information in the Maine State Archives when the study was completed.[36] It was so privileged that even I was unable to access it myself later.

Highly Significant Findings From the Maine–Vermont Comparison Study

Three major cross-sectional findings stood out in stark relief. Vermont, with its comprehensive, coordinated system and innovative model demonstration rehabilitation program, appeared to have produced *significantly more employ-ment (p. < 0.0009), fewer symptoms (p. < 0.002) and much better community func-tioning (p. < 0.001)*.[37] These are highly significant statistical findings which no one could quibble with. Getting our first glimpse of the findings was exciting. Knowing these very important findings, it seems more appropriate to place rehabilitation strategies at the top of the treatment regimen for current pa-tients than to consider rehabilitation as only an adjunctive plan after all symp-toms have abated. This is where the biomedical model of mental disorder has led us off in the wrong direction. For most people, rehabilitation gets them back to work or school, helps them to find a home and a place in the com-munity with friends and intimate others, and, in the process, reduces symp-toms and poverty. Best of all, rehabilitation can restore a sense of personhood.

Some Expected Findings With a Twist

It is critical to remember that the people under study were now middle-aged or much older and had been hospitalized for long periods of time. So when we say that people, who were younger and better educated, had managed to get out of the hospital earlier, it is an extremely relative matter because of everyone's general chronicity. But younger people did better in both samples, being able to take care of themselves with no differences be-tween states. Younger, better-educated women without schizophrenia but with other more chronic forms of major affective disorders, and who were discharged earlier, did better with social functioning, as expected based on the literature, without significant differences between states. The interest-ing fact to point out is that this combination persisted across three decades. Psychological research has consistently found that, in general, more women than men with schizophrenia do better with social functioning, but this is also true in society in general.[38]

People with relatively shorter hospital stays and fewer symptoms also did better in general across both states. No surprise there either; nor was it a surprise that people with no diagnosis of schizophrenia, relatively shorter hospital stays, and who were better-educated did better in community func-tioning across both states. However, people with that same profile and an acute onset did less well in community and global functioning in Vermont but better in Maine.[39] This finding was a surprise and may be a fluke given the difficulties in establishing the original point of real onset.[40]

Another surprise slipped in the door with the Mini Mental State Examination (MMSE).[41] Those people who were better-educated and relatively younger in both states and who had been diagnosed with schizophrenia scored better on this cognitive test. For many years, research with long-term hospitalized patients had found that people with schizophrenia experienced cognitive slippage,[42] and this turned out not to be the case in either of our samples.[43] This finding is important, and recent research has reported similar findings. As such there is currently a growing appreciation of the continued growth of synapses in the aging brain,[44] the care of people outside of an institution, and the development of cognitive therapy and cognitive remediation techniques for both schizophrenia and affective disorders.[45,46]

What Else Did We Learn About People With Lived Experience From the Time of Discharge Until Now?

As in the Vermont Longitudinal Study, we not only collected information on how subjects were faring at interview but also about how they had lived their lives since Index Release or Discharge. We used the VCQ-L described in detail in Chapter 8, including the Life Chart derived from the work of Professor Adolf Meyer, one of the fathers of American psychiatry, and Professors Alexander and Dorothea Leighton, one a Harvard psychiatrist and the other an anthropologist, respectively. We also double-checked the information given by primary interviewees about their own history against other sources. In general, we found that people were actually fairly accurate, as Manfred Bleuler had found in his detailed follow-up of 22 years.[47] This surprised many colleagues who had routinely viewed personal histories given by patients as mostly spurious. For deceased subjects, the special interview was used with family and friends.

Intraproject and interrater trials were successfully completed between Maine and Vermont clinicians. The data reduction process was described at length in a DeSisto et al. paper on the longitudinal part of the study.[48] The four areas focused upon were residence, work, income source, and use of community resources. Findings revealed that Mainers spent considerably more time in the hospital (50% to Vermont's 13%) while Vermonters were either living independently (46%) or in half-way or board-and-care housing as spots opened up. Vermonters also worked a great deal more (35–60%) because (1) they were provided with vocational assessment, training, placement, and after job supports, and (2) they were out of the hospital and could work in the community a great deal longer. Only 12.5% of the Vermonters used community resources (e.g., community mental health centers [CMHCs]) across the years, which is very different from expected.[49]

The Maine team determined that "the longitudinal course comparisons demonstrate clearly that the Vermont programme [sic] had a significant impact on the course for Vermont subjects compared to the Maine subjects."[50] By spending much less time in the hospital and having been given opportunities to live in the community, help with finding and keeping work, and provision of social activities, these Vermonters were able to get back to their lives. "The Vermont programme [sic] was an eclectic programme [sic] that integrated the knowledge from social psychiatry, including principles of milieu therapy, therapeutic community, and interpersonal psychiatry, with the use of medicine and vocational rehabilitation."[51]

DeSisto et al. made a strong statement at the end of their paper, stating that the Vermont legacy "is in the values and principles which guided it . . . a pervasive attitude of hope and optimism about human potential, through a vision that if given the opportunity, persons with mental illness could become self-sufficient."[52]

What was startling was the fact that there was a shift, even in some places in Vermont, from rehabilitation in the 1950s and 1960s to a new era of deinstitutionalization in the early 1970s. But, in fact, many CMHCs across the country paid little attention to people struggling with serious symptoms until the mid-1990s and only after Public Law 99-660 forced them to provide care. Given the nation's new preference for regionalization and provision of reimbursement for the medical model, mental health centers opted not to use low reimbursable psychiatric rehab and switched to higher reimbursable strategies such as diagnosis, medication, and entitlements. This shift in Vermont created a loss of "continuity and comprehensiveness," and the focus became reducing symptoms rather than trying to regain life itself.[53] As discussed in Chapter 5, Brooks, in the Vermont transition, dealt with this situation with a grant called IMPACT and sent clinicians out into the community to set up and connect ex-patients with multiple community resources. Maine's approach was focused on transinstitutionalization to

board-and-care or nursing homes. In 1979, Medicaid covered case management and the Community Support Program enhanced the development of
new residential programs.[54]

Re-emphasizing an Important Message for Today's Policymakers and Program Planners

In light of these highly significant findings, it seems even more critical to
place rehabilitation strategies at the top of the treatment regimen for current patients than to consider them as only an adjunctive or minimal plan
until most or all symptoms have abated. For most people, rehabilitation provides important and validating occupations, helps them find a place to live
and a role to play in the community, reconnects or forges new relationships
with friends and family, and, in the process, reduces symptoms and relieves
poverty and estrangement. Best of all, rehabilitation can restore a sense of
personhood. As an example, when I worked in New York City, I found a
center just outside of the city that had decided on a "teaching model." The
"students" went to classes instead of "treatment," and the clinicians were
"teachers." It was run like a college. Students were participants not just re-
cipients. It brought into care many younger people who had resisted having
anything to do with a mental health center and was quite successful. Indeed,
the last two chapters of this book are filled with examples of ideas that work
from all over the world.

Examples of Two Mainers Who Were Matched to Vermonters

"Bill" the Lobsterman was 70 years old and retired when the Maine team
interviewed him. Bill was born in Portland in 1918, into a rambunctious
household of five brothers. His mother had been a barmaid at a local pub
when she met a lobsterman at the bar who had a boat out in the harbor.
Together they worked hard and had little extra money. Being a lobsterman was a long and tiring day job, putting the baited traps out and then
hauling them back in, hoping the lobsters trapped were big enough to
keep and throwing back the small ones. The Atlantic was a tough mistress,

unpredictable and demanding. This Lobsterman drank a lot, yelled often, and used his belt to corral his unruly brood and sometimes his temperamental wife.

Bill was the youngest child and took the brunt of the abuse from everyone. When he was about 14, he began to withdraw into the room that he shared with four others. It was hard to do, so he hid in the one closet. Everyone was frustrated with him, but his mother said that he would come around sooner or later. He rarely talked to others but was heard jabbering to himself. He stopped bathing and wore the same jeans and old tee-shirt day in and day out. Finally, by the time he was 16, Bill had not been to school for quite a while so Social Services came by to find out why. He was taken to Augusta Mental Health Hospital. He was in and out until 1950, then stayed in until 1973.

Bill listened to his voices more and more. Often combative, he was given chlorpromazine (Thorazine), then haloperidol (Haldol), and several other antipsychotics, sometimes in combinations, which calmed him down but didn't lessen the voices. Electroconvulsive therapy (ECT) was proposed but he was so resistant to that treatment that the staff decided it wasn't worth putting up with his tantrums. He retreated into his own world. He scuffed around in slippers, hardly took a bath, became grizzled, and stayed unkempt. He watched television often and became disgruntled when someone wanted to change the station. No one came to visit anymore, not even his mother. He became convinced that the government was listening and recording everything that everyone was talking about, especially him. He wanted foil to put on the cardboard hat he had fashioned for himself to fend off the interference.

As he grew older, things started to settle down. He yelled less, ate more food, took a shower more often, started talking to volunteers about his days helping his father on the lobster boat. By the early 1970s, Maine had begun, along with other states, to transinstitutionalize patients to board-and-care and nursing homes. Bill was transferred out of the hospital to a much smaller place in Portland. There were women there, too. He cleaned himself up even more.

Eventually, while walking out on the docks listening to the local lobstermen talk about their day, he went up to a couple and asked if they needed any help. He had been on his father's boat as a kid, he told them. Soon he began working on a boat called the *Mary Adele*, with a kindly old skipper who helped him relearn the trade. Bill became more of who he was meant to be, and although he still had the voices, he learned to put them into the background. He hung out with the lobstermen and found a couple of friends. He had been matched to a Vermonter who, in the end, had almost fully recovered; Bill had definitely improved and had more of his life back.

As another illustration of a comparison, "Catherine" had been matched to Helene in Vermont, described earlier. They were matched in age, sex, diagnosis, and length of hospitalization, as they were in 1955. Catherine was an inpatient at AMHI in Maine, where there was little to no rehabilitation offered to back-ward patients. Helene's history has been described in Chapter 11. When the Maine research team first met Catherine in 1987, she was living in a board-and-care home in Portland. Like Helene, Catherine had been hospitalized at age 20, full of rage and anguish about the abuse she had suffered at home for many years. Both she and Helene were diagnosed as having schizophrenia because of their convictions that they were being followed by police and family members, spoke repeatedly to themselves regardless of who else was in the room, yelled at people who were not in the room, were usually unkempt, were generally unable to take care of themselves, and had been found wandering in the streets. While Helene participated in the Vermont rehabilitation program in 1955, Catherine was given no such opportunity. She finally was released from AMHI 12 years after Helene, in 1972, when most hospitals in the nation rushed to deinstitutionalization. Catherine was sent to a board-and-care home that housed 30 other patients. This move from one institution to another was considered a step forward in returning people to the community, but for many the move to the real community stopped there. This stalled process—or worse—happened across the nation. Many patients were simply let out of state hospitals with no place to go and with no other supports. It was a national disaster.

What was of great interest to the clinical investigators was that Catherine had slowly begun to shed most of her hospital behaviors and symptoms, even though she had been expected by her traditionally trained clinical team to continue with marginal levels of functioning. When the Maine team interviewed Catherine, they found that she dressed neatly, had regained a sense of humor, and spoke of the part-time job she had recently acquired making lobster rolls in a nearby restaurant. She no longer yelled or spoke to herself but she did show some of the side effects of years of medications and institutionalization, such as slowed movements, stooped posture, and an inexpressive face. Her anger had mellowed into an acceptance of her past, but she still felt retraumatized by the repeated use of restraint and seclusion when she was in the hospital and the staff felt she was out of control. She grieved over the loss of so many years of her life. But in a system of care that had not provided rehabilitation, Catherine was improving anyway and had regained considerable functioning.

A Look at the Impact of Historical Policy and Program Decisions

We also started exploring the differences between the way the two states had developed policy and program implementation by creating life histories of the preceding 35 years for both states.[55] Although Maine and Vermont had similar distributions of age, gender, household size, and per capita and household incomes during the period under study, Maine was much larger, with twice the population; it had four metropolitan areas and was mostly conservative in political leaning. Vermont was geographically small, had a much smaller population, and was liberally minded. If you wanted to get things done in Vermont, you just walked across the street to talk to the governor, who was out mowing the grass, or went to the local legislators up the hill. The Vermont rehab program started long before a similar movement across the country to change from hospital care to community mental health and community support systems. In addition, Vermont had a rare collaboration in those days between its single psychiatric hospital and the Department of Vocational Rehabilitation.

DeSisto, in a genius move, decided that, across three decades, many policy and program changes had occurred which might further impact the lives of people under care as well as our own data. He put together a team of policy and program makers who documented a year-by-year history in both states using the idea of our Life Chart for patients.[56] The group in Maine consisted of Walter Rohm, MD; William Schumacher, MD; Roy Ettlinger, MHA; Walter Lowell, EdD; and Ann DeWitt, and, in Vermont, John Pandiani, PhD; John Pierce, Rodney Copeland, PhD; and Vasilio Bellini.[57] We suggest that any longitudinal study needs to do these analyses to account for policy and program changes affecting the lives of patients in systems of care.

The life histories of these states revealed that Maine had significantly lagged behind Vermont in many ways across time. These challenges made Maine less comprehensive in its mission and design, not as coordinated, and much slower in its implementation of programs.[58] The comparison of the study participants from both states revealed that Vermonters had been released much earlier and had benefited from significantly more time being supported in the community. "This opportunity, when combined with an array of residential, work, and social opportunities, resulted in a more diverse and favorable course compared to the Maine group across the domains studied."[59] Thus, we began to add another explanation of the difference in outcome. However, William Deane and George Brooks of Vermont in 1963, Norman Cousins of UCLA in 1979, Shari Mead and Mary Ellen Copland in 2000, and Michael DeSisto et al. in the Maine–Vermont Matched Comparison Study in 1988 all added strong caveats about the importance of hope and optimism.[60,61,62] DeSisto et al. stated that

> The Vermont legacy is not to be found, as Bachrach (1989) suggested, in the details of the program or the methods used, all of which were exemplary. Instead, its legacy is the values and the principles which guided it. . . . Perhaps, the most important value was that the program had a pervasive attitude of hope and optimism about human potential, through the vision that, if given the opportunity, persons with mental illness could become self-sufficient.[63]

What Did We Do With All These Findings?

The overall findings had shown that the global positive outcome difference between Maine and Vermont was highly significant, at 49% versus 68%.[64] We jubilantly went about the world talking about the impact of rehabilitation for people who are struggling with substantial emotional distress. However, 49% of the Mainers had improved anyway (as illustrated in the two life histories), despite being in a struggling system with caregivers expecting marginal levels of functioning or a downward course.

Finally, we looked at the findings of the 9 other long-term studies from across the world, in which over 2,700 patients with serious and persistent illness had been followed for at least two to three decades after first admission. These results showed a range of 46–68% to even 84% of persons significantly improved or recovered across time, no matter what programs had been available or how cohesive (or not) their system of care had been or what theoretical model had been applied. In the back of my mind, there was a gnawing sense that perhaps we were missing something important.

Putative Roles of Neuroplasticity and Epigenetics

Something very interesting was going on, and it hit me like a lightning bolt. Could there be some self-correcting mechanism in the brains and bodies of people who significantly improved or recovered? In 1991, I began talking about something I had learned about as a nurse 16 years earlier having to do with *plasticity*, the process by which the brain and body change constantly in interaction with the internal and external environments during a natural push toward health. Many colleagues thought I had lost my own mind and would argue with me while I was giving presentations. Once such person was a professor at Johns Hopkins University who declared that I was "either a revolutionary or a romantic." I suspect that he thought I was the latter.

Another was the eminent neuroscientist Nancy Andreasen, MD. To her credit, after years of looking at brains with functional magnetic resonance imaging (MRI) and investigating on her own, she found that a psychologist, Donald Hebb from Canada, had been writing about neuroplasticity since the late 1940s.[65] Hebb had written that the brain was the most plastic organ we have and that it was in constant flux and change in response to the inner and outer environments in which it is located. Associated with his work is the now well-known phrase, "Cells that fire together, wire together."[66] In 2003, Brown and Milner pointed out that Hebb's work has influenced developmental psychology, neuropsychology, perception, and the study of emotions.[67] I ask, "Why not rehabilitation and recovery from serious and persistent mental disorder, too?"

Andreasen wrote about the disordered brain in the early 1980s, dubbing it "The Broken Brain."[68] But, in 2001, she excitedly told me about her new book, *The Brave New Brain*,[69] while we were both on a plane headed to a schizophrenia meeting in Vancouver. In this new book, Andreasen wrote this stimulating paragraph about neuroplasticity as the brain interacted with the mind:

> The essence of psychotherapy is to help people make changes in their feelings, thoughts and behavior. This appears to occur through a multiplicity of techniques . . . which can lead to changes in a plastic brain which learns new ways to respond and adapt that are then translated into changes in how a

person feels, thinks, and behaves. It, in its own way, is as biological as the use of drugs.[70]

I would now add that perhaps self-help and rehabilitation are also "just as biological as the use of drugs"![71] Many schizophrenic brains and bodies seem to be able to slowly but surely correct themselves over time. Perhaps neuroplasticity reflects what the epigeneticists have found, that we can turn on and off how genes are read in interaction with our environment, how brain cells read changing DNA messages.[72] Those interactions mean that medications, psychological interventions, and rehabilitation—all external modifiers of DNA, can affect or interrupt the natural push toward health. Whatever is going on, we need to support that process and not get in its way.

16

Northern New England

Perfect Environments for
Longitudinal Research

Environment Matters

The environment—time, place, and local culture—always has an effect on research. It shapes the decisions made, the opportunities and resources to be had, the type of questions to be posed, the availability of study participants, and the spirit of inquiry.[1] Therefore it is important to know about the environments within which a truly remarkable rehabilitation program evolved, as well as those in which its comparison study and our two three-decade follow-up studies were conducted.

This chapter is a love letter of sorts to Vermont and Maine because living and working in these states has been such a delight for our research teams. The natural beauty of both states, the sense of community, the collection of fair-minded citizens, the accessibility of people who run the government and services and make the rules and laws, the general kindness in the air, and the sense of stewardship about the environment have made our lives as longitudinal investigators much easier.

Until recently, few people ever moved out of either state, so we were able to locate a remarkable 97% in the Vermont sample and 94% in the matched sample in Maine, even decades after people left the hospitals.[2] As we waded through all the procedures seeking approvals here and there, gatekeepers were problem-solvers and did not erect unnecessary hurdles along the way. Participants in our studies, their families, designated friends, and current and past clinicians opened their doors to us and were willing to teach us

Recovery from Schizophrenia. Courtenay M. Harding, Oxford University Press. © Courtenay M. Harding 2024.
DOI: 10.1093/oso/9780195380095.003.0016

what they knew. We had incredibly low refusal rates (4–5%).[3] Thanks to this generosity, Northern New Englanders brought the world some important information about working together to better understand what happens when a person gets caught in an avalanche of problems affecting mental and physical health. They educated us about the impact of innovations, the persistence toward resilience, and about remarkable recoveries from schizophrenia spectrum and other psychotic disorders, and more serious forms of major affective disorders. And yet, many clinicians in today's mental health systems still think improvement—never mind recovery—is impossible.

Although health, census, and catchment area data suggested all of Vermont and the lower half of Maine were good matches for our comparison study, these states were, and still are, somewhat culturally, geographically, and often programmatically different from one another.

Vermont: The Green Mountain State

Vermont has been imbued by Hollywood with magical qualities of snow-laden trees and horse-drawn sleighs, with Bing Crosby crooning holiday songs.[4] As a small northern New England state, it lies between New York and along Lake Champlain (which dreams of being America's next Great Lake) and New Hampshire, with its other borders on the Canadian Province of Quebec and the state of Massachusetts. (I am describing the geographical locations of these two states because of the not infrequent response I received when telling people that I was working on studies in Vermont and Maine. "Oh, aren't they near Detroit?")

There are ancient rolling hills for which Vermont is named, *les monts verts*, from the French, who roamed around in the 17th century and claimed it; or, if you prefer, the Latin, *veridis montis*, so christened by the British who fought the French for it.[5] These foreign names became as Americanized as the Green Mountain State but the old versions explain why my alma mater, the University of Vermont, is also referred to as UVM.

Small villages with white church steeples are surrounded by deep but unexpectedly newer forests, rolling farmland, and crystal lakes. These lakes and related streams were created when heavy Ice Age glaciers broke off the tops of the mountains, gouging out waterways as the receding ice melted. Even today, water in Vermont streams is apt to be frigid even in the summertime.

Originally, indigenous peoples lived by the shore of both sides of Lake Champlain in the lush green valleys left behind when the lake water receded to its current level. Folklore has it that there were many rocks dotting the land inland from the valley. There was so many in fact, that the Mohawks, once known as Mahawks, part of the Iroquois Nation from the New York side, and Abenakis, part of the Wabanaki Confederation of the Algonquin Nation on the eastern side to the shores of Maine, both hunted in the interior.[6] They reportedly thought that white settlers in the 1700s were very strange to try to actually live there, except perhaps in the Champlain Valley. Indeed, every time it rains today, more rocks emerge as if by magic from the depths of the soil, making farming tougher for everyone. This also explains why Vermont is full of hand-made stone walls that crisscross the landscape.[7]

Early on, much of Vermont was full of pastureland kept nearly treeless (about 80%) by Merino sheep, over a million of which helped create the woolen industry in the first half of the 1800s.[8] The mills had too much competition from elsewhere though, and eventually the sheep were replaced by cows. "By 1899, Vermont was producing 35 million pounds of butter" for the Boston market.[9] Current "cowscapes" show that the environment is still an agricultural state, although dairy farming has dropped significantly in recent years. People now outnumber cows, a situation that causes consternation in many older citizens. Unused pastures revert to soft wood growth within 5 years, and now forests cover nearly 75% of the state's rolling green hills and valleys.[10] Vermonters now produce apples, cheese, knitwear, Ben and Jerry's ice cream, very fine granite and marble, and more maple syrup than anywhere else in the United States. All the white marble markers in Arlington National Cemetery come from Vermont. The winters, with few exceptions, have always been long and hard, with heavy snow, ice, and very cold temperatures. The 6–8 weeks of warmer summer weather have been held dear by cabin-fevered Vermonters for the intense growing season full of tomatoes, hay, corn, and flowers along with outdoor picnics, hiking, and biking. The local joke is "And on that warm day, we cram it all in."

The capital, Montpelier, has a population of only 7,966 people and is the smallest but most picturesque capital in the United States.[11] There are at least 13 larger towns in Vermont, including Burlington, which is the largest at 44,703.[12]

Vermont was an independent republic from 1777 to 1791, having declared its liberation from New York and the British. It then became the 14th state in the Union as an antislavery state to counterbalance the admission of Kentucky. Even today, as the state with the second smallest population in the nation (647,064 estimated for 2022),[13] Vermont continues to carve out its own path. During the Nixon and Trump administrations, many Vermonters seriously considered seceding from the Union. It was thought that these "freedom fighters" could hold off the National Guard at the old Vermont State Hospital, built on the model of an 1890s French fortress, for at least 30 days.

Many outsiders feel that Vermont is the most liberal-minded northern state, while Maine is less conservative than New Hampshire, whose license plates are imprinted still with its slogan, "Live Free or Die." Defying Yankee stereotyping, Vermonters have been known for advanced perspectives about the world (alternating with a few periods of conservatism). They ratified the first state constitution, a document that permitted the first universal suffrage for all males (landowners or not) and outlawed slavery in 1777.[14] Later, the legislature endorsed the first stamp, passed the first anti-billboard law, the first Head Start Program, the first bottle return law, as well as one of the first laws to allow abortions. More recently, the state was the first to approve civil unions and the second to approve of same-sex marriage after Hawaii. The first US patent was signed by George Washington, himself, and given to a soap-making entrepreneur in Vermont. The state has the next to lowest carbon footprint in the United States, and Vermonters are justly very proud of all these landmark achievements.

These tendencies to promote creative and pioneering approaches help to explain why Vermont was one of the first places to develop modern rehabilitation and why it follows that it was the state in which it was discovered that persons with serious and persistent psychiatric problems could and did significantly improve and that many even experienced full recoveries.

The state Chambers of Commerce are always unhappy when a dark side of any state is reported. In years past, Vermont has been one of the poorest states in the Union, at 36th in per capita annual income, with an average of $9,979 in 1982, when we were collecting our data.[15] Sections of the state known as the Northeast Kingdom received electricity only in the mid-1980s. Seventy-plus years ago, the state also had some of the highest rates of alcohol use, suicide, and incest, much of which has been ameliorated in recent years through state and local efforts.[16,17]

In the past three decades, Vermont has become a destination. In 2021, the state had a per capita income of $67,674.[18] Vermont environmentalists are now focused on building clustered housing to protect green spaces. Higher education is much valued, and there are 23 colleges and universities nestled among the natural habitats and wildlife. The UVM was the fifth institution of higher education built in New England after Harvard, Yale, Dartmouth, and Brown and was chartered in 1791. General Lafayette of the Revolutionary War laid the cornerstone, and the university started admitting women in the 1870s long before the others. The Medical School at the University of Vermont was the seventh to be built in the new nation.

Many urbanites think that rural people are usually hard-working and primarily focused on solving local issues. However, among the many Vermonters who have made contributions to the broader United States are two US Presidents, Calvin Coolidge and Chester A. Arthur; the inventors John Deere (tractors) and Elisha Otis (elevators); Admiral George Dewey of the Spanish-American War; philosopher and educator John Dewey; US Senators Steven A. Douglas, Bernie Sanders, and Patrick Leahy; psychiatrist George Brooks; Alcoholics Anonymous originators William Wilson and Robert Smith; photographer Wilson "Snowflake" Bentley; Ethan and Ira Allen of the Green Mountain Boys in the American Revolution; author Dorothy Canfield Fisher; and Rudy Vallee, singer; as well as businessmen Charles Orvis for his fly fishing enterprise and Henry Wells of Wells Fargo & Co. Surprisingly, Robert Frost, whose poems often reflected on the life and landscapes of Vermont, was actually born in California, but he had a summer home in Ripton, near Middlebury College.

Maine: The Pine Tree State

Though probably "discovered" first by Viking voyagers and many others from France, Spain, and England, one of the first recorded European mentions of the land that would become Maine was as early as 1498, by the Cabots. The first settlement in Maine territory was not established until 1607, in Sagadahoc, at the mouth of the Kennebec River on the coast, about 25 miles north of what is now Portland. "By October, Fort St. George mounted 12 cannon and enclosed 50 log cabins, a church, and a storehouse."[19] Pioneers were entranced by the prospect of fur trading, the availability of trees, delicious wild game, and an abundance of fish. 1607 is the same inaugural year as that of the more famous and longer-lasting settlement at Jamestown, Virginia, but the harsh winter and the loss of the settlement's leaders ended the experiment in Maine a year later.[20] Maine also suffers from an average snowfall of 50–70 inches a year and occasionally sees avalanches in Baxter State Park on Mt. Katahdin.[21]

The French and English fought over the territory, and the indigenous peoples, especially the Abenakis, lost most of their lands and lives. King Charles I became irritated that there were so many proposed names for his land grant. His 1639 charter reads that it "shall forever hereafter be called and named the Province or County of Mayne and not by any other name or names whatsoever."[22] It is good to be king (at least for the next 10 years), and clearly there were barristers aplenty in his day as well. Today, the descendants of these European forebears are still primarily situated along the coast and inland rivers, and somehow the (y) in Mayne became an (i) in Maine during statehood discussions much later.

During the Revolutionary War, the first American–British naval battle occurred off the coast of Maine, in 1775, and Portland (then called Falmouth) was burned. The first lighthouse in America is called the Portland Light and was commissioned by George Washington in 1791. Long considered to be an appendage or northern district of Massachusetts, a rebellious Maine still took another 29 years to declare itself an independent state. At the time it was thought to be more liberal than Massachusetts. It was admitted to the Union as the 23rd state in 1820, balancing the slave state of Missouri due to Maine's strong antislavery sentiment.[23]

Although it took a while for its population to grow, Maine is more than three times the size of Vermont (35,387 vs. 9,615 square miles)[24] and has more than twice the population (1,385,340 vs. 647,064).[25] Now, Maine is the 43rd state by population although its geographic size is just about equal to that of the other five New England states combined. The government was staunchly Republican for a century until the arrival of Edmund Muskie and the Democrats. The most northern country of Aroostook is still predominantly Republican. Today, politics are still considered unpredictable, and many residents have identified themselves as Independent.

Maine is bounded by the Canadian border, Massachusetts, New Hampshire, the Gulf of Maine, and the Bay of Fundy in the Atlantic Ocean. There are five distinct geographic regions: Southern Maine, Downeast

(Washington County), The County (Aroostook), Western Maine, and Central Maine, each with its own distinct character. Augusta is the capital, with a population of 18,968 as of 2021, and it is the third smallest capital in the United States after Vermont's and South Dakota's.[26] There are about seven cities in the state which are larger, with Portland being the largest at 68,313, as estimated by the US Census for 2021.

To the north of Augusta is the larger city of Bangor, almost twice the size at 31,921, and, beyond that, the state becomes increasingly sparsely populated. This region even boasts of the only frontier area in the eastern United States with six or fewer people per square mile; this is called the Unorganized Region of Northwest Aroostook County. This part of the county has only a few, mostly French-speaking, people near the Canadian border. Ironically, all of Aroostook County is the largest county east of the Mississippi. People in Aroostook and Washington Counties are often poorer than those living in the south. Aroostook County industry is based on potatoes, which the county grows in great abundance. At harvest time, the children are let out of school to help dig them out of the ground.[27]

I was very curious about Washington County, whose inhabitants were called "downeasters" by people "who live away." After conducting considerable research, I discovered some fascinating and unexpected history. During the late 1700s and most of the 1800s, the county was a very busy place, building big sailing vessels called schooners that carried cargo not only to the lower states but also to India, in the China Trade. They were in strong competition with captains in Salem and Boston, Massachusetts, and New York.

Their schooners also plied cargo from Boston back to wharves along the Maine coast. They were generally fortunate in the summer to have what is called a "downwind," which is most desirable, easily filling the sails from one's stern or back of the boat. Ships from Boston had to sail east to go north because the Maine coastline flows east toward Canada, therefore they were dubbed "downeasters." It is complicated, I know. But it is important to know that early Washington County contained worldly, sophisticated businessmen, not just rural folk.

In Augusta and south, the story is quite different. There are many industries, such as the remnants of textiles, shipbuilding, lobstering, and deep-sea fishing along the rugged and rocky coastline. There are also many ski areas and other tourist attractions, such as L.L. Bean with its trademark large

Maine hunting boot out front. There are picture-perfect towns strung along its tidal coastline of nooks and crannies now measured by satellite at 3,478 miles and longer than California's 3,427 tidal coastline miles.[28] And, as in Vermont, artists and other crafts people in Maine have set up shops cheek to jowl with the local hardware and grocery stores.

The best description I have found of Maine was written by Bill Roorbach and published in the *New York Times Book Review*. It turns out that there are two sides of Maine.

> There is the Maine of coast and towns, of wealth and leisure (or at least job security and weekends), of education and solid middle-of-the-road values: mowed lawns, and clapboard siding, and pavement. And then there's the interior, more rural Maine, blue tarps and old washers in the yard, underfunded schools, cable-spool kitchen tables, poverty, and lack of opportunity often teaming up with social and civic failures to drive radical values, some of these tending to the right on the face of the political clock, some to the left, all meeting at six on the dial: *kaboom.*[29]

This state, like many others across America, also has its share of poverty, alcoholism, drug abuse, incest, and suicide. But, like Vermont, the state has invested some resources in alleviating these public health problems.

Maine is about 90% forested land, which promoted lumbering and pulp industries in the past. The state has been the second leading producer of paper and wooden toothpicks. There are about 2,000–2,500 lakes and ponds and 5,000 streams, depending on who's counting. The state also produces 98% of the nation's supply of sweet lowbush wild blueberries, and tons of sardines and lobsters are fished out of the ocean each year.[30,31]

Mainers recreate themselves as needed as a defense against economic downturns by having diversified trade and industry. The shipbuilding (with the exception of Bath Ironworks), lumber, and textile industries have been largely supplanted by trade, service, and finance businesses. Lumber mills have been transformed to papermaking and other wood products on a small scale. Granite, sand, gravel, zinc, and peat are being exported. Visitors and retirees have been drawn to the recreational and outdoor life. Maine also has several well-known colleges and universities (Bates, Bowdoin, Colby, and the five campuses of the University of Maine) plus an additional 20+ other institutions.

Many people have become increasingly worried about environmental issues, particularly the salmon population, which are now considered to be endangered. To help with the situation, dams have been dismantled and logs on the river have been banned. Clear-cutting forests and the cultivation of fish farms have been debated.

Northern New Englanders are sometimes known for their accented terseness which began, in all probability, with the cold weather demanding that one be short and quick in any discussion. They never mince words.[32]

Native Mainers tend to lean toward the more austere northern Yankee conservatism in general, unlike Vermonters who still have a somewhat liberal bent. However, like Vermonters, they also pride themselves on self-sufficiency and hard work.

In spite of its general ruralness, a frontier county, and the erroneous assumptions about being from the "back woods," some of the famous people from Maine to make contributions to the nation include the legendary Colonel Joshua Chamberlain of the 20th Maine Regiment at the Battle of Little Round Top in Gettysburg; state hospital builder Dorothea Dix; the composer Walter Piston; novelists Kenneth Roberts and Stephen King; poets Henry Wadsworth Longfellow and Edna St. Vincent Millay; US Senators George Mitchell, Margaret Chase Smith, and Edmund Muskie (later US Secretary of State in the Carter administration); US Representative Edith Nourse Rogers (author of the GI Bill); publisher John Hay Whitney; film director John Ford and producer David E. Kelley; Hannibal Hamlin, 15th Vice President of the US during the first Lincoln presidency; and William Cohen, Secretary of Defense in the Clinton administration.[33]

People in both states value their deep green forests, wildlife, and blue-gray lakes for hunting and fishing and their land for grazing cows, growing crops, and raising children. They are similar in many ways, but the significant difference in size and population adds considerable complexity in the pursuit of policy and pragmatic on-the-ground programmatic changes. In addition, differences in political views have made Maine much slower to address the social inequities that drive some of its most pressing public health problems.

Further Caveats About the Population, Policies, and Programs Under Study

Since almost all the population in both Maine and Vermont are still of Caucasian descent, any research done in Northern New England, even today, has very few, if any, people from other ethnicities under study. Strict research protocols unfortunately limit any generalizations to be made for other populations. However, I would venture to propose that the basic findings on significant improvement and recovery from serious and persistent psychiatric problems, such as schizophrenia, other psychosis spectrum disorders, and chronic forms of major affective disorders, may very well hold true for people of any ethnicity. But they must first be offered the opportunity.

The prospects for all people to reduce suffering from psychiatric distress seem to depend less on ethnicity itself and more on a wide variety of other factors, including social determinants of health and mental health (of course these have much to do with poverty, and minority populations are disproportionately impacted by poverty in the United States today, much to our shame). Improvements in health and mental health rates would include access to the following:

- Living in safe housing, neighborhoods, and access to transportation
- Freedom from racism, discrimination, and violence
- Opportunities for education, jobs/careers, and income
- Extinction of physical, verbal, and sexual abuse
- Access to nutritious foods and physical activity
- Living with in unpolluted air and drinking water
- Learning enhanced language and literacy skills.[34]

The Next Question to Be Addressed

The results of our two studies provided us with strong hints about improvement and recovery from schizophrenia. But nine other studies in the world literature, conducted thousands of miles from the rolling pastures and wooded hillsides of Vermont and Maine, have also addressed the long-term outcomes of people diagnosed with serious emotional and cognitive disturbances. The next chapter will review these findings. It appears that many others snowed under by avalanches of profound mental suffering have dug themselves out and reclaimed their lives.

PART FOUR

Nine Other Very-Long-Term Studies From Across the World

17

Worldwide Evidence of Recovery

If we had only the Vermont and Maine studies with which to declare that many people with severe emotional and cognitive distress can and do get their lives back, I would have been much shyer challenging people to understand what the possibilities are. But there are now nine additional two- and three-decade-long studies from across the world indicating the same thing. They have found significant improvement *or recovery* in 46% (very narrow criteria) to 68% of people with criteria from the *Diagnostic and Statistical Manual of Mental Disorders*, third edition (DSM-III; closest criteria to the current DSM-5), and in 85% (with broad criteria) with schizophrenia or severe versions of affective disorders.[1] And yet there is still skepticism. Why?

Recognizing Individual Trajectories

These studies continue to support the need for a new paradigm and for a new, entirely different kind of environment for this population—one that promotes hope, reclamation of selves, and recoveries. First and foremost, however, it should be emphasized that although this chapter is focused on very-long-term outcomes, people can and often do start recovery as early as 18 months to 7years after onset of the symptoms and dysfunctional behaviors associated with schizophrenia and other psychoses.[2,3] Others take 10, 12, 15 years, or more. It seems that length of time to significant improvement and recovery has to do with several factors, among them:

- Access to opportunities to re-engage with education, work, and other people

Recovery from Schizophrenia. Courtenay M. Harding, Oxford University Press. © Courtenay M. Harding 2024.
DOI: 10.1093/oso/9780195380095.003.0017

- Encouragement and the availability of supports
- Personality style of all parties
- Ability to cope with psychosis, and degree of severity
- Comorbidities that make recovery more complicated, and
- Just plain luck!

The Nine Other Long-Term Studies

These nine studies from across the world, along with the Vermont and Maine projects, shed light on what might be possible for struggling people. One, by Manfred Bleuler in Zurich, followed people every year after admission, for 23 years.[4] Bleuler was known for decades as a preeminent figure in European psychiatry. The new Chicago Study in the United States followed people into their 20th year, having conducted baseline plus six interviews across time from admission to several hospitals.[5] Other projects include the Enquête de Lausanne Investigations,[6] the Gumma University Study in Japan,[7] the Bonn Investigations in Germany,[8] the Innsbruck Psychiatric Clinic Study in Austria,[9] the Iowa 500 Study,[10] the Bulgarian Clinical Psychiatric Hospital Study,[11] and the National Dispensary Lithuanian long-term study.[12]

All of them looked at the long-term outcome of what is called "the schizophrenias." Nearly 2,700 people (including those from Vermont and Maine) were assessed on who they were, how they were, and what their outcomes were at points in time across decades. Much to everyone's surprise, nearly one-half to greater than four-fifths of people diagnosed as having schizophrenia, in one form or another, were eventually able to reclaim their lives. They represent a major challenge to commonly accepted pessimistic assumptions about chronicity. This chapter provides a brief overview of each of the remaining studies, considering them all in one place even though they have been scattered across the world literature for years.

The Burghölzli University Psychiatric Clinic
Study In Zurich, Switzerland: M. Bleuler

Manfred Bleuler's father was Eugen Bleuler, the Swiss physician who took Emil Kraepelin's dementia praecox and renamed it "*die Gruppe de Schizophrenien*."[13] He was the superintendent of Burghölzli Psychiatric

University Clinic in Zurich from 1898 to 1927. The Burghölzli has been one of Europe's finest training institutions for over a century.[14] E. Bleuler was the first superintendent to be from the Canton of Zurich; he spoke the language of its inhabitants and understood local customs. Palmai and Blackwell wrote of him,

> One of Eugen Bleuler's most practical contributions lay in his management of schizophrenia, where he realized the deleterious effects of prolonged confinement in an institution and advocated early discharge as soon as acute symptoms subsided. He created the beginnings of community care by organizing a service to follow up discharged schizophrenics [sic] and facilitate their rehabilitation . . . as "active" occupational therapy.[15]

But Manfred Bleuler wrote, too, about how his father became more pessimistic over time. Every summer he attended the Rheinau Clinic in the small community at the bend of the Rhine River, the site of his early work as a psychiatrist. He saw that a few of his old patients were still there, and he became increasingly discouraged.[16] This happens to many clinicians and is one reason[17] why the long-term studies are so important.

M. Bleuler took over as superintendent at Burghözli in 1942, and he became even more curious about what happened to his patients. He began following a group of 208 people who were admitted to the hospital in 1942 and 1943.[18] Aiming for half men and half women, he started out with the admission of 103 men and 109 women to compensate for future dropouts. With a dropout rate of only 1.75%, these admissions became his famous cohort of 100 men and 108 women. Their ages ranged from 16 to 67½ years, and, for a third, it was their first admission. Then Bleuler did something his father and most other superintendents neglected to do, with George Brooks of Vermont being an exception. He followed his cohort personally for an average of 23 years, whether they were in or out of the hospital, using a systematic and comprehensive approach with structured instruments and clinical interviews.

For his long-term study, M. Bleuler used a combination of his father's and Kraepelin's diagnostic criteria, which together were closer to our own DSM-III and which were used by both studies in Vermont and Maine. M. Bleuler's criteria included confused train of thought, no emotional empathy, stupor or excitement, hallucinations and delusions, plus abrupt changes and keeping a "double set of books," meaning that "a normal degree of intellectual accomplishment potential was evident along with severe psychotic manifestations."[19] He excluded from his selection criteria brain disease, endocrine disorders, schizoaffective disorders, poisoning, latent schizophrenia, and neurosis.

Such criteria were vitally important because Kraepelin had mistakenly included a wide variety of other disorders under his umbrella of dementia praecox. He unknowingly involved tertiary syphilis, encephalitis lethargica, other dementias, and numerous other neurological disorders, all of which had a clear downhill course at the time.[20] By the time M. Bleuler was working, these conditions had been recognized as different from dementia praecox or the group of schizophrenias.

Furthermore, Kraepelin's hospital in Heidelberg tended not to discharge people and encouraged admissions to the point of serious overcrowding so that he could collect enough cases (enough "Zahkartens," small cards with patient information on them) to study. He began to target prognosis as an indicator of diagnosis even though he actually had some difficulty in following life courses.[21] He followed an administrative rule that if one could not get better and leave the hospital within 2 years, the keys to these individuals' freedom were basically thrown away. All of these factors predisposed Kraepelin to declare that those people diagnosed with more episodic affective disorders improved and those with dementia praecox deteriorated.[22] Eventually Kraepelin did come to see that many different entities emanated from a similar set of symptoms in dementia praecox. Much to my own surprise, apparently even he found that some people with dementia praecox recovered, according to M. Bleuler.[23] I believe it amounted to about 10%.

The findings from M. Bleuler's study were published in 1972, in German, and were translated into English in 1978. They were bound in a large red book and were very significant. Sixty-eight percent of first admissions and 53% of multiple admissions were rated as significantly improved or recovered.[24] Surprisingly, M. Bleuler found none of the subgroups of the schizophrenias proposed by his father. These were finally dropped by the DSM-5 in 2013[25] and by the International Classification of Disease (ICD-11)[26] in 2022 due to "little clinical utility, low diagnostic stability, no heritability and little influence on treatment."[27]

There were no causal linkages with family disturbances, and genetics appeared to play only a partial role in becoming ill. Social functioning was determined by the ability to work, independence from care, and living in a nonsheltered environment. There was no social impairment for 46% of the overall cohort, with 59% of the first admission group having decent social functioning.[28] Therapy may or may not have been helpful, although M. Bleuler did find that many recoveries began with exposure to new therapies and strategies perhaps by engendering more hope?[29]

M. Bleuler also found differences among the sexes. There was more improvement in women compared to men, and they also held a slight edge in recovery.[30] Early experiences such as loss of a parent, a difficult family life, and changes in relationships appeared more prevalent. Women also had more parents and siblings with some form of schizophrenia.[31]

In 1984, considering the study results, M. Bleuler wrote, "I have found the prognosis of schizophrenia to be more hopeful than it has long been considered to be,"[32] and "Easily half to three-quarters of all schizophrenics [sic] about ten or more years after onset, attain reasonable, stable states that last for many years."[33] (pg. 141) Despite M. Bleuler's prestigious position and careful investigations, European psychiatry believed not a word of it.

Visiting With Manfred Bleuler

In 1986, a group of us went to Bern, Switzerland, at the behest of Professor Luc Ciompi to give presentations at a conference. I was there with Professors John Strauss, Bonnie Spring, and Joe Zubin. Ciompi hired a van to drive us to his lovely home in Lausanne, a renovated former winery with white stucco walls and large windows letting in as much sunshine as Switzerland was willing to share. The house's design was radically different from the tiny-windowed chalets typical of Switzerland and much preferred by an Italian psychiatrist married to a Greek dancer. Ciompi's wife Mairi laid on a delicious lunch on their deck overlooking Lake Geneva and the Alps. It was one of those moments now referred to as having "flow," with wonderful company and scenery.[34] Next, we were driven to a smaller suburb of Zurich to meet with Manfred Bleuler. He appeared pleased to meet our group, all of whom had challenged the prevailing pessimistic attitudes about schizophrenia. I, myself, had shown, with much more rigorous methodology and design, that his original data and findings from the longitudinal study had been correct. (I heard later that he had said to friends in Montreal that he could die happy now). This touched me deeply because he had spent his entire 50 years learning from his patients, being tough on his residents, and immensely curious about the vagaries of the schizophrenias.

While we were together in Switzerland, Zubin and Bleuler began reminiscing about people that most of us had only read about. They told stories about Bleuler's father Eugen, and about Langfeldt, Schneider, Leonhard, and Kraepelin. These were many of the people who, in the late 19th and early 20th centuries, had shaped the field of psychiatry as we know it today. We were entranced by these unpublished stories of psychiatry's quest to unlock the secrets of schizophrenia. One story led to the next and the next; I wish we had had a tape recorder. I do recall Professor Bleuler's story about how his father brought patients home to have Sunday supper with the family and how Manfred had grown up sitting on the laps of patients as a little boy. He also said his father would hand-write drafts of his original contributions at the dinner table.

The Bonn Investigations in Germany: Huber et al.

Across Europe in the 1800s, medical schools began to set up psychiatric clinics to study and treat people for a multitude of illnesses. The University Psychiatric Clinic in Bonn, Germany, was one of those and has since become highly regarded. Between 1967 and 1973, three faculty members, Gerd Huber, Gisela Gross, and Reinhold Schüttler, began interviewing 502 of the 758 patients admitted after World War II, between 1945 and 1959.[35] These study subjects were considered a representative sample of the clinic population.

One hundred and forty-two (19%) died before follow-up. This left 209 men and 293 women, and, of those, 67% were first admissions. The group was diagnosed with a combination of K. Schneider and M. Bleuler's criteria for schizophrenia, which was closer to the DSM-III criteria than Bleuler's alone. However, the German team wrote,

> We agree with Bleuler and Müller, in that no symptoms or syndromes at the time of onset could be used to predict, with any certainty whatever, the differentiation between malignant or benign, process or nonprocess, genuine or pseudo-schizophrenic, and schizophrenia or schizophreniform psychoses.[36]

The research team conducted personal interviews with an average follow-up of 22.4 years. Thirty-four were lost and six were found to have a brain disease. Forty-eight refused to be interviewed but were found to have good prognostic factors such as higher IQ and upper-class status. Information was provided by relatives of 26 members of the study sample.

The findings revealed that 65% significantly improved or recovered. Of those study subjects, 22% were fully recovered and an additional 43% had what their team called "noncharacteristic residual syndromes." "The rather high rate of social recovery in the total sample—56 percent—is all the more remarkable when one considers that only 13% of these patients had participated in any outpatient rehabilitation programs."[37] In fact, of the 435 probands not in hospital, two-thirds were *not* under care. Thirty-five percent were considered to have "characteristic syndromes" of schizophrenia and were not doing well.

Positive social outcome was correlated with improvement in psychopathology. Women, as usual, did better at 60% compared to 51% of men.[38] Although they usually had more florid symptoms than did their male counterparts, women had later onsets with more complete remissions and social recovery.[39] Patients who were treated for psychoses soon after their first break did much better than those treated later. Early intervention with better outcomes was mostly expected. The research team identified 76 course types but thankfully collapsed those categories finally into 12.[40] All of these categories displayed the hidden underlying heterogeneity and possible multiple etiologies within the global diagnosis of schizophrenia.

In the end, Huber (1980) wrote the following, agreeing with M. Bleuler: "Schizophrenia does not seem to be a disease of slow, progressive deterioration. Even in the second and third decade of illness, there is still the potential for full or partial recovery."[41]

And still the world paid little attention.

The Enquête de Lausanne in Switzerland: Ciompi and Müller

Two Swiss psychiatrists, Luc Ciompi and Christian Müller, were at the Psychiatric University Hospital of Lausanne, a French-speaking canton, They became very curious about the final long-term outcome for schizophrenia posited by E. Bleuler. "Reichtung Prognose" stated that no one ever recovered to their baseline self. But I, myself, have been told by recovered persons that they are much *better* than their baseline selves, that they have grown and learned considerably more about themselves and the world, much in the way many other people have after having survived crises such as cancer, for example.

Like the whole state of Vermont, the catchment area for Lausanne held about a half a million people with very low mobility and excellent records in all health facilities. Ciompi and Müller were able to find 96% of their cohort of people, who were now at least 65 years of age.[42] These investigators studied 289 people (92 men and 197 women) who were considered to be representative of the 1,642 admissions during that time. The average follow-up time was 36.9 years, ranging up to 64 years after first admission, making this project the longest follow-up in the world's literature. Twenty percent of these histories were more than 50 years in length. The average age of men at follow-up was 75.2 years; for women, 75.8 years.[43]

People were diagnosed using a combination of E. Bleuler and Kraepelin's criteria for schizophrenia, which again brought them closer in line with the DSM-III in the United States. Disturbance was marked by disorders of thought and emotions, autism, ambivalence, loss of contact, and depersonalization. The investigators conducted a 2-hour semi-structured interview in each person's home. Record reviews, correspondence, and interviews with family, friends, and other clinicians were also undertaken.

Findings were very close to the others described. Sixty-three percent were considered significantly improved or recovered.[44] Fifty-seven percent had become free of conflicts, calm and peaceful. "Sixty-two percent of all individual symptoms observed upon initial hospitalizations had completely vanished in old age."[45] Only 20% had intensified symptoms. This team found that some of expected predictors had held.

> Good premorbid social, familial, and professional adaptation, few premorbid personality disorders, a marriage, completion of vocational training, and a higher premorbid functional level had predicted better outcome. On the other hand, gender, intelligence, education, family relationships during childhood (investigated retrospectively), and surprisingly family history of schizophrenia or other types of mental disorders, as well as constitution, did not significantly influence long-term course.[46]

On the other hand, 66.3% of women and 61% of men were in the recovered or mild categories. Ciompi concluded that there were eight course types within his data, with each assigned a percentage; suddenly, wherever I went, I found clinicians jumping to the conclusion that those course types were written in stone. In 1980, Ciompi wrote about the studies from Bonn and Burghölzli.

> Bleuler and Huber both concluded that schizophrenia is in no way "basically" or even "predominately" [an] unfavorable "disease process" running an inexorably deteriorating course. Its course is as vulnerable to change as life itself, and is obviously subject to a multitude of influences.[47]

But he was not listened to very much about his findings on recovery.

Three Other Long-Term Studies From Europe Employing Wider Diagnostic Criteria

There emerged from farther east a trio of studies from Austria, Lithuania, and Bulgaria using much more inclusive criteria and including affective components in their diagnostic profiles—all of which are known to be even more positive in long-term outcome.

The first was completed by H. Hinterhuber, in 1973, and studied patients first admitted to the Innsbruck Psychiatric University Clinic in Austria between 1930 and 1940.[48] Hinterhuber started with 157 people and conducted follow-along interviews at 30, 33, 35, 37, and 40 years after original admission. Average length of follow-up time was 30 years. However, only 37% (or 58 people) were still alive and the other 63% (99 people) had died or were presumed to have died. (Remember that World War II had intervened.)

Hinterhuber utilized structured interviews and medical records, as well as talking with relatives, and he acquired biographies of 87 women and 70 men. The findings were nevertheless striking: 77% were working full-time with another 20% part-time. Only 3% were in family care. Forty-five percent had come from a poor family situation. The modifiers leading to poorer outcome were psychological trauma, genetic loading, and onset after age 40.[49] The author found that 30.5% were considered to be chronically ill. However, 40.3% were improved, leaving 29.2% considered "cured." Most clinicians these days call this state "recovered," but not "cured" by psychiatry or medications. Thus, 69.5% were considered improved or recovered.

These figures have generally held true no matter what diagnostic criteria were used and regardless of the strength of the methodology applied in the various long-term studies.

In the study "Late Catamnesis of Recurrent Schizophrenia with Prolonged Remissions," conducted in Lithuania and published in 1977, Kreditor completed a 20-year observational study in five regions of Riga at the National Dispensary.[50] He found 115 patients with episodic schizophrenia (48 men and 67 women). Their ages ranged from 35 to 82 years of age with 54% over the age of 50. Again, the diagnostic criteria were broader than the US DSM-III. Ninety-seven (or 84%) had long-term remissions from 8 to 40 years with 61% sustaining remission. Kreditor identified two types of episodic disorders (multiple or prolonged). Prolonged status included 39% with 20–40 years' worth of dysfunction. Only 18 people became worse. The predictors of long-term remission included "harmony of premorbid personality," lack of or low occurrence of character pathology, late onset (30–40 years), and affective stability. These two course types (multiple or prolonged) differed in premorbid personality, age of onset, and illness course. Therefore, Kreditor announced that *the difference between the two groups was so clear that clinicians did not need to guess the future.* This pronouncement also provided further indication that there is indeed plenty of evidence of multiple etiologies lurking beneath diagnostic labels. (Thanks to Professor Zlatka Russinova of the Center for Psychiatric Rehabilitation at Boston University for her translation of this work from the Russian.)

In 1971, A. Marinow published his results from the Clinical Psychiatric Hospital in Bela, Bulgaria. He wrote about a study of 405 men admitted with schizophrenia between 1946 and 1950. They were followed up in 1957 as a 10-year study.[51]

He then decided to do a prospective follow-along study of 280 men from that same group after discharge from hospitalization, at an average of 20.2 years.[52] He assessed symptoms, work, and social functioning every 5 years. He found that education, getting married, and going to work, although considered to be social factors, were really affected by clinical ones, such as symptoms and onset.[53] Furthermore, he pointed out that people who stayed in the hospital longer and who were considered chronically ill were more likely to be affected by social factors than by clinical ones.

As far as long-term outcome, Marinow found that getting back to work was far more complicated than he had thought. He found what Strauss and Carpenter had found earlier with their well-known "open-linked" systems.[54] Their results revealed that social functioning before illness better predicted later social functioning; prior work functioning predicted post-episode work function, and symptoms and hospitalization did not cross over to predict anything. The only crossover was social skills predicting better work functioning given the need for social interaction in the workplace. (I wonder how this finding might have changed since the inception of computers, social media, Zoom, and the 24-hour workday.)

Using wide diagnostic criteria, Marinow wrote about favorable outcomes in 72.5% (50.7% good and 21.8% improved) with 27.5% experiencing poor outcome.[55] He found that, "At the onset of illness, no specific criteria are present which could be used as 'prognostic predictors,'"[56] as had several other studies.

The Gumma University Study in Japan: Ogawa et al.

It was important to get beyond European thinking and find out whether similar findings were available from Asia (although this next study did eventually use the criteria of the ICD-9).[57]

Kazuo Ogawa, Mahito Miya, Akio Wataral, Masao Nakazawa, Shuichi Yuasa, and Hiroshi Utena published their 21- to 27-year study in 1987.[58] Of the original 140 participants, 81% were younger than 30, and 79% were first admissions. They were provided with neuroleptics, an open-door system, and intensive aftercare. This program was called *Seikatasu-rinsko*, translating to "clinical work in everyday life."[59] It also included case management and individual counseling. Monthly assessments were conducted over time.

At follow-up more than two decades later, 91% of 140 people were assessed. One hundred and five were still living at an average of 23.6 years after Index Hospitalization (range 21–27 years).[60] They were rediagnosed using the ICD-9 criteria and Eguma's Social Adjustment Scale.[61,62] At long-term follow-up were 48 men and 57 women. Patterns revealed many fluctuations in recovery status early on, while later the courses differentiated themselves between self-supporting and chronically institutionalized groups. Nineteen people were in semi-supportive groups. Thirty-four percent were either hospitalized or considered "maladjusted cases." Social recovery was considered greater than psychiatric status. Forty-five percent were married. Thirty-one percent were considered recovered, with 46% improved.[63] Findings also revealed that 47% were fully self-supportive. This status meant that the person was fully productive; 96% were living in their own homes; 82% were married; and 77% were psychologically recovered, with a return to premorbid levels of functioning as well as maintenance of a normal family life.[64]

Changing the Name of Schizophrenia

In 2002, Japanese psychiatrists found that so much stigma and poor expectations surrounded a person diagnosed with schizophrenia that they relabeled this experience "integration disorder," partially based on work done by M. Bleuler, Ciompi and Müller, and Harding et al.[65,66] A 12-year follow-up found that stigma had been considerably reduced.[67] Since then, psychiatry in South Korea has renamed schizophrenia "attunement disorder."[68] Hong Kong, China, and Taiwan are also in the midst of considering renaming schizophrenia, moving from a word that means "splitting of the mind" to something indicating the "dysfunction of thought and perception."[69,70]

Of course, renaming schizophrenia has caused a commotion within US psychiatry, but some stalwart psychiatrists, families, patients, and governmental entities, including the World Health Organization, are pushing for change. For example, William Carpenter, Editor-in-Chief of *Schizophrenia Bulletin*, has, along with others, tried to rename the publication *Psychosis Bulletin* but the change was outvoted by the publication's editorial board because they did not want to sacrifice its historical authority. They did, however, add a subtitle: *The Journal of Psychoses and Related Disorders*.[71]

The Iowa 500 Study in the United States: Tsuang et al.

In the early 1970s, John Feighner and others at Washington University in St. Louis were determined to help American psychiatry become more reliable, particularly in the context of schizophrenia and 13 other psychiatric diagnoses.[72] The St. Louis team assembled a list of tighter criteria based on clinical description, laboratory studies, exclusion of other disorders, family studies, and a follow-up study to see if, indeed, the diagnosis held true. This project was a challenge to the authority of the DSM-II,[73] current at the time, and the St. Louis group meant to provide tighter controls on the diagnosis of patients by psychiatry in the next edition of the manual.

With this very narrow view of schizophrenia, people selected must be single and have poor premorbid social adjustment, a family history of schizophrenia, an absence of alcoholism or drug abuse at least 1 year prior to diagnosis, and an onset of illness prior to age 40. They were looking for "true or core schizophrenia." George Winokur was part of the St. Louis team as a resident before he went to Iowa. (This is the same Winokur, mentioned in an earlier chapter, who claimed he "did not believe a word" I said at my first presentation of the Vermont findings at the National Institute of Mental Health (NIMH) concerning improvement and recovery. Our data challenged the prediction of outcome possibilities for schizophrenia written in the DSMs as well as the findings of the Iowa 500 study.[74,75]

The authors claimed that the Iowa 500 was a *naturalistic* follow-up of schizophrenia, saying that there was no treatment available to these patients in the 1930s to 1940s.[76] I beg to differ. These people were locked up in a state hospital, terrified and feeling helpless, with no hope of getting out nor much respect for their humanity. There were cold water baths and strait jackets, and they were tied to their beds. Although these investigators denied it, a historical account of the Iowa hospitals produced by an arm of the American Psychiatric Association (APA) in 1937 told of pentylenetetrazol (Metrazol) administration, shock treatments, and insulin shock from the mid 1930s through the 1940s.[77] This was considered "treatment" at that time. The study definitely did not trace the "natural history" nor "natural outcome" for schizophrenia. There was nothing natural about how these patients were treated. Moreover, the hospital being used for the Iowa 500 long-term research was attached to the university's medical school, and many research projects were carried out simultaneously, including spinal cord permeability, acetylcholine, psychopathic effects of certain drugs, experiments on frustration with "maniacs" [sic], and psychoneurotics, hydrotherapy, use of narcotics, etc.[78] Certainly these strategies were available and are recorded in the history of the hospital during that period.

Iowa Research Strategies

The long-term portion of the Iowa 500 study began in 1972, was completed by 1976, and was published in 1979.[79] The lead investigators were

Ming Tsuang, Robert Woolson, and Jerome Fleming, with Winokur and many others joining in over time. Of the 3,800 charts available from the 1930s and 1940s, those of 874 people were reviewed, with 63% of those with a chart diagnosis of schizophrenia rejected because these investigators used their newly proposed Feighner criteria, described earlier; given American clinicians' propensity to overdiagnose the disorder, it was probably a good idea.

However, the Iowa 500 sample ended up with 325 affective disorders, 160 surgical controls, and 200 in the schizophrenia subsample. Psychiatric subjects were selected from consecutive admissions at University of Iowa Psychopathic Hospital from 1934 to 1944.[80] The study was able to trace more than 90% of all people at the time of long-term follow-up, ranging from 30 to 40 years.

In the end, the basic number shrank from 200 to 186 people with schizophrenia, and, within that group, 77 (or 41%) of people were found to be deceased. One hundred and nine were rated as 53% of the original sample. Of the original 100 people diagnosed with mania, 33 (or 38%) were rated; of the 225 persons with depression, 50 (or 24%) were rated; and of the 160 control patients from the general hospital undergoing surgery, there were 90 (or 62%) rated.[81]

Because of constraints in the Feighner criteria, which focused on men, there was an effort to rebalance the study in the schizophrenia group with 48.5% women and 51.5% men. Twenty percent were married, 50% had poor premorbid adjustment, and 28% were high school graduates. Median age of onset was 25, and age at admission was 27. Only 26% were discharged to the community.[82] There was no community care available.

The Iowa team conducted an average of 37 years of follow-up on 86 people of the 139 patients with schizophrenia. Letters were sent by social workers to families and study members with follow-up and structured telephone interviews. Current diagnoses were based on the Iowa Structured Psychiatric Interview given by nonmedical interviewers. The research team listed interrater trials in every paper, but, in tracking back through them all, it turned out these were clinical agreements by three senior clinicians sitting together. Interrater trials are quite different from clinicians sitting around arguing over what the diagnosis should be. Real research interrater reliability has to do with clinicians rating independently and using statistics to weed out the chance effects.

Patients who had died, who had refused to be interviewed, or who had no first-degree relatives who could be found were given "approximate" diagnoses based on records.[83]

Only four major outcome domains were measured: marital, residential, occupational status, and psychiatric symptoms. Sex differences were not studied. Good outcome included being married or widowed; living in one's own home or a relative's; being employed, retired, a homemaker, or student; and having no psychiatric symptoms. Fair outcome included being single or divorced, living in a nursing or county home, incapacitated due to physical illness, and some symptoms. A poor outcome meant that the person never married, lived in a mental hospital, was not working due to a mental illness, and had incapacitating symptoms.[84]

Even with all the cards stacked against them, the long-term outcome findings of 30 to nearly 40 years after index hospitalization revealed that 21% of people, once diagnosed as having schizophrenia, had good marital outcomes, and an additional 12% were fair. Thirty-four percent had good residential outcome, while 48% were fair. As far as employment went, 35% had good work outcome, with 8% being fair. Twenty percent demonstrated good psychiatric status, with 20% being fair.[85]

The two predictors of poor outcome were disorientation and memory deficits at admission. These investigators found more good outcomes in their adjacent studies, which ranged in descending order from affective to schizoaffective disorders to paranoid subtype to the disorganized subtype of schizophrenia, as expected by the field. Fifty-four percent of persons diagnosed as having schizophrenia were found to be doing poorly and were always portrayed as such in all their publications, *yet 46% had fair to good outcomes despite their asylum care and the application of new diagnostic criteria.* One of my slides showing these results was later endorsed by Iowa coauthor Ming Tsuang at an APA annual meeting.

The New Chicago Study

A psychologist, a psychiatrist, and a statistician walked into . . . a building on the University of Illinois at Chicago campus in the late 1980s and early 1990s just as all the rest of us had completed our long-term studies. Investigators Martin Harrow, Thomas Jobe, and many others in the Department of

Psychiatry within the Medical College at the university began to collect data on and study 274 young people (average age 23 years) who were admitted to one of two local hospitals, one public and one private.

One hundred and thirty-nine people had been diagnosed as having either schizophrenia spectrum disorders (61 plus 9 schizoaffective disorders) with 69 persons with psychotic affective disorders. Forty-one percent were first admissions, and an additional 25% were in their second admission.[86] Sixty-percent of the patients diagnosed with schizophrenia, and 42% of those with affective disorders were men.

Structured interviews were conducted at baseline, then at 2, 4.5, 7.5, 10, 15, and 20 years and are still continuing forward. Interrater trials were conducted, again successfully. The DSM-III was used to determine diagnoses, and the interviewers were not told of their subjects' diagnoses at follow-up. Sixty-one percent were determined to be middle to upper class in socioeconomic levels, and sex was split half and half for the entire sample.[87] Not only were prescriptions for psychiatric drugs tracked but also well-known instruments were used to record positive and negative symptoms, periods of recovery, levels of work, and times back in the hospital.[88]

At the 15-year mark, 145 participants had been studied five times. In this cohort, 110 people were the 15-year follow-up participants (75.9%). One of the key questions under discussion was "Can unmedicated persons with schizophrenia do as well as those who are medicated?"[89]

Sixty-four people were determined to have schizophrenia at baseline, with more men (56%) in this category. The average age at initial admission was 22.9 years. Forty-six percent were first-admission patients, and 21% had a previous admission at Index 15 years earlier.

Study participants had been diagnosed at Index as having schizophrenia, schizophreniform disorder, psychotic affective disorders, and nonpsychotic disorders. In this study, the schizophrenia/schizophreniform group on antipsychotic medication was compared to the group that had dropped their medication, as well as to once-psychotic nonschizophrenia patients who were also using or not using antipsychotic medications.

The assessment targeted symptoms, work performance, self-support, social and family functioning, life adjustment, and rehospitalization with or without medications. Recovery was defined as absence of major symptoms, paid work (half-time or more), good social function, and no rehospitalization.[90] As with many other long-term studies, these investigators also wanted to know if there was anything that could predict long-term out-come from a long list of good and poor pre-illness factors.

Sixty-five percent of people with schizophrenia who were no longer on antipsychotics were working at 15 years; 73% at the 20-year interview. People with negative symptoms from schizophrenia or who once had psychotic mood disorders and who were still on antipsychotics were not doing as well with work and in many other ways. Neither were patients with good premorbid scores who were still on antipsychotics.[91] The study revealed that the assumption that antipsychotics make life easier after the first 2 years is significantly flawed. Furthermore, people who stopped their medications were more apt to feel more in control of life and of themselves than were those who stayed on antipsychotics.[92] The nonusers also came from a place of more strength in their backgrounds, known as classic good prognostic factors, such as acute onset, having mood and positive symptoms, being female, and having good pre-illness social and work functioning. Fifty percent were considered well.

I should point out that many of the people in Vermont had very poor prognostic factors and extreme long-term disability before the rehab program. But most participants significantly improved or fully recovered after discharge, without antipsychotic medications, in the domains of work, living independently, and relating well to others. All of these findings change the valence, as Kurt Lewin once pointed out.[93] Those rehab programs that aim to help people expand their sense of self, power, and horizons support many more positive outcomes. The Chicago group found that, at the 15-year follow-up, "Over 50% of the schizophrenia patients did not have a disorder that was chronic and continuous."[94]

The 20th year of the Chicago follow-up included 139 people from the original sample, with 61 people with schizophrenia spectrum disorders, 9 with schizoaffective disorders, and the remaining 69 with affective disorders. Those participants included 38 bipolar patients with psychosis and 31 with psychotic unipolar depression.

The Chicago investigators again found that there was a shift after Index Hospitalization plus 2 years. Many people either left treatment or dropped their antipsychotics from 2 to 4 years after psychosis. Those with either schizophrenia or affective psychotic disorders had more periods of recovery and better levels of functioning than did those who stayed adherent.[95]

The repeated finding across multiple study points from Year 3 onward, and even more amplified at 20 years out, was the following:

> Regardless of diagnosis (schizophrenia and affective psychosis) participants not prescribed antipsychotic medications are more likely to experience more episodes of recovery, increased GAF [Global Assessment of Functioning] scores, and less likely to be hospitalized. Further, participants not on antipsychotic medication were about six times more likely to recover than participants on medication regardless of diagnosis status, prognostic index, race, sex, age, education and other factors.[96]

Prior to this statement in 2010, the past director of the NIMH, Thomas Insel, had already written the following comment:

> Pharmacological treatments have been in wide use for nearly a half a century yet there is little evidence that these treatments have substantially improved outcomes for most people with schizophrenia.[97]

The Vermont findings revealed that 16% of subjects in the study had no further medications prescribed in later years after hospitalization; another 34% were prescribed medications but they were put away, unused; 25% only used them when the person was feeling out of sorts and were then put away again. Only 25% declared that they used them consistently. I wonder if the Chicago investigators realized how few of their subjects who were prescribed meds were actually using them and not storing them away in a drawer somewhere. The research team suggested that

> With the lack of efficacy of antipsychotics reported in maintenance antipsychotic treatment over time and concerns over side effects and serious health detriments with prolonged antipsychotic exposure, the field of psychiatry has reason to pause and reexamine the first line treatment guideline regarding prescribed maintenance or continuous antipsychotic medication.[98]

A Study of Reducing and Discontinuing Psychiatric Medications

This necessary re-evaluation is already taking place. In 2019, Joanna Moncrief and associates in the United Kingdom began a multicenter randomized controlled trial ($N = 253$) of antipsychotic medication reduction and discontinuation, called RADAR, to determine the balance of risks and benefits of such guided strategies.[99] More and more discussions are now circulating among leading psychiatrists, psychologists, and other clinicians, as well as state and national entities, about how to change and shorten medication protocols (e.g., no, low, slow approaches and tapering strategies).[100]

The next chapter reviews what we have learned from the very-long-term studies just described; differences in views of what recovery means; the challenges suffered by consumers of services; changes in the profession; and a list of some of ordinary, everyday, and well-known people who suffered from illness of one type or another but who did and are making contributions to society, as well as some critical lessons learned from conducting this research. These are my last hurrahs. This will be followed by two chapters providing examples of exciting US and worldwide programs helping to make recovery a reality for more people, right now.

18

Eating Humble Pie

Summary of Findings

The 11 very-long-term studies from across the world have shown us a remarkably different picture from the general assumption of past 125 years that expects only marginal levels of functioning or a downward course. In other words, what was observed during the era of total institutionalization and in the era of outpatient treatment (primarily applied as stabilization, maintenance, medications, and entitlements) added to the perception of chronicity and has been significantly challenged by these very-long-term follow-up studies. These studies of nearly 2,700 people diagnosed as once having schizophrenia-like symptoms found that 20–30% or more of study participants (with one outlier at 50%) had fully recovered and an additional 21–49% had achieved improvement or significant improvement at two to three decades.[1] To add to these accomplishments, one-half to three-quarters of study participants had achieved restoration of social functioning.[2]

- Switzerland: Bleuler (1972/1978), after 23 years, found 53–68% improved and/or recovered, with 46–59% socially recovered.[3]
- Austria: Hinterhuber (1973), after 30–40 years, found that 40.3% were improved and 29.2% were recovered, equaling 69.5% neither marginal nor downhill, with 77% working full-time and another 20% part-time.[4]
- Switzerland: Ciompi and Müller (1976), after 37 years, found 57–63% improved or recovered, and 57% with good social functioning.[5]
- Lithuania: Kreditor (1977), after 20+ years, found that 84% had long-term remissions from 8 to 40 years, with 61% complete remission across time (but not enough information on social functioning).[6]

Recovery from Schizophrenia. Courtenay M. Harding, Oxford University Press. © Courtenay M. Harding 2024.
DOI: 10.1093/oso/9780195380095.003.0018

- Germany: Huber et al. (1979), after 22.4-year follow-up, found 22% recovered and 43% improved (which equals 65%), with 56% socially recovered and only 19% in treatment programs.[7]
- United States: Tsuang et al.'s (1979) Iowa 500, after 35–37 years, found 46% improved or recovered, with 21% married as the only good social outcome indicator.[8]
- Bulgaria: Marinow (1986), after 20.2 years, found 50.7% considered to have achieved good outcome, with an additional 21.8% with improved status, making a total of 72.5% (with not enough information on social recovery).[9]
- United States: Harding et al. (1987) in Vermont, with an average of 32 years follow-up of the most chronic cases plus intensive rehab as well as being rediagnosed with DSM-III criteria, revealed that 62–68% significantly improved or recovered, with 68% recovered socially as well. (It is surprising that Brooks's chronic cohort ended up with findings similar to those of M. Bleuler's mostly first-admission group.[10])
- Japan: Ogawa et al. (1987) found, at 22.5 years, 31% recovered plus 46% improved; 77% were considered psychologically recovered with social functioning even better, and another 47% were fully self-supportive.[11]
- United States: DeSisto et al. (1995) in Maine, in the matched comparison research with Vermont, at 36-year follow-up reported 49% improved, with no statistical difference in social functioning without rehab.[12]
- United States: Harrow et al. (2017/2021), in the Chicago Study, at 15–20 years follow-up, found 50–60% both with schizophrenia and affective psychosis doing well, working, and functioning significantly better while *off* antipsychotics (73%) compared with those who were still on them.[13,14]

Although long-term studies of two to three decades from across the world often used diagnostic criteria that were broad or narrow and different research protocols (some stronger than others), findings indicating significant improvement and recovery have persisted. Most of the studies targeted first or second admissions while others, such as those in Vermont and Maine, focused on heavily chronic and profoundly disabled patients. "Recovered" was defined by those two studies very strictly as people who had totally reclaimed their lives. They worked, had a home they desired, enjoyed friends and family, and had no further symptoms or medication use. By our criteria, "significantly improved" meant success in every domain except one of the variables listed in the previous sentence. These were the most stringent research criteria to meet for outcome.[15]

Observations, and More Lessons Learned

This book covers more than 40 years of learning, investigating, caring, and observing people with the lived experience of psychosis, their families, the field of psychiatry and other caring professions, plus public mental health systems. Listed below are some of the most important things I have learned from them, and from studies, colleagues, literature, and conferences over all those years.

The good stuff is

- Many more people significantly improved or recovered from a diagnosis of schizophrenia than is currently expected by most clinicians, program managers, and government officials.
- Even the most chronically disabled persons can also recover or significantly improve; therefore holding out hope and expectations is a good idea. Clinicians must share this research evidence with those they serve.
- Those people with only one episode (about 20% of the treated population) often seem to do better more quickly and may have a different combination of factors helping them, or have different versions of illness.[16]
- One-half to three-quarters of patients reacquired social skills after having been run off the rails by symptoms.
- Women with spectrum-like diagnoses generally show much faster turn-arounds than do men, who struggle much longer to return to health, but the long-term studies reveal that eventually many can and do recover or significantly improve[17,18]
- Diagnosis of schizophrenia should have been a cross-sectional "working hypothesis" only and probably not a lifetime label for most people.
- Schizophrenia may be more accurately conceptualized as an umbrella term with many unknown causes lurking underneath. It is now

known as schizophrenia spectrum disorder in the *Diagnostic and Statistical Manual of Mental Disorders* (DSM-5) and in the International Classification of Disease (ICD-11).

- The original subtypes (paranoid, disorganized, catatonic, undifferentiated, and residual) of schizophrenia used for years in psychiatry have been discarded by the current DSM-5.[19]
- The use of the label of "schizophrenia" is being replaced around the world with help from families and psychiatrists in efforts to reduce stigma and redefine the problem.
- Finding a career or a job depends on educational opportunities to finish high school or college. Accommodations for such students are simple things costing little, such as seating a student up front, providing a key to the elevator, establishing a closer parking spot, rescheduling exams if needed, and help with applications and financial aid.
- Social functioning can and did reconstitute and develop further for one-half to three-quarters of people studied, as shown in long-term studies. It often *improved* before some psychiatric symptoms receded.
- People treated as individuals and provided with the hope of improvement and recovery are challenging behavioral health systems to replace older models of care.
- Being able to work was not predicted by symptoms, diagnosis, or hospitalization. Being sociable helps but is perhaps less important in "work from home" situations.
- Many people who eventually discontinued antipsychotic medications had significantly better long-term outcomes in both the Vermont and Chicago studies. The Chicago Study has shown that patients appear to do much better without antipsychotic and antidepressant drugs after the first 2 years. The group known as Critical Psychiatry is developing protocols for carefully tapering people off their medications.[20]
- Many more people went to work, if given the opportunity, and being off antipsychotic medications helped significantly.
- Some clinicians and researchers became humble about their knowledge and more willing to genuinely work together with people with lived experience. They learned how to cross-train one another to find some of these surprising new insights.[21,22]
- Models of rehabilitation, self-sufficiency, and community integration have worked in combination to help people reclaim their lives.

- Some of the many variables that seem to increase resilience, improvement, and recovery include a focus on a person's strengths, not on damage, pathology, and dysfunction. Choices in decision-making, wellness, function, hope, rights and privileges, interdependence, and a life with meaning can all be embedded in a treatment plan. Or how about a joint action plan for both sides of the equation instead?

- Kraepelin's 1897 pessimistic notions about outcome finally need to be set aside. In fact, Engstrom and Kendler write that "A careful rereading and historical contextualization of his works reveals that, compared with his popular iconic image in North America, the real Kraepelin was: 1) much more psychological in orientation, 2) considerably less brain-centric, and 3) nosologically more skeptical and less doctrinaire."[23] For me to acknowledge Kraepelin in any way after fighting with him all these years is remarkable.

Recognizing Current Limitations of Knowledge

- Biomedical strategies have not been as helpful as hoped by the field of psychiatry, although most psychiatrists have insisted on telling parents and patients that schizophrenia is a "brain disease" or a "neurochemical disorder." Both are claims for which we have neither concrete data nor real understanding. These labels also imply lifelong illness. Families often are relieved to receive what they think is a definitive diagnosis but are slowly learning that the field is still in its pioneering phase.

- There are no blood tests, no brain scans, no genetic markers to aid in the diagnosis of schizophrenia, simply a broad set of symptoms and behaviors, many of which can be found in at least 26 other disorders. For affective disorders there are at least 43 other disorders that mimic the symptoms displayed. The diagnostic manual has been designed for reliability, not validity. Therefore, teaching all clinicians to cope by providing a course of "Gray 101" instead of seeing diagnosis in terms of black and white, might be helpful to get them to do more than check the boxes and see more of the whole person underneath.[24,25]

- Predictors of both good and poor long-term outcome often lost power across time as other factors intervened.

- It has been my observation, both directly and through reading, that about 50–80% of patients presenting with schizophrenia-like symptoms have either physical, emotional, and/or sexual abuse in their backgrounds, issues that are often not treated, in addition to other social determinants. Investigations are ongoing.
- Antipsychotic medications appeared to help people with schizophrenia-like symptoms and psychotic affective disorders for a short time (the first 2–3 years) only by dampening down positive symptoms not curing them.[26]
- Co-occurring disorders are often treated separately by different clinicians using different models and getting paid by different funding streams. Integrated approaches have been shown to work better in most cases.[27,28]
- When a mind is in chaos being treated in a chaotic environment, such as a noisy inpatient unit instead of a quiet outpatient setting (e.g., Soteria House with little to no medication), the noise may not be helpful; it also explains why neuroleptics are used to settle a person down in an inpatient unit and thus why the chaos takes longer to subside.[29]
- Some clinicians, especially psychiatrists, have not recognized that work might be helpful to reduce symptoms because of the stress and inability to concentrate. But Marone and Golowka asked, "If work makes people with mental illness sick, what do unemployment, poverty, and social isolation cause?"[30]
- We found that factoring in the role of behavioral health policies, funding, and program availability as some of the critical environmental factors that people with the lived experience and their clinicians face during their work together impacts outcome, but this is often left untouched by researchers. The longer the study, the more important it is.[31]
- Other important variables seem to play roles in impeding improvement and recovery, such as medication side effects, socialization into the patient role, living in isolation or institutionalization, poverty, and, again, low staff expectations, as well as being told one has a lifelong illness.
- It takes a government an unbelievably long time to make changes in programs and policies, and, when it does, there are often unpredicted side effects.

More Things That Get in the Way

Professors Mike Slade in England and Michaela Amering in Austria and many others worked together to bring to our attention the fact that the word "recovery" has been much abused in the service sector. They found at least seven "mis-uses or abuses" prevalent in policies and programs. They are:

- "Recovery is just the latest model" and solved by adding peers. Next year, we will have a new model so why change our main practices?
- "Recovery does not apply to my patients." They have lifelong illnesses."
- "Services can *make* people recover through effective treatments," instead of working together to figure out what the person wishes for their own life and ways to achieve it.
- "Compulsory detention and treatment aid recovery," but they rarely have.
- "A recovery orientation means closing services," but, unfortunately, there will always be new customers to work with and brief flare-ups in old ones.
- "Recovery is about *making* people independent and normal," but the target is ideally having a self-selected life and become a contributing citizen. Most people in the community are interdependent, and the range of what is normal is considerable. One doesn't "make" someone do something anyway.
- "Contributing to society happens only after the person is recovered"[32] (see the later list of people who challenge this assumption).

Slade and his team went on to identify 10 programs which prioritize "connectedness, hope, identity, meaning and empowerment."[33] Many are listed in the last two chapters of this book. Staff members at recovery programs often tell me that they are already incorporating most of these aspects in their clinical work. What I have discovered, however, working in numerous hospitals and centers over time, is that the following is the reality in many programs, and this was also found by Slade and his team:

- There is still a residual one-up and one-down mentality;
- Still doing things *for or to* and less doing things *with*;

- Not much talk about real recovery because staff often doesn't believe that is possible for the struggling person in front of them;
- Believing that they know more than the person in care and failing to acknowledge that the person might have some wisdom to offer and might know what helps; and
- Not fighting to offer access to critical programs proven to help people recover; instead, program administrators are more worried about the bottom line than the values they espouse.[34]

In interviewing those who have recovered, LeRoy Spaniol and his colleagues at Boston University's Center for Psychiatric Rehabilitation discovered that they were not focusing on their illnesses, per se, but rather on getting over

- the loss of self, connection, and hope;
- loss of roles and opportunities;
- devaluing and disempowering programs, practices, and environments;
- prejudices and discrimination in society; and
- internalized oppression and shame.[35]

These additional challenges take one's breath away! Across that study and many more that we did ourselves, recovering people told us their own stories about what helped them most: "Somebody believed in me," "A friend with similar problems helped me get better," "I got a job that made me feel competent," "My parents stuck with me," "My own persistence," "Some people held up a mirror so that I could see that I was a worthwhile person," "Someone told me that I had a chance to get better," "Just plain stubbornness," "When I helped other people who were suffering, it helped me," "Someone really listened to me," "It really helped to know that each person might be able to recover and find a place in the world." Note that no one mentioned medication nor professionals specifically.

It is time for all of us to make clear and strong decisions about how we do our work, how we see persons with the lived experience of profound disabling pain and suffering, and how much we must change ourselves to be more helpful.

In 1961, the Vermont Study revealed that changing from a hierarchical system of care to a horizontal one turned out to be more effective for all parties, including professional, nonprofessional, and patients alike. As early as the 5-year follow-up, data revealed recovery and improvement was possible in the most chronic of cases using rehabilitation and community care. In addition, the approach of participatory action research protocols and the implementation of collaboration between the Departments of Mental Health and Vocational Rehabilitation made the difference in restoring lives.[36,37]

After *The Vermont Story* was published in 1961, the Joint Commission of Mental Illness and Mental Health (American Psychiatric Association, American Medical Association, American Academy of Neurology, and the Department of Justice) published *Action for Mental Health*. In this document was the statement "'Hopelessness,' and 'incurability,' should be attacked and the prospects of recovery and improvement through modern concepts of treatment and rehabilitation emphasized."[38] It bears repeating again and again. In spite of this, as of this writing in 2023, the National Institute of Mental Health (NIMH) reported that there remain millions of lives being lived out without much mitigation or remediation.[39]

In 2001, I joined with Pat Deegan and Priscilla Ridgway (two people with lived experiences) to create a vision statement for a university institute on human resilience. This declaration included the following: "People facing serious life challenges (such as severe illness, disability, and/or disadvantage) are resilient and can significantly improve and often recover when they have access to knowledge, self-help resources, skilled professionals, sustaining environments, and social justice." We keep saying things like this over and over.

A Slightly Different View of Recovery

Some people with lived experience, along with psychologist Bill Anthony at Boston University's Center for Psychiatric Rehabilitation (BU/CPR), have challenged the idea that people could not be considered recovered if they had residual symptoms. Anthony wrote a touching soliloquy on the subject and I repeat it here.

> Recovery is a deeply personal, unique process of changing one's attitudes, values, feelings, goals, skills, and/or roles. It is a way of living a satisfying, hopeful, and contributing life even with the limitations caused by illness. Recovery involves the development of new meaning and purpose in one's life as one grows beyond the catastrophic effects of mental illness.[40]

People with the lived experiences of digging out of such cataclysmic events and reclaiming their lives have begun to talk openly about their new realities,[41,42] raising their voices, starting in the 1970s, louder and louder worldwide; now they are beginning to receive the attention they wanted.[43] Many do attain full recovery while others get their lives back in bits and pieces while growing forward into the future. By the way, in medicine very few problems are cured with the exception of a few surgeries and some antibiotics. Most physicians will admit that they are helping the person to heal themselves.

Ordinary and Famous People Making Contributions Despite Having Suffered From Serious Emotional and Cognitive Problems

In an earlier chapter, I wrote about getting phone calls from engineers, professors, high school teachers, lawyers, and others after talking about the possibility of recovery from schizophrenia during a National Public Radio interview in the late 1980s. They all spoke about the persistent stigma in society that had restrained them from telling their own stories, but they were glad that I had talked about these data.

Many well-known people around the globe have made substantial contributions to community and society despite having suffered from severe depression, bipolar disorder, and schizophrenia. Such a very long list includes politicians (e.g., Winston Churchill and Abraham Lincoln), scientists (e.g., Sir Isaac Newton, Nobel Prize mathematician John Nash, and Leon Rosenberg, pioneering geneticist), playwrights (e.g., Eugene O'Neill and Tennessee Williams), authors (e.g., Ernest Hemingway and Leo Tolstoy), composers (e.g., Ludwig von Beethoven and Peter Ilyich Tchaikovsky), professors (e.g., Kay Redfield Jamison of Johns Hopkins School of Medicine and Elyn Saks of the University of Southern California Gould School of Law), newscasters (e.g., Jane Pawley and Carol LeBeau), actors (e.g., Marlon Brando and Carrie Fisher), singers (e.g., Charlie Pride and Bette Midler), comedians (e.g., Roseanne Barr and Jonathan Winters), athletes (e.g., Lionel Aldridge of the Green Bay Packers football team and Jimmy Piersall of the Boston Red Socks baseball team), artists (Michelangelo and Vincent Van Gogh), and even an astronaut (Buzz Aldrin). The list goes on and on. Many of these well-known and other lesser-known heroes have spoken out to help others understand their struggles and victories and reduce stigma and discrimination.

Discussions Ensued During the Past Decade With Practice and Research Moving Forward

Psychologists began to look at ways they could make more contributions other than research to the care and understanding of very seriously distressed patients. Finally, in 2009, the Serious Mental Illness (SMI) Task Force, working with the American Psychological Association, endorsed a formal resolution (a public announcement and a big shift from earlier days) regarding the possibilities of recovery for persons with serious mental illness, partially based on the findings from long-term studies.[44]

In 2014, the American Psychological Association also announced that, together with Mary Jansen, it had published a 400-page document that included a section "Recovery to Practice Curriculum: Reframing Psychology for the Emerging Health Care Environment."[45] The main emphasis was placed on "health, home, purpose, and community." The recommended critical ingredients for all treatment programs are "hope, self-directed, individualized and person-centered, empowerment, holistic, non-linear, strengths-based, peer support, respect, and responsibility."[46] Other national groups also followed suit—nurses, social workers, peer groups, and substance abuse counselors—all funded by the US federal Substance Abuse and Mental Health Services Administration (SAMHSA).

The British Psychological Society published their version in 2014 and revised it in 2017, "Understanding Psychosis and Schizophrenia: Why People Sometimes Hear Voices, Believe Things That Others Find Strange, or Appear Out of Touch with Reality, and What Can Help."[47] It is chock full of comments and contributions from persons with lived experience, including families, to guide the way for professionals.

Starting on December 1, 2020, the whole nation of Norway began to shift from a psychiatric approach, which focused on psychopathology, damage, and deficits to treat mental illness, with a psychological model in order to redesign and run its care system. This effort was led by Professor Anne-Kari Torgalsbøen, an investigator into recovery, resilience, and the care of

seriously ill people. The field of psychology in Norway is using subspeciali-
ties such as clinical, developmental, cognitive, and personality approaches to
offer different approaches to promote recovery.[48,49]

Reducing Avalanches in Care Systems

After a half-century (1950s to 2000s), things are trending in a positive new
direction in many quarters around the world. However, many lives are being
lived without much remediation as people wait for the "silver bullet": the
cause of the illness, and its *cure*. For the past 50 years, hardworking neuro-
scientists, geneticists, pharmacologists, and biologists have been looking at
neurotransmitters, neurochemical imbalances, genes, epigenetics, positron
emission tomography (PET) scans, magnetic resonance imaging (MRI),
functional fMRIs, and neuropsychological tests in order to diagnose, understand, and treat schizophrenia and other disabling disorders. Bigger diagnostic manuals have been published, and more and more pharmaceuticals are
being prescribed. On the surface, reading the brief headlines, it looks like we
are getting somewhere, but the complexities within the brain and mind, and
the physiology of these systems interacting with a person's emotions, cogni-
tions, neuroplasticity, epigenetics, social interactions, and community conditions are almost infinite. It is time to be humbler about what we know and
don't know, and I suspect that it will take much more time to figure it all out.

In his blog, Thomas Insel, a former director of the NIMH, outlined the
challenge and this bears repeating.

> Terms like "depression" or "schizophrenia" or "autism" have achieved a reality
> that far outstrips their scientific value. Each refers to a cluster of symptoms,
> similar to "fever" or "headache." But beyond symptoms that cluster together,
> there should be no presumption that these are singular disorders, each with a
> single cause and a common treatment.[50]

Funding has targeted pharmaceutical and biomedical models yet there are
substantial numbers of biopsychosocial programs all over the world that
have been developed and successfully applied. These approaches have been
shown to work in helping people recover. But our efforts are still severely
underfunded, not widely available geographically, and underutilized where
they are.

I often wonder how many clinicians tell people living with the challenges of schizophrenia spectrum disorder and other complicated problems about the positive data from the long-term studies? People need to know they are "still loveable,"[51] still part of their communities, and learn about the future with possibilities of improvement and recovery. The focus should be on a home of choice, finishing school or finding a job they like, friends, and a date for Saturday night. While they are figuring all that out, the symptoms often start to settle down because, otherwise, they get in the way of other things people wish to do. In addition, setting up programs in which helping others as a struggling and still symptomatic person also turns out to be a healing process for all parties. Having collaborative input into how the programs are run is critical as well. These down-to-earth and common-sense approaches have had considerable success in helping people reacquire a sense of control and an image of a positive future, get a life back, and reduce symptoms along the way. Remember that psychiatrist George Brooks lived in one of the poorest states in America, as described at the beginning of this book. He admitted that he did not know what to do next, and so everyone (the patients and staff on the most disabled wards, vocational rehabilitation, and the community) all pitched in, and, slowly, most of his most severely disabled patients grabbed their lives back![52] His approaches can still be used today.

If we could only radically change public policies, funding mechanisms, and maintenance programs, many more people experiencing psychoses could start to reclaim their lives. There are always activist family members, ex-patients, some clinicians, and a few lawyers working together with dedicated organizations and sympathetic legislators to make needed changes. Read the book *Fighting for Recovery*.[53] It has taken more than 70 years to get to where we are today, and we have more to fix.

However, since change is remarkably slow, it behooves what little staff and dollars we have to set up environments that provide encouragement to the very patients we are supposed to be helping to pick themselves up and help change a good many things for themselves. Set up real patient governments to help run organizations, as they did in Vermont. Grab back control from current policies, reimbursement criteria, and biomedical approaches. Inculcate hope, kindness, trial-and-error stubbornness, and a view of the future. Pay attention to local culture. As an example, paint the place. I once visited a mental health center south of San Diego. The walls were vibrant colors. There was food laid out and music in the air. Families were included in treatment strategies, and so were parish priests and local healers known as *curanderos* (who, by the way, were paid by insurance). All conversations were conducted in Spanish. These changes to match a culture and needs are some of the secrets of real rehabilitation.

The last two chapters of this book are devoted to specific descriptions of programs initiated by multiple caring disciplines, families, patients, and ex-patients from across the world, as well as in America, and they provide new ideas for energetic directors, clinicians, their patients, and family partners to change what is going on in clinics, centers, hospitals, courts, and communities. The new and exciting ideas behind such programs bring mental health and substance abuse services into the 21st century and encourage more struggling people to achieve recovery.

PART FIVE

Rehabilitation Programs for Recovery

19

World Programs

The last two chapters of this book provide descriptions and stories of modern programs and practices designed by enlightened multidisciplinary clinicians in collaboration with people with the lived experience of psychosis and other serious problems. These pioneers attended closely to the challenges involved in the process of recovery from severe emotional and cognitive distress. They either expanded the traditionally narrow biomedical paradigm, left it behind entirely, or never ascribed to it in the first place. These projects from around the world created environments that were safe enough, collaborative enough, and respectful enough to enable most struggling people find their way back to health and happiness—in their own way and in their own time. Many of these ventures incorporated some of the same ingredients found in the Vermont Study of the 1950s.

Italy: Social Cooperatives

The Italian story has been quite remarkable. In 1991, I was invited by the World Health Organization, along with Professor Richard Warner of Colorado (who had written a book on recovery and economics[1]), to give lectures in Florence, Trieste, and Genoa. "It was a tough job, but somebody had to do it!" as the tongue-in-cheek saying goes. From Florence, we took to Trieste a train that was headed for war-torn Sarajevo, still in the former Yugoslavia. Trieste is located at the far reaches of Italy and is often described as the eastern part of the boot top. A war was raging across the border, and we saw bullet holes in the train cars. We were very glad to get off before the train entered the battle zone.

Recovery from Schizophrenia. Courtenay M. Harding, Oxford University Press. © Courtenay M. Harding 2024.
DOI: 10.1093/oso/9780195380095.003.0019

We were picked up by a hotel car and taken to a small boutique hotel sitting beside large chain hotels on the Adriatic. This hotel was owned and run by a social cooperative that employed a high proportion of people with mental health problems. Everyone from the manager down to the chamber maids was part of the cooperative. To paraphrase another common American saying, "We knew we weren't in Kansas anymore." (Although, it should be also noted that the state of Kansas has been successfully working on the "strength-based approach.")[2]

On our first night, the deputy head of the system of care, Giuseppe Dell'Acqua, took us to a social cooperative-run restaurant and bar downtown. The next day we went up the hill to the former state hospital (closed more than a decade earlier) and found it was now corporate headquarters for more than 40 social cooperative businesses. These enterprises included a moving company, a construction company, leather and fancy paper-making companies, a dance troupe, a documentary-making group, and much more, including two beauty parlors, which were so booked that I was unable to get a badly needed appointment there. In addition, there was a computer training school located in one of the former psychiatric units. This school was run by a middle-aged lady who had once been a patient in that hospital.

It turned out that, in the early 1960s, a young psychiatrist named Franco Basaglia, having just graduated from residency, was sent to supervise a state hospital in Gorizia. He found deplorable conditions, with patients walking around with shifts and scuffs on, sleeping in rows of beds in the hallways, and sitting on wooden benches all day with nothing to do. He took the bars off windows and made semi-private rooms for patients to sleep in, each with a locked cabinet for personal belongings. He begged and borrowed from the townspeople to reclothe his patients and provide hairbrushes and toothbrushes, because his patients had none. He encouraged students from the nearby town to come and read to the patients. He reduced restraint and electroshock therapy and opened the doors.[3]

After all this effort, the Italian psychiatric establishment "encouraged him to leave" and sent Basaglia to Trieste, situated as far from the powers-that-be as possible. Meant to be an exile, this was the only mental hospital in the province, whose population was about 250,000 people in a geographical area less than one-half of the size of Vermont. He found similar circumstances in that hospital and proceeded to make improvements—but this time he went even further. He decided that people should actually be living downtown and not in a hospital for the rest of their lives. With staff and patients, Basaglia built a huge Trojan horse, which I actually saw when I visited, still sitting on the hospital's front porch. They rolled it down to the town square and gave a theatrical performance with the theme of bringing patients back into the community. It was a very Italian thing to do. Then Basaglia began to build a comprehensive community mental health system, and he made a deal with the general hospital for acute care only. He slowly and carefully emptied the hospital.

As the story went, Basaglia knew that his patients needed jobs. So he and a group of disabled people and other unemployed workers applied for a government contract to take care of the beautiful city parks. They won that contract and so sought the next one, which was cleaning government office buildings. They won that one, too. The status of social cooperatives was then formalized into state law and eventually into regional law. The growing collection of social cooperatives in Trieste won other contracts to run the cafeterias in the city office buildings and in the former mental hospital, open a restaurant in the city, and, finally, run the Opera House Café.

The co-ops grew from there and made more than $US7.6 million by 1991—$16,692,214 million in 2023 money! We wondered why they had invited us to lecture them on rehabilitation and recovery. Later, when the world went into an economic slump, I heard that people from downtown Trieste came up to corporate headquarters to inquire about job possibilities and that the co-ops now were now staffed by approximately 70% people with and 30% without psychiatric histories. What irony.

The next day of our visit, Warner went off with Roberto Mezzina to see the comprehensive community mental health system.[4] I asked to see the Women's Club (now somewhat regrettably called the Women's Mental Health Center). I had heard about it the night before at dinner from a young female psychologist. Dell'Acqua had never seen it and was not interested in seeing it, as he said it seemed quite unnecessary as a service. But as I was his guest, he capitulated and took me there.

The Women's Club was in a brownstone in the middle of a shopping district downtown. There were two co-op–run stores on the street level—one a dress shop and the other offering arts and crafts. On the second floor was the Club. It had a large main room with furniture built by that co-op and side rooms containing another beauty parlor (also too booked for an appointment), a jazzercize room, and a kitchen. There was also an apothecary

shop in which older women would teach younger ones how to make traditional herbal medicines.

About 45 well-dressed and coiffed women came for the day, and we all
partook of expresso and sat around a large table. I asked them to tell us what
their lives were like before the Club opened and afterward. These stories
were initially heartbreaking because many women had been ejected from
their families; now they had an extended family and a place to see their
children. These women also looked after one another, and, if one did not
show up when expected, then a couple of other women would go find out
what the situation was. Dell'Acqua had to translate for me, and, during one
particularly poignant story, he started to tear up. We all did. He was a sturdy
man from Naples with a thick gray moustache, and he turned to me and
said, "And now, I have to cry again in English!" (He approved this story
before press.)

Trieste has since become a World Health Organization Collaborating
Center for Research and Training focused on building social cooperatives, deinstitutionalizing psychiatric hospitals, and replacing them with
integrated community care (including 24-hour mental health centers).
Recently a conservative government wished to privatize the mental health
system, and this caused a public and professional uproar.[5]

Some Efforts in the Rest of Italy

Eventually the Italian psychiatric establishment began to shut down all the
state hospitals and transinstitutionalize patients to small homes across the
nation, similar to the plan described in an earlier chapter about the Maine
Project. I was invited to the celebration in Torino for the 30th anniversary
of this transition in 2008, and I dared to suggest that the Italians had forgotten the key last step. This crucial final stage should have placed as many
people as possible back into the real community, living in a place of their
own choice and with employment opportunities. Caterina Corbascio, a
local psychiatrist working as director of the Departmenti Salute Mentale in
Asti e Alesandria, and others, took on this task, and so the torch was passed
to a new generation.[6] Nevertheless, despite their best efforts, the plan came
to a screeching halt when private companies took over the running of the
small houses, and patients' final transition to the community did not occur.
Corbascio and colleagues are working to make the best of the situation. It

has now been 40 years since this transinstitutionalization—and these houses are still separate from the communities in which they sit.

Finland: Community Living and Working, Need-Adapted Treatment, and Open Dialogue

While presenting at a fall meeting of the Finnish Psychiatric Association in 1995, I had the opportunity to meet a pioneering psychologist, Erik Anttinen, from Tampere, a city which lies northwest of Helsinki. In the 1970s, he began telling the psychiatrists at the hospital where he worked that their patients really needed to be out of the hospital.[7] The members of the faculty threatened him with expulsion. He persisted and managed to get private funding to build handsome housing in the community. He also established work opportunities, such as a business that restored antique furniture, for people who gradually became ex-patients. We took the train north after the meeting and Anttinen proudly showed me some of his programs.

Need-Adapted Treatment

In the far west of the country I met another Finn, Yryö Alanen, Professor of Psychiatry in Turku, along with members of his team K. Lehtinen, V. Räkköläinen, and J. Aaltonen. In 1976, they began to develop what is known today as "need-adapted treatment."[8] It was created and used by both hospital and community psychiatrists and their teams. The program was designed to be flexible and "case-specific" for persons with the diagnosis of schizophrenia and their families. Alanen decided that a "one-size-fits-all" strategy did not make sense for this population because there were so many competing theories and approaches to treating schizophrenia. Whatever was accomplished was done with psychotherapeutic goals in mind: treatment needed to consider an individual person's development and the ways the individual's clinical picture presented itself, instead of using a more generalized institutional approach. The clinical team met jointly with each patient and his or her family to help them "conceive of the situation as a consequence of the difficulties the patients and those close to them have encountered in their lives [rather] than a mysterious illness that the patient has developed as an individual."[9] Treatments offered, therefore, were based on individual needs and could include individual, couple, and family approaches. Low-dose medications, given for a short time, were the goal. This helped to reduce the patient population by 60% in Finnish hospitals.

Open Dialogue

Over the past 20 years, emerging from the far north of Finland in Tornio, Western Lapland, has been an expansion of the concept of need-adapted treatment, led by Jaakko Seikkula and his team. It is called "open dialogue."[10] This approach sends a team of clinicians to visit with the family in which there is a struggling person, sometimes as early as 24 hours after an acute crisis. The meeting includes not only the person and family but often members of their social network as well. Everything (the discussions, the clinical impressions, and eventually a joint problem-solving plan) is spoken about openly, with nothing hidden from view. Medications are used if needed but not right away. This form of very early intervention, which is part of an already established system of care and embedded within psychiatry and the community, often reduces the duration of psychosis to 3 weeks instead of the usually much longer process. Employment of seven principles within the open dialogue approach (immediate help, social network perspective, flexibility and mobility, responsibility, psychological continuity, tolerance of uncertainty, dialogue, and polyphony) helped participants put words to the stress of a psychosis and enabled family members to express themselves a well. Success rates have been impressive, and the approach is now being tried in the United States, in Vermont and elsewhere. In addition, a treatment manual has been developed, along with an extensive training program, more research, and clinical trials.[11]

Sweden: The Parachute Project

In Sweden, I met with Johan Cullberg, a professor of psychiatry in Stockholm who has written many books and conducted extensive research. He began to study how crises could strengthen and mature a person. He later began to think about how noxious environments in both hospital and community were not helpful to a person's sense of self, nor was overmedication. He focused on kindness and respect. He established a plan with

Sonia Levander and others in the public health department and called it the "Parachute Project."[12] In this approach, first-episode patients and others were removed from the noisy atmosphere of hospitals and placed into small, quiet suburban homes with mobile crisis teams for support. The teams followed the Finnish approach of need-adapted treatment, alongside a comparison group which received treatment as usual (high-dose medication and hospital care). There were six principles of care: (1) early intervention, preferably at the family home; (2) need-specific intervention; (3) ongoing meetings with patient and family; (4) access to a stable team for 5 years; (5) lowest optimal dose of antipsychotic medication (but only after a 2-week trial of no antipsychotics or only antianxiety medications); and (6) access to a small overnight bed if the family home situation was untenable.[13] Mixed-method studies targeted the 1-, 3-, 5-, and 13-year outcome status of 253 people as well as 246 comparison subjects. Among their many findings, results indicated significantly less use of the hospital and medications in the Parachute group and better outcomes, including work.[14]

Building on the work in Sweden and Finland, and funded by the Innovation Center in the Federal Centers for Medicaid and Medicare, New York City funded a project to implement an integration of the Parachute Project, open dialogue, mobile crisis, and respite bed programs from 2012 to 2015. This amalgamation seemed to make a great deal of sense, and the challenge was to see how it would work in one of the largest cities in the world. After a 3-year trial, the project ceased. Kim Hopper, project ethnographer/anthropologist at Columbia University School of Public Health, suggested that one of the problems, among many, was that the models of care were often competing and getting in the way of one another due to their own design structures, the need for time to train in new techniques, and the managed care environment.[15]

Switzerland: Soteria Berne

In 1985, I was lecturing in Berne and visiting with Professor Luc Ciompi, who conducted the Enquête de Lausanne, the very-long-term study of 37 years described in an Chapter 17. We discussed his work on the interaction between thinking and feeling known as "affect-logic."[16]

As Ciompi took me for a drive to see "something special," he told me the following story. He said that he had been sitting at a luncheon one day held by a private organization composed of relatives, professionals, and people with the lived experience of mental illness. This organization had garnered substantial funds for improving healthcare services. The person sitting next to him asked Ciompi what his dream was. Ciompi said that he had a plan, called Soteria Berne,[17] to help young people struggling with psychosis— but that the house and program would cost about 1.2 million Swiss francs. The person listening said, "Okay, I will give you the money!" Six months later the organization fully funded the project. Ciompi admitted that he would never again complain of having to go to formal lunches.

The "something special" was Ciompi's new treatment center. It was a large, beautiful house with a walled garden in the middle of a residential neighborhood near downtown. The garden was a delightfully quiet place with a few tables and chairs scattered about. Inside the house there were rounded corners, and, unlike many European homes, there were neither paintings on the walls nor tchotchkes on the many flat surfaces. A low stimuli atmosphere was the goal, to help quiet unruly minds and emotions coping with an early episode of psychosis. The staff, often nonprofessionals, spoke in soft voices and had the aim of "being with" the struggling person.

Unlike the early days of his friend and colleague Loren Mosher's original Soteria project in San Francisco, which used no medication,[18] Ciompi admitted to using sleep aids and antianxiety medications to help people through the rough patches. The atmosphere at the house was very tranquil, and most of the young people were cleared of psychotic symptoms within about 6–8 weeks. Their need for services continued after discharge but generally only for the next 2 or 3 more years.

Soteria Berne has been in existence for more than 32 years. Eventually the ideas embedded within this program spread to Germany, where there are 13 Soteria-like programs, with more in the Netherlands, Israel, Japan, and elsewhere. The approach has now been reproduced in the United States, where it had been derided for many years, and one is now located in Vermont.

Colombia: Fungrata and "Accompanied Self-Rehabilitation"

In South America, a professor and psychiatrist born in Philadelphia but raised in Colombia sees things differently as well. Alberto Fergusson started out as an aide in an asylum and was fired after a couple of weeks for daring to organize group discussions in the evening for patients who were otherwise just sitting around. He went on to receive his medical training and was dismayed to find that so many discharged patients were walking aimlessly around the streets of Bogotá. In response, he set up a village called Fungrata, which offered not only a home to live in but work opportunities in a bakery, a library, a pottery, a laundry, and a town meeting hall.[19]

After 20 years Fergusson concluded that he had actually created his own community but that it was not "the real community." He began to rethink his entire strategy and decided that people needed to be in charge of their own rehabilitation—but with supports. So he invented "Accompanied Self-Rehabilitation"[20] and moved everyone into the nearby suburb of Sopo. If someone wished to have a job, they went to where everyone else was looking for jobs. If someone needed to change his or her apartment, they went to where everyone else went to find one. Clinicians and community volunteers took a backseat, but they were available to share what we know about psychiatric distress, help to discern triggers, identify ways to cope better, and also learn what people have discovered themselves. Only very recently did Fergusson see that there were a few people who really needed the environment of a Fungrata. About a third of patients continue to not respond well to all these programs. We still do not know what their problems are and how to help. We still do not know who will and will not respond to recovery programs over time because some of the very worst cases do turn around and some of the good-looking cases do not.

The Netherlands and the United Kingdom: Hearing Voices Movement, Networks, and Groups

About 30 years ago the psychiatrist Marius Romme of Maastricht University and a patient, Patsy Hage, went on local TV and spoke about how she heard voices. They asked whether there was anyone out there who had figured out how to live with such hallucinations. The patient and psychiatrist were unable to figure it out by themselves. Much to their great surprise, a large number of people of all ages later called the assigned telephone number to report that they also heard voices.[21] The first conference on the subject was attended by 700 people, of whom 500 were voice-hearers. One-third had no history of contact with the psychiatric establishment or mental health system. The efforts of Romme and his partner, science journalist Sandra Escher, led to the development of a broad hearing-voices movement that has spread internationally.[22] This movement has enabled national networks of peer-support groups to be established in 30 countries on five continents. Such groups offer an important alternative to traditional psychiatric treatment. The fifteenth World Hearing Voices Congress will be held in Copenhagen, Denmark in November, 2024.

Instead of being castigated and shunned for rampant psychopathology, people like Jacqui Dillon in the United Kingdom revealed that these voices could become guides, helping people to defuse overwhelming inner turmoil caused by trauma, bullying, racial inequities, fears of being different (e.g., as a LGBTQ or an overweight person), or some other societal concern foisted on them as unwitting victims.[23] Groups of voice-hearers and those with other unusual perceptions (e.g., other hallucinations and delusions) plucked solace and guidance out of their nightmares in the company of other voice-hearers. They discovered that by talking together they could heal and share experiences in safe places of mutual respect while learning and practicing new strategies. Learning what these perceptions had to teach them helped people regain power over their lives. Clinicians, families, and people with these lived experiences are being trained to provide such group environments despite the psychiatric profession's insistence that hearing voices and the behaviors they can generate are symptoms always in need of medication.[24]

Eleanor Longden, one of the founders of the UK groups, said in her 2016 TED talk that psychiatry should not keep asking, "What is wrong with you?" but instead ask, "What has happened to you?"[25,26] In fact, pathologizing and medicating to suppress voices have not worked very well, and many people remain miserable. This new approach seems more successful.

As a student, I thought I was doing quite well with this situation myself. When working with a person listening to a voice instead of paying attention to me, I said, "Please tell your voice to go away for a short time so that I might talk with you, because I will have to go soon." It worked, and I was pleased with myself. Now I understand what I missed—and what so many other professionals have missed—in not talking about the voices. We missed the opportunity to help the person relate the voices to their own life story, to learn their triggers and learn how to express emotions in a more balanced way.

A psychology professor at Mount Holyoke College, Gail Hornstein, working with the UK network, has developed a US national research project designed to empirically analyze the functioning of hearing-voices groups.[27,28]

A Couple of Brief Examples of Social Psychiatry in England

In my travels to the United Kingdom, I have had the honor of meeting some very innovative activists who fought for patient rights and better care and who trained other psychiatrists, family doctors, and nurses to see those with psychosis as people. A stellar example was Jim Birley, Dean of the Royal College of Psychiatrists for many years. He and George Brown, a well-known professor of medical sociology, wrote a classic paper arguing that stressful life events could contribute to psychosis.[29] It was met with great resistance, but this perspective is now incorporated into everyone's thinking. Birley fought for rehabilitation and decent housing, among many other means of making life better. He and his wife Julia invited me and my youngest daughter Ashley, then 17, for supper one evening. They were down-to-earth, caring, and kind. The talk of the evening was not about schizophrenia but of the recent hurricane that had hit London. I didn't know London had them. The storm had taken down their prized magnolia tree that they had carefully nurtured for 19 years in the hope of finally seeing it bloom in its 20th year. Those people were patient but persistent gardeners, just as they were patient but persistent activists with systems of care.

And then there was Julian Leff, a social psychiatrist of many talents who had helped us understand the social and emotional impact of deinstitutionalization and culture on people. After his so-called retirement, he invented a treatment for hearing voices. He had people develop avatars for them to talk to on their computers and help resolve many of the issues involved.[30] He had fun and was an imaginative genius.

Australia: Reducing the DUP with Early Interventions for Psychosis in Melbourne Plus Creating a Ruckus in Sydney Fighting for Improvements

Reducing the long gap between when psychosis begins and when treatment is obtained (called *duration of untreated psychosis* or DUP) has been a major concern and of interest in psychiatry.[31] Across the world, the gap between a person becoming increasingly upset, scared, and psychotic and then finding people to help them has been usually more than 2 years. In 1984, Irish immigrant, psychiatrist, and professor, Patrick McGorry established a specialty psychosocial recovery unit in Melbourne for young people and their families. In 1991, while visiting, I witnessed firsthand one of his first outpatient strategies. McGorry set up a small clinic and told high school students that if they were becoming upset about the stresses of homework, trouble with their parents, or being disappointed by friends, they could come in, talk, and get some support. During that process, if the young person was found to be on the brink of collapse, significant intervention could be proposed. By 1992, McGorry had established the first Early Psychosis Prevention and Intervention Centre (EPPIC).[32]

By 1997, this program and its research had expanded across many neighborhoods of Melbourne (population now more than 5 million), and, by 2001, a foundation had been established to fund longer-term support. The programs Orygen and headspace (the National Youth Mental Health Foundation) were established in 2002 and 2006, respectively, to provide acute and continuing care as well as psychosocial recovery. EPPIC went national and then international during the next decade.

A particularly interesting research project has been conducted in Melbourne, funded by the US National Institute of Mental Health (NIMH). Called the STEP Study (Staged Treatment in Early Psychosis), it is characterized by many clinical and research steps. Participants in the study consist of high-risk, below-threshold, and brief psychotic symptom groups of young people (ages 12–25) as well as a comparison group.

- Step 1: Support and problem-solving for 6 weeks with a behavioral focus provided to all participants.

- Step 2: If people need more help, they are randomly split into two groups—one receives continued supports and the other cognitive behavioral therapy (CBT).
- Step 3: If more help is needed, then groups are randomly split; one receives placebo therapy and the other an antipsychotic medication. Participants are always randomized at various stages after the first 6 weeks.
- Follow-ups are planned at 4, 6, 9, 12, 18, and 24 months.

What I especially like about this protocol is that it recognizes that these kids are quite variable in their levels of distress. They are suffering, and instead of the "one-size-fits-all, rush to fix it!" approach, with psychiatrists tending to order medication as a matter of course,[33] we could all learn a great deal more about how to better triage and provide support.

In the past, there have been major delays worldwide in treating first-episode psychosis because it can be difficult to deduce whether a young person is experiencing garden-variety adolescent or early 20s turmoil or is, in fact, becoming psychotic. Early intervention was considered key to nipping the psychosis in the bud and ameliorating suffering sooner. McGorry traveled the world to advocate for more early intervention. For a while, he was affectionately teased and called "The Qantas Professor of Psychiatry" (Qantas is Australia's national airline). Eventually, EPPIC blossomed into an expanded worldwide network using varied approaches. Other centers in many other countries also came into being, such as those in Norway, Denmark, and the United States (including the Departments of Psychiatry at Columbia, Yale, and the University of California at Los Angeles, which employ a protocol called RAISE with some now also employing STEP).[34]

Sydney: Highlighting Yet Another Courageous Psychiatrist

In Sydney, the largest city in Australia, Alan Rosen has battled local, state, and the federal government in Canberra, working on behalf of others for excellence in the care and understanding of patients with significant distress and impairment and their families. For more than four decades, as a psychiatrist and professor, he has raised a ruckus and caused commotions everywhere. He has pursued his cause through commissions, standards, writing, teaching, conferences, research, service development, and as Director and Clinical Director of the Royal North Shore Hospital and Community Mental Health Services.

From the time I met Rosen in Sydney, back in 1991, I had to put on my roller skates just to keep up with him. He has softly and persistently spoken and written about recovery, healing, interdisciplinary teamwork, the importance of destigmatizing, the value of culture, the loving care of kinship networks, and reverence for Australian Aboriginal people and their land—the list goes on. Although eventually he did receive some local, state, and federal awards for his work, Rosen continues to fight the good fight because governments and belief systems are extremely difficult to change and sometimes even go backward.[35]

Every country has at least a handful of doctors and other professionals who fight for their patients like Roman gladiators, often at the risk of losing their jobs and reputations. They do it to improve care and services, joining with many voices of consumers and their families in tenacious battles.[36,37] Many such fighters have been covered in this book. I wish that we had many more such heroes, and I hope that the next generation will also take up the cause. We seem to be on the cusp of change.

20

US Programs

For 40 years, I had the great pleasure of periodically sitting at a table in New York City while eating delicious dinners and listening to clinicians from all over the world. These dinners were hosted by social worker Margaret Newmark and psychiatrist Christian Beels. They both spent a lifetime helping individuals and families in a wide variety of ways.[1,2] Beels was the founder of the Fellowship in Public Psychiatry at the New York State Psychiatric Institute (NYSPI), which still gives newly graduated psychiatrists a year of experience in their choice of programs in the New York area. Beels also taught psychiatry residents about the social context of their work. "This was the only place in the curriculum where the psychiatric effects of race, poverty, and immigration were taken up" (personal communication, C.C. Beels, March 19, 2021). The lack of training on these issues in the past, in favor of the mainstream biomedical curriculum, was unfortunate because understanding these influences is key to the recovery process. This fellowship has helped to integrate a wider curriculum across all years of training in psychiatry.[3]

Beels helped devise many changes in existing systems, including converting an old Bronx post office into a community mental health center (CMHC). As a member of the Board of Project Renewal, Beels worked with the director, Ed Geffner, to convert a central Manhattan hotel into a residence for mentally ill homeless people, including a program in the dining room where they could learn to work in the food industry (personal communication, C.C. Beels, March 19, 2021).

Margaret Newmark worked with another group at NYSPI, under the direction of psychiatrist William McFarlane, which tested psychoeducation with multifamily groups as a vehicle for hospital discharge for patients with schizophrenia. This project showed the superiority of such

Recovery from Schizophrenia. Courtenay M. Harding, Oxford University Press. © Courtenay M. Harding 2024.
DOI: 10.1093/oso/9780195380095.003.0020

groups over those families with unsupported discharge plans for their loved ones.[4] In addition, Newmark in New York City and Carol Anderson in her Pittsburgh family studies[5] also noticed that helpful support and sharing between families often goes on during breaks between sessions in the cafeteria, lobby, or the hallway—any place they could find.

Beels and Newmark introduced me to many other pioneers in rehabilitation and recovery programs, as well as to new clinical practices that have evolved over time. I had the opportunity to meet some of these innovators and then often to see their programs, both in the United States and abroad, firsthand. The rest of this chapter will briefly describe just a few of the many successful recovery strategies that have emerged in the United States. It is definitely time to rethink how we do things, especially for community care with its usual focus on stabilization, maintenance medications and entitlements, and here are some guiding examples.

Boston, Massachusetts: Psychiatric Rehabilitation

In a modest two-story building on Commonwealth Avenue in the heart of Boston University's campus is a remarkable group of independent people who are complementary thinkers. The Center for Psychiatric Rehabilitation (CPR) was built, idea by idea, and guided by the vision of psychologist William Anthony. Since the early 1970s, the Center has wielded worldwide influence.[6]

Anthony started out as a young Army officer working at Walter Reed Hospital in Washington, DC, in the late 1960s, with soldiers coming back from the Vietnam War. He noticed that men with physical wounds were being provided with rehabilitation, including occupational training. He wondered why his patients in the psychiatric unit were not provided with the same opportunities.

Having been exposed to the thinking of Carl Rogers,[7] Viktor Frankl,[8] and Abraham Maslow,[9] all humanistic psychologists, Anthony began a lifelong career of carefully piecing together the new field of psychiatric rehabilitation. In the Davidson et al. book mentioned in an earlier chapter, the authors wrote,

> Rogers was certainly a pioneer in the pursuit of active, reflective listening. Frankl understood the importance of having a sense of purpose and meaning

in life and Maslow appreciated the urgency of meeting an individual's basic need for home, income, food, safety, and companionship.[10] (pg. 17)

Anthony incorporated all of those understandings into a comprehensive approach and was always influenced by the voices of people with lived experience. He was supported by Art Dell Orto, then Chair of the Department of Rehabilitation Counseling, and encouraged to break new ground in the area of rehabilitation for individuals with psychiatric conditions. Anthony wrote the first grant, and the Center was funded. After all, professors also need a kind and helpful environment in which to build a life for themselves and others.

The Center is now led by Dori Hutchinson, Zlatka Russinova, Sally Rogers, Marianne Farkas, Larry Kohn, Kim Mueser, and many others, past and present. Researchers at the Center devised eight value-laden comprehensive components essential for any rehabilitation strategy. These critical approaches include

- *Person orientation* (a focus on the whole person with talents and aspirations as well as limitations),
- *Functioning* (performance of everyday activities),
- *Support* (for as long as needed or wanted to reach a self-defined goal),
- *Environmental specificity* (a focus on functioning in the domains of living, learning, working, and socializing),
- Full *involvement* (a real collaboration),
- *Choice* (the person's right to self-determination),
- *Outcome orientation* (evaluation determined by impact on person), and
- *Growth potential* (an inherent capacity for success and satisfaction that particularly emerges in a hopeful and supportive environment).[11]

These values are infused into the services delivered by the Center as well as into all of its research, training, and dissemination activities. Since 1979, the Center has been funded as a rehabilitation research and training center by the federal government, as well as by philanthropists for direct services.

Anthony himself had always been less focused on models and more on his vision of a deeply personal and unique process.[12] (pg. 15) One of Anthony's favorite poems by Robert Frost has a line which reads, "Something there is that doesn't love a wall."[13] He practiced the art of speaking simply and quietly about very complicated matters and felt that supporting hope and choice was absolutely non-negotiable.

The CPR also practices what it preaches to the world in its own clinical program, called the Learning Center, which is run on the first floor of the Center. It has successfully implemented the abovementioned eight essential ingredients. One of the inspiring projects within the Learning Center began in 2000 and caused much excitement, drawing city-wide attention. A young and creative teacher named Sasha Bowers was trained in an empowering technique called Photovoice.[14] She had interested students use instant cameras to take pictures of what recovery could look like. Off they went around Boston, returning with amazing photographs of people, places, and things (such as an open gate). Next, they were taught how to narrate their photos. The pictures and stories were put together on poster boards and mounted on the Center's walls to share their images of recovery with others. This Photovoice project was opened to the public so that others could learn about recovery from the very people who were striving to recover. Soon there was press coverage of the initiative. Others, including me, began to use Photovoice as a tool to empower recovery in participants and to help professionals learn what recovery means to those who are living with mental health conditions, as well as to affect social change. I had a group of visiting clinicians from Denmark take cameras and do the same thing. I remember a touching photo of a vibrant yellow dandelion emerging from a steel manhole cover as an example.

Springfield, Vermont: The Diner Project

I came upon another example of people integrating back into the community in Vermont, one unconnected to Dr. Brooks's work at the state hospital. In the early 1980s, Jerry Cutler, a young pre-care/aftercare services manager, was approached by four participants at the local mental health center (Mental Health Services of Southeastern Vermont) in Springfield. This center was located in an old mill building sitting next to the roaring Black River, slightly back from the main street of this small town. Four men bemoaned the closure of a very small local cafe that sat just in front of the center on Main Street. It was so small that the building was just a bit wider than the width of its front door. Called "Ma's Diner," this had been the only place to hang out when people were not at the center. It was owned by a negligent landlord who had let it fall into significant disrepair, and the

Health Department had posted a notice on the door that the café was to shut down.

Cutler was inspired to drive up to Montpelier, the state capital, and plead with the Department of Vocational Rehabilitation to give him $3,000 to teach these four men how to paint and help renovate the diner. Next, he approached townspeople such as the manager of a local motel, the head of a busy department store, and local contractors asking them to join an advisory board for the project. He convinced the landlord to give him three rent-free months to fix up the place. Cutler had never rehabilitated a building before, and so having knowledgeable people coach him was a wise idea. He also discovered that some of the clinicians at the center had relevant building skills and would volunteer to help. The contractors on his Community Board also provided left-over lumber.

I have pictures showing the inside of the diner both before and after the project. It was filthy, dark, and gloomy at the beginning but the end result was light, bright, and airy. The rehab team uncovered a skylight and painted the walls white with red trim. A furniture-making group, composed of other so-called disabled people from across the river, made new booths and stools for the counter. Another group wove colorful placemats and a wall hanging out of old but clean fabric strips from cast-aside woolen skirts, coats, and pants—a traditional New England recycling strategy.

There was now a need for cooks, food managers, servers, and cashiers. Slowly but surely, more and more people were pulled from the Day Room at the Center, where they had previously spent their days smoking and watching TV, to learn these jobs. As soon as they were trained by Margaret (aka Marnie) Smith, a day-treatment specialist, some were hired by the motel or the department store down the street, and so more people had to be trained. Staff came to have their coffee breaks, and the waiters got practice doing their jobs, too.

The painters formed a business in the community. The carpenters began rehabbing people's garages into recreational rooms. A famous New York department store gave contracts to the furniture workers for some Danish-inspired chairs and to the weavers for more of their placemats.

The governor of the state at that time, Richard Snelling, came down to cut the ribbon at the reopening ceremonies for Ma's Diner, which now had a fancy new sign, "The Diner by the Falls." Having the governor come to town certainly drew the attention of the townspeople, and the occasion was written up in a glossy magazine and in local newspapers.[15] Whereas community members used to shun the old diner, now grandmothers and children came there to eat. The entire Mental Health Center staff was rejuvenated, as were people once seen only as patients. Everyone was truly integrated into the fabric of the town—thanks to $3,000, remarkable ingenuity, and energetic effort. I have since heard of a derelict motel in the middle of a Wyoming town rehabbed into eight apartments for and by people at the local center, as well as bakeries, restaurants, and art galleries in other states.

Brooklyn, New York: The Mental Health Court

While working in New York City sometime around 2010, I discovered the Brooklyn Mental Health Court and had the honor of sitting in the jury box with visiting judges from Delaware and Pennsylvania to watch how it worked. The Brooklyn judge, Matthew D'Emic, who seemed to be a natural clinician, and the District Attorney (DA)'s office had struck a deal.[16] The DA could offer a deal to some defendants, usually a young person who had committed a nonviolent crime and who had exhibited significant mental health issues. If the person would agree to attend a clinical program and receive help for 2 years, then the DA would expunge the judicial record and the person could start life fresh and untainted by a criminal record.

The person was expected to come to court regularly with a court-appointed attorney, and the DA's office would also be represented. The courtroom was often full of family members and friends. The judge would call the defendant up to the bench, along with the two lawyers, and have a quiet discussion about how things were going. The clinic and social service providers would also send reports, and their work demonstrated accountability. This Court also had its own social workers and other trained staff. They initially assessed the person and coordinated appropriate resources in the community. The Court designated three levels of success. When the judge announced a successful completion of one level, the entire courtroom, including the bailiff, would break into applause and cheers.

These courts were "dedicated to improving safety, court operations, and the well-being of justice-involved individuals living with mental illness by linking them with court-supervised, community-based treatment."[17] There are 29 such Mental Health Courts in the state of New York, and they have served more than 9,000 people. In the entire United States, there are at least 300 Mental Health Courts, and a training curriculum has been created.[18]

New York City: Fountain House

When I worked in New York between 2009 and 2012, I also hung out at the famous Fountain House project, started in the late 1940s by a group of six patients from Rockland State Hospital, in New York state, where they had devised a social group. These six left the hospital for New York City but continued to meet on the steps of the New York Public Library. Later they found a place to hang out on West 47th Street. Jim Beard, a social worker, worked hand-in-hand with them, painting the place alongside these "members." Fountain House eventually became world famous and has replicated itself in 40 states and across the globe at least 320 times.[19,20]

Members essentially run the place in real collaboration with a small professional staff, many of whom have recovered from serious emotional distress. There is a cafe, a daily newspaper, a research department, a place to grow plants, and many other jobs to be had. The programs there teach social and work skills, provide tutoring and mentoring, offer literacy and computer classes, and make scholarships and financial assistance available. The Transitional Employment Program provides members with job coaches and helps them to begin working outside the program; it also provides opportunities to pursue a GED high school diploma, return to school or college, or be placed in a permanent job.

Other programs there provide affordable housing (a neat trick in New York City), and evening and weekend social, cultural, and sports activities. Programs include health and substance abuse initiatives and visits to High Point Farm in nearby New Jersey. This is another place where "everyone knows your name."

I went to Fountain House to help mount a pilot research project on youth in transition, employing some of the members as emerging investigators. We first looked at the questions for which we wanted some answers; then we looked at inclusion and exclusion criteria. We decided on a rich mixed-methods design, picked the instruments (some structured, some objective, some subjective), and saw what variables they assessed. Procedures were important, including the rules of confidentiality and privacy, as well as Institutional Review Board review. Training was provided on sticking to research questions as asked and recording answers accurately, with practice and more practice. Then we followed with data collection and analyses, with Sally Rogers at Boston University helping to analyze the answers. There was a vivid description of the sample as well a comparison with the rest of the Fountain House members. The size and density of social networks, supports, and relationships was assessed using an instrument called the Star Chart, developed by this author.[21] This effort was considered an important collaborative pilot study for its time and engendered much discussion about the findings and implications for behavioral health services. This study also revealed that people with the lived experience of mental disorders could indeed learn to do serious research projects.

Long Beach, California: The Village ISA

Another special place is The Village, a program of Mental Health America of Los Angeles.[22] Martha Long, the founding director,[23] and Mark Ragins, the chief psychiatrist, were determined to create a different kind of place than the typical CMHC.[24] In 1997, within an hour of arriving for a visit, I felt at home. Staff members and I ate in the Village Cafeteria run by members, used the same bathrooms, found administrative office doors open and welcoming, and saw that police or security guards were not stationed at the front door. Such practices communicate a welcoming tone rather than a mistrustful or suspicious one. These strategies have not often been used in other CMHCs, where there is a deliberate separation and hierarchy between those serving and those being served.

New members were provided a laminated "menu" of recovery-based options in employment, education, and housing, along with an explanation of each option from which they were encouraged to choose. Before that, Ragins spent time with each new member, asking specific questions and listening to their answers. He took down a history and showed it to each person asking, "Did I get this right?" How many contemporary clinicians do that? Working with people who had often been experiencing homelessness and/or incarceration in addition to serious mental illness, Ragins and the member's personal service coordinator (case manager) would help members find a home, a job, get back to school, reconnect with family, and/

or find a church, synagogue, mosque, or temple for their spiritual growth. All of this was done prior to efforts to reduce alcohol and drug use, not as a prerequisite to services. This last strategy is often reversed by other systems of care and with less functional success.

The Village and its nurses, social workers, peer advocates, administrators, and psychiatrists had to learn to be person-centered and not illness- and medication-focused. Yes, medications were prescribed, but identifying and supporting "quality of life" outcome became the emphasis. Ragins has written extensively on the obligation of recovery-oriented programs to help members attain "hope, empowerment, self-responsibility, and meaningful roles" in their lives.[25] Ragins and Mental Health America Los Angeles' CEO Dave Pilon also found that traditional outcome measurements sought by the state did not support this kind of growth. Pilon and his team created a tool to chart the movement of members from one stage of growth to another, giving staff a clearer picture of each member's level of risk, current engagement with the mental health system, degree of functional skills currently possessed, and need for support. They then helped programs and agencies from around the country apply this tool to their everyday mental health services.[26]

The Village also provided sold-out training sessions on recovery-based services for mental health professionals and clinicians of all stripes, including supervisors. Supervisors are particularly crucial to success; I have personally seen staff get excited about changing to recovery-based services only to be told, upon return to their agencies, "Well, that is all very well and good but we have no time to make these program changes, and how would we get reimbursed?"

On the employment front, the Village offered an array (or menu) of work options. Employment was available in one of the agency-owned businesses. There were the "Try Work for a Day" option, and there were part-time and full-time work available in the community. Numerous job developers were on staff to secure more options for members.

And there was the Village Cookie Shoppe.[27] This business was developed to provide further real work experience to people in recovery for whom employment was foreign. Cookies were sold on site and through the internet, and were not inexpensive. This was one of many creative ideas encouraged by Martha Long. The work that members did was competitive; the wages members were paid were real. The Village Cookie Shoppe was voted in a Long Beach newspaper's readers poll to be "The Best Dessert" in Long Beach.

In the beginning, employment director Paul Barry said staff would refer to all of these working menu options as "vocational services." But "vocational" did not invoke the recovery concept the Village wanted to promote. Vocational services are often busywork activities that prepare people to consider the possibility of perhaps working *some day*, at some time in the future—often a day that never comes. Barry wanted the services to be called "employment opportunities" because that's what they were. In fact, Barry walked around with a roll of dollar bills in his pocket, and, whenever someone used the word "employment" to describe these Village services, he would give them a dollar (and yes, he also charged a buck every time "vocational" was used). He eventually ran out of dollars but by then the Employment Department was born. This is but one example of how awash the mental health system is with language that should be reconsidered and replaced.

More functional real-life accomplishments were also recognized and should be in all programs that call themselves recovery-based. Recovery services, in the mental health field, have little to do with targeting symptoms. Instead, this means that great efforts are made to help people create (or recover) an identity that is not defined by the diagnosis and related behaviors. This often significantly reduces pain and suffering. At the Village, people receiving services are encouraged to set goals and take on an array of new roles (and new identities). Such new roles could include being a worker, a student, a church/temple/mosque member, a substance-free individual, a family member, or many combinations from this list.

Based on the nearby Hollywood's Oscars, the Village held an annual "Golden Ducky Award" ceremony during which functional accomplishments and new roles were recognized and celebrated. Everyone got dressed up for the event, strolled past a rented limo parked out front, and walked up a long red carpet to the entrance of the church borrowed for the evening. Attendees were met with cameras with flashbulbs recording this occasion as they enter the building. Instead of an Oscar, a little yellow rubber duck, chosen in honor of the Muppet Ernie from the *Sesame Street* television program, was awarded to each person who had achieved and maintained a goal for 6 months or more. In *Sesame Street*, Ernie took his ducky everywhere until one day he put down his comforting ducky to learn to play the saxophone.[28]

Denver, Colorado: How the Religious Community and Psychiatry Got Together

While I was working at the med school in Denver during the 1990s, I was part of a team training and supervising senior residents about public psychiatry.[29] Most of these almost-graduated physicians were unhappy about this because they really wanted to be in private practice as soon as possible. They thought that Gordon Neligh, Ruth Ryan (now Myers), and I were delusional in our obvious enthusiasm for working with the people who had the most complicated lives. We gave these residents double supervision, one at the mental health clinic to which they were assigned for a year and one at the university. We gave them a year's seminar series as well. About 80% stayed in the public sector after graduation as I recall.

One of our invited seminar lecturers was working at the University Hospital as a chaplain. She raised our awareness about the gaps in training for religious communities about mental health as well as in psychiatry about religion. To address this gap, one Saturday we were able to gather together members of the Denver Council of Churches and our department in order to spend the day teaching one another. The Council members spoke about how often they were the first line of approach for families and individuals. They were uneasy about their abilities to determine who needed a referral and how to make one. The psychiatrists had been uneasy about differentiating between what was religious thinking and what was religiosity as a symptom, and they had often misinterpreted these conversations in clinical assessments. In fact, research has shown that at least 50% of patients considered that relying on something "larger than they were" (e.g., through a formal religion, Mother Nature, art, or music) which was very important to the healing process.[30] This collaborative, reciprocal training was important and proved helpful for both sides, as well as for individuals and their families.

Monterey, Massachusetts: Gould Farm

One of the oldest, most straightforward approaches to recovery is to form a community in which each person is an essential element and has a contributing role to play. This structure is radically different from that of a general mental health program in which one group provides care to another who, suffering, passively receives it.

Gould Farm is the oldest version of a true community of this type in the United States. It began in the beautiful Berkshire mountains in Western Massachusetts more than 100 years ago.[31] Everyone who participates has a critical job to do and is expected to perform it consistently so the farm can continue to thrive. There are cows to tend, loaves of bread to bake, and vegetables to grow. Nearly all of the 120 multigenerational participants live on campus, and everyone brings skills and interests to enrich the community. Modern concepts of treatment are provided, when needed, such as cognitive behavioral therapy (CBT), dialectical behavioral therapy (DBT), or open dialogue, and include the lowest possible dosages of medications if they have not already been tapered off. Music is employed as another way to bring people together, and every day begins with music performed right after breakfast. People who were once considered patients with serious and persistent problems in the outside world now see themselves through the work they do, not as patients.

Everyone relies on everyone else, as a farm family demands. People with lived experience are on equal footing with staff to help make the farm a success. Diagnosis is less important than the person. A strength-based approach is used, and significant improvement generally occurs within 6–24 months. Transition back to the community at large is also part of the continuity of care. It should be noted that Gould Farm, like other similar programs, is not a residential treatment center that focuses primarily on symptom reduction, but targets instead a more natural process of healing. This helps a person once severely alienated from him- or herself and society to reintegrate with a renewed sense of self and place in the world.

Portland, Oregon: Dual Diagnosis Anonymous

Dual Diagnosis Anonymous (DDA) is an authorized version of a 12-step program with five additional steps adapted to the needs of people who have co-occurring problems with both alcohol and drugs and mental health challenges. This is a critical peer support service because approximately 50% of people with major mental health challenges also struggle with substance use problems, and only about 10% receive help.[32] DDA was founded in 1996, by Vietnam War veteran Corbett Monica, who had experienced mental health problems due to trauma experienced in the war and which had led him to a heroin addiction. Upon getting clean and sober, he began taking others with co-occurring disorders to Alcoholics Anonymous (AA) and Narcotics Anonymous (NA) meetings, but people with both problems were often asked not to return. As a result, Monica developed the "12-Step Plus 5 Program" in 1998. Upon moving to Oregon in 2005, he obtained public funding from the new Commissioner of Mental Health, and Addictions, Robert Nikkel, MSW, who was previously an addiction counselor. The extra five steps involve acknowledging both illnesses, accepting help for both conditions, understanding the importance of a variety of interventions, combining illness self-management with peer supports and spirituality, and working with the program by helping others. Each DDA group has one primary purpose—to carry its message of hope and recovery to those who still suffer from the effects of a dual diagnosis. Meetings allow for "cross-talk" in ways that AA and NA tend to not approve. Meetings use the 12-Step Plus 5 as a framework but focus largely on peer supports, personal acceptance, and practical ways to cope with mental health and substance use problems.

There are in-person meetings throughout Oregon in prisons, the state hospital, community mental health programs, peer support organizations, residential facilities, churches, and other settings. Online meetings were established during the COVID crisis, which expanded access greatly for members who could not attend the in-person meetings. DDA has steadily evolved to include community activities like picnics, bowling events, and other drug-free social opportunities for members and others. There has been a steady growth in meetings, sites, and activities. Meetings have become available in many states and internationally in the United Kingdom, Ireland, the Netherlands, Italy, Germany, and South Africa. Qualitative studies conducted in the United Kingdom at the University of West London[33] and in the United States[34] showed themes expressed by members that included acceptance of and from others, self-development for improvements in social interaction and employment, and hope for future aspirations and sense of purpose. Program materials, such as the handbook written by Monica, have been translated into Italian and other languages. Responses to the DDA supports have been enthusiastic and widespread. Many DDA members tell of dramatic improvements in their lives and even life-saving effects of the supports.

Vermont: The Wellness Recovery Action Plan

Many other clinical contributions have come directly and independently from people with the lived experience of mental disorders, such as Mary Ellen Copland, who had dealt with major depression. Many years ago she asked her Vermont psychiatrist what she could do to help herself get better. To his credit he told her that he was not aware of any activities, at that point in time, but that he would look into it. He returned to say he could not find any. So Copland developed the Wellness Recovery Action (WRAP) Plan for herself; now it is helping many others worldwide. The Plan aims to help people figure out for themselves what triggers crises, how to avoid them, how to cope, how to stabilize oneself in a preplanned way, and much more.[35,36]

Massachusetts: Common Ground

Dr. Patricia Deegan, who was labeled with schizophrenia and languished in a hospital for more than 17 years, decided to leave the facility and become a psychologist. She has provided valuable insights into the emotional lives of people, their strengths, and the battles with stigma and discrimination, especially coming from staff, of all people. Among her many projects, she devised a computerized method (called Common Ground) to help people better explain themselves to psychiatrists about their medications, how the meds make them feel, and what else is helping to reduce symptoms.[37] This work was accomplished in the psychiatrist's front office with a peer aide. Her entire website offers a myriad of helpful workshops, webinars, and keynotes on recovery oriented practices, peer supports, personal medicine leading to empowerment, personal reflection, and self-discovery.[38]

Kansas: Supported Housing

Dr. Priscilla Ridgway, in Kansas, received her doctorate in social work and has led many federal efforts to revise care systems based on one's strengths rather than psychopathology and to make care more responsive to the needs of people. Her many contributions include not only helping the Maine–Vermont Comparison Study get off the ground with me and Michael DeSisto, but also projects like Supported Housing, developed with Paul Carling,[39] the reshaping of clinical and scientific responsibilities[40] and the application of the Capabilities Approach with Larry Davidson.[41] The Supported Housing approach entailed finding the best setting for a person's desires and wishes and bringing supports to them based on their changing needs—rather than making them move every time their needs changed, leaving friends and having to adjust to new environments.

All of the programs discussed in these last two chapters, and many more not listed here, have been created either by persons with the lived experience or in conjunction with other inventive and caring clinicians and researchers. These investigators have listened with a large degree of respectful humility to the individual needs expressed by receivers of services and their families. The most crucial ingredient has been this multicollaboration on the invention of new approaches, new understandings, and new pathways and the focus on weaving mental health back into the healthy fabric of a person, their family, and community.

Celebrating Every Step Forward

If only state block grants and behavioral healthcare companies would understand that by helping people reclaim their lives, rather than saddling them with medications and few options, such individuals would eventually leave the system of care, contribute to their communities, and save dollars. It would be more helpful and better for the bottom line if behavioral health with state and federal legislators would underwrite pathways out of the system by creating more flexible monetary supports for approaches based on real recovery models and using the large number of innovative and successful programs we already have developed. Currently, even those programs touted as evidence-based are rarely among the services offered—let alone those successful enough to be considered as practice-based evidence. Unfortunately, without societal imperatives; a renewed emphasis on social, psychological, and environmental aspects of psychiatry; and with an integrated public health model in place, these behavioral health managed care companies and other agencies will always have many new customers and overwhelmed budgets. They should be happy to let go of their current programs, but *only* when they have been provided with other ways to help patients get their lives back and repair the iatrogenic damage caused by keeping people chronic.

Thanks to the kinds of projects described in this chapter, the Centers for Medicaid and Medicare Services (CMS) are beginning to pay attention and understand how different these types of programs are from the narrow biomedical model. In 2018, Congress passed the SUPPORT Act, and, in 2021, it passed the American Rescue Plan Act (ARPA). However, these funding mechanisms are being used to target previously cut or underimplemented basic services, such as more mobile crisis teams in some states and telehealth services in others, Now some legislators are also beginning to understand that people can become taxpayers rather than economic liabilities when they get their lives back. They are starting to understand that reallocated funding will be necessary to target recovery-focused programs.

It is high time to weave the whole person back together. Rehabilitation, psychology, psychotherapy, education, peer-related activities, nursing, social work, and a newly minted biopsychosocial psychiatry have many skills and benefits to offer—including, incidentally, symptom reduction—and should no longer take a back seat to biomedical psychiatry, long-term medications, and community quasi-institutionalization. We need to embrace, instead, an integrated biopsychosocial approach to both mental and physical health, with psychiatric medicine used only as an adjunct, in smaller doses, for much shorter durations, and only for better understood and newly redesignated subgroups. Remember, even one-half to two-thirds of the most chronic cases, once labeled as suffering from schizophrenia, got their lives back when given a chance.

It cheers me to see an energetic new coterie of young clinicians from across disciplines beginning to step up, rethink everything, walk the path with people who are struggling rather than being apart from them. They will all find joy in their work helping people and their families reclaim their lives, and help create and sustain truly vibrant and integrated communities of healthier and happier people.

Notes

CHAPTER 1

1. D'Agostino, L. (1948). *The history of public welfare in Vermont, no. 198.* St. Michael's College Press, 131–138.
2. Deutsch, A. (1937). *The mentally ill in America: A history of their care and treatment from colonial times.* Doubleday, Doran.
3. Ponzio, R. (1981). *Madness, law, and medicine in Vermont: 200 years of institutionalism.*
4. Hemenway, A. M. (1886). The poor house. *The Vermont Historical Gazetteer.*
5. Dain, N. (1964). *Concepts of insanity in the United States, 1789–1865.* Rutgers University Press, 5.
6. U. S. Census Bureau Report. (1895).
7. D'Agostino (1948), 93.
8. See also Ponzio (1981).
9. See also Swift, E. M., & Beach, M. (1984). *The New England System. Brattleboro Retreat, 1834–1984: 150 years of change.* The Retreat, 31–37
10. Gerard, D. L. (1998). Chiarugi and Pinel considered: Soul's brain/person's mind. *Journal of the History of the Behavioral Sciences, 33*(4), 381–403.
11. Ibid.
12. Bockhoven, S. (1963). *Moral treatment in community mental health.* Springer.
13. Ibid.
14. Ibid.
15. Ibid.
16. Anthony, W. A., & Liberman, R. P. (1986). The practice of psychiatric rehabilitation: Historical, conceptual, and research base. *Schizophrenia Bulletin, 12*(4), 542–559.
17. Bockhoven (1963).
18. www.historyofyork.org.uk/themes/georgian/the-retreat
19. www.theretreatatyork.org.uk
20. Millon, T. (1969). *Modern psychopathology: A biosocial approach to maladaptive learning and functioning.* W. P. Saunders.
21. Swift & Beach (1984).
22. Ibid.
23. Ibid.
24. Ponzio (1981), 69.

25. www.dhhs.state.nc.us

26. Brown, T. J. (1998). *Dorothea Dix: New England reformer.* Harvard University Press, 123.

27. www.dhhs.state.nc.us

28. http://www.PBS.org./teacher/horace.html

29. Deutsch, A. (1937). 177.

30. www.kirkpridebuildings.com

31. Sarason, I. G., & Sarason, B. R. (2004). *Abnormal psychology: The problem of maladaptive behavior.* Prentice Hall.

32. Woodward, S. B (1850). Observations on the medical treatment of insanity. (Read at a meeting of the Association of Medical Superintendents of American Institutions for the Insane, May 1846.) *American Journal of Insanity, 7,* 1–34.

33. Draper, L. C. (1887). *The Vermont asylum for the insane: Its annals for fifty years (1836–1886).* Hildreth & Fales. In Ponzio, R. (1981), 172.

34. Deutsch (1937), quoted by Ponzio (1981), 152.

35. Ibid.

36. Godding, W. (1890). Aspects and outlook of insanity in America. *American Journal of Insanity, 47,* 1–16.

37. Wing, J. K. (1962). Institutionalism in mental hospitals. *British Journal of Social and Clinical Psychology, 1*(1), 38–51. https://doi.org/10.1111/j.2044-8260.1962.tb00680

38. Goffman, E. (1961). *Asylums: Essays on the social situation of mental patients and other inmates.* Anchor Books.

39. Ludwig, A. M. (1971). Chronic schizophrenics as behavioral engineers. *Journal of Nervous and Mental Disease, 152,* 31–40.

40. Grob, G. N. (1991). *From asylum to community: Mental health policy in modern America.* Princeton University Press.

41. https://history of Massachusetts.org/danvers-state-hospital-cemetery

42. Swift & Beach (1984).

43. Ibid.

44. Kincheloe, M. R., & Hunt, H. G. (1989). *Empty beds: History of Vermont state hospital.* Northlight Studio Press, 4–5.

45. Ibid., 4–5.

46. Ibid., 5.

47. Ibid., 29.

48. Ibid., 30.

49. Ibid., 182–183.

50. Ibid., 100.

51. Perkins, H. F. (1931). *Eugenics survey of Vermont.* University of Vermont Press.

52. (2020). *The future of the human: A confluence of genetic medicine & eugenics.* University of Chicago, 2020.

53. Kincheloe & Hunt (1989), 36–47.

54. Ibid., 47.

55. Deutsch, A. (1948). *The shame of the states: Mental illness and social policy. The American experience* (1st ed.). Harcourt, Brace, 177.

56. Kincheloe & Hunt (1989), 106–107.

57. Chittick, R. A., Brooks, G. W., Irons, F. S., & Deane, W. N. (1961). *The Vermont story: Rehabilitation of chronic schizophrenic patients.* Queen City Printers (out of print).

CHAPTER 2

1. Tillotson, K. J. (1932). Some newer trends in psychiatry. *New England Journal of Medicine, 207,* 8–12.

2. Murphy, R. Vermont Historical Society-Leahy Library Reference Desk, Montpelier, Vt. Personal Communication, January 29, 2019.

3. American Psychiatric Association (APA). (1980). *Diagnostic and statistical manual of mental health disorders* (3rd ed.). American Psychiatric Press.

4. Taintor, Z. 11th World Congress of the World Association of Psychosocial Rehabilitation in Milan, Italy. He took part in the original APA survey. Personal Communication, November 11, 2012.

5. Kincheloe, M. R., & Hunt, H. G. (1989). *Empty beds: A history of Vermont State Hospital.* Northlight Studio Press, 104.

6. Grob, G. N. (1991). From hospital to community: Mental health policy in modern America. *Psychiatric Quarterly, 62*(3), 187–212.

7. Williams, R. H., & Ozarin, L. D. (1968). *Community mental health: An international perspective.* Jossey-Bass.

8. Reed, K. L. (1992). History of federal legislation for persons with disabilities. *American Journal of Occupational Disabilities, 46*(5), 397–408.

9. Anthony, W. A., Cohen, M. R., & Farkas, M. (1990). Curriculum for the core disciplines for professional preservice training in working with the long-term mentally ill. In Dale L. Johnson (Ed.), *Service needs of the seriously mentally ill: Training implications for psychology* (pp. 51–58). American Psychological Association Press.

10. Foley, H. A., & Scharfstein, S. S. (1983). *Madness and government: Who cares for the mentally ill?* American Psychiatric Press.

11. Ibid.

12. Deutsch, A. (1948). The *shame of the states: Mental illness and social policy-the American experience* (1st ed.). Harcourt, Brace.

13. Grob, G. N. (1991).

14. Ward, M. J. (1946). *The snake pit.* Random House.

15. Foley & Scharfstein (1983).

16. Beers, C. W. (1908). *The mind that found itself: An autobiography.* Longmans Green.

17. Shakow, D. (1969). *Clinical psychology as science & profession.* Aldine.

18. Strother, C. R. (Ed.). (1956). *Psychology and mental health.* American Psychological Association. https://doi.org/10.1037/10791-000

19. Roe, A., Gustad, J. W., Moore, B. V., Ross, S., & Skodak, M. (Eds.). (1959). *Graduate education in psychology: Report of the Conference on Graduate Education in Psychology.* American Psychological Association. https://doi.org/10.1037/11398-000

20. The Commission for the Recognition of Specialties and Proficiencies in Professional Psychology (CRSPPP) recommended the Serious Mental Illness Psychology Specialty to the Council of Representatives on August 7, 2019. The recommendation was approved. American Psychological Association.

21. Eldred, D. M. (1957). Problems opening a rehabilitation house. *Mental Hospitals, 8*(5), 20–21.

22. Cox, L. E., Tice, C. J., & Long, D. D. (2019). *Introduction to social work: An advocacy-based profession* (2nd ed.). Sage Publications.

23. Deane, W. N., & Brooks, G. W. (1967). *Five-year followup of chronic hospitalized patients.* Vermont State Hospital & University of Vermont Press.

24. Peplau, H. (1989). Future directions in psychiatric nursing from the perspective of history. *Journal of Psychosocial Nursing and Mental Health, 27*(2), 18–28.

25. Kincheloe & Hunt (1989), 106.

26. Brooks, G. W., Deane, W. N., Lagor, R. C., & Curtis, B. B. (1963). Varieties of family participation in the rehabilitation of released chronic schizophrenic patients. *Journal of Nervous and Mental Disease, 136*(5), 432–444.

27. Kincheloe & Hunt (1989), 230.

28. Ibid., 231.

29. George Brooks, Personal Communication, October 10, 1980.

30. Fromm-Reichman, F. (1948). Notes on the development of treatment of schizophrenics by psychoanalytic psychotherapy. *Psychotherapy, 11*, 263–273.

31. Alexander, F. G., & Selesnick, S. T. (1966). *The history of psychiatry: An evaluation of psychiatric thought and practice from prehistoric times to the present.* Harper and Row.

32. Ozarin, L. D. (1954). Moral treatment and the mental hospital. *American Journal of Psychiatry, 111*(1), 371–378.

33. Greenblatt, M., Levinson, D. J., & Williams, R. H. (1957). *The patient and the mental hospital.* Free Press.

34. Cumming, J., & Clancy, I. L. W. (1956). Improving patient care through organizational changes in the mental hospital. *Psychiatry, 19*, 361–369.

35. Goffman, E. (1957). The characteristics of total institutions. Symposium on preventive and social psychiatry. Walter Reed Army Institute of Research, 43–84.

CHAPTER 3

1. Grob G. N. (1994). *The mad among us: A history of the care of America's mentally ill.* Free Press.

2. Spargo, M. (1989). WCAX Vermont radio report on April 4, 1951. In M. R. Kincheloe & H. G. Hunt, H. G. (Eds.), *Empty beds: A history of Vermont state hospital* (p. 64). Northlight Studio Press.

3. Kincheloe, M. R., & Hunt, H. G. (1989). *Empty beds: History of Vermont state hospital*. Northlight Studio Press, 68.

4. Ibid.

5. Ibid., 71.

6. Ban, T. A. (2007). Fifty years of chlorpromazine: A historical perspective. *Neuropsychiatric Disease Treatment, 3*(4), 495–500.

7. Ibid.

8. Uhrbrand, L., & Faurbye, A. (1960). Reversible and irreversible dyskinesia after treatment with perphenazine, chlorpromazine, reserpine, and electroconvulsive therapy. *Psychopharmacologia Journal*, 408–418.

9. Ibid.

10. Ibid.

11. www.cochrane,org/CD007655/HTN_reserpine-lowe. Accessed February 6, 2019.

12. www.wedgewoodpettrx.com/learning-center/.../reserpine-for-veterinary-use.html. Accessed February 6, 2019.

13. Gardner, D. M., Baldessarini, & Waraich, P. (2005). Modern antipsychotic drugs: A critical overview. *Canadian Medical Association Journal, 172*(13), 1703–1711.

14. Braslow, J., & Marder, S. (2019). History of Psychopharmacology. *Annual Review of Clinical Psychology, 15*(1), 25–50. http://dx.doi.org/10.1146/annurev-clinpsy-050718-095514. Retrieved from https://escholarship.org/uc/item/5qp5h8qs

15. Chittick, R. A., Brooks, G. W., Irons, F. S., & Deane, W. N. (1961). *The Vermont story*. Queen City Printers, 18–19.

16. Harding, C. M., Brooks, G. W., Ashikaga, T., Strauss, J. S., & Breier, A. (1987a). The Vermont longitudinal study of persons with severe mental illness: I. Methodology, study sample, and overall status 32 years later. *American Journal of Psychiatry, 144*(6), 718–726.

17. Chittick et al. (1961), 29–30.

18. Harding et al. (1987b), 728.

19. Chittick et al. (1961), 29–30.

20. American Psychiatric Association (APA). (1952). *Diagnostic and statistical manual: Mental disorders* (1st ed.). American Psychiatric Press.

21. Harding et al. (1987b), 728.

22. Ibid.

23. Cooper, J. E., Kendell, R. E., Gurland, B. J., Sharpe, L., & Copeland, J. R. M. (1972). *Psychiatric diagnoses in New York and London: A comparative study of mental hospital admissions*. Institute of Psychiatry, Maudsley Monograph Number 20. Oxford University Press.

24. APA (1952).

25. American Psychiatric Association (APA). (1980). *Diagnostic and statistical manual of mental disorders* (3rd ed.). American Psychiatric Press.

26. Harding et al. (1987b), 730.

27. Kraepelin, E. (1899). *Psychiatrie. Ein Lehrbuch für Studierende und Ärte*. Barth.

28. Chittick et al. (1961), 30.

29. Ibid., 29–30.

30. Ibid., 31.

31. Ibid.

32. Sullivan, H. S. (1953). *The interpersonal theory of psychiatry.* W. W. Norton.

33. Chittick et al. (1961), 65.

34. Ibid.

35. Ibid.

36. Harding et al. (1987b), 730.

37. Ayd, F. S. Jr. (1977, October). Ethical and legal dilemmas posed. *Medical-Moral Newsletter, 14*(8), 29–32.

38. Chittick et al. (1961), 65.

39. Public Law (PL) 789-113 – Barden-LaFollette Act (1943). USC. Washington, DC. US Govt. Printing Office.

40. PL 789-113 (1943).

41. Chittick et al. (1961), 5.

42. Ibid., 8–9.

43. Jones, M., Baker, A., Freeman, T., Merry, J., Pomryn, Sandler, J., & Tuxford, J. (1953). *The therapeutic community: A new treatment method in psychiatry* (1st ed.). Basic Books.

44. Jones et al. (1953).

45. Sullivan (1953).

46. Chittick et al. (1961), 17–20.

47. Ibid., 70.

48. Harding, C. M., & Keller, A. B. (1998). Long-term outcome of social functioning. In K. T. Mueser & N. Tarrier (Eds.), *The handbook of social functioning* (pp. 134–148). Allyn & Bacon of Simon & Schuster Educ. Gp.

49. Chittick et al. (1961), 15–16.

50. Ibid., 69.

51. Fromm-Reichmann, F. (1948). Notes on the development of treatment of schizophrenics by psychoanalytic psychotherapy. *Psychiatry, 11*(3), 263–273.

52. Chittick et al. (1961), 69.

53. Caplan, G. (1966). *Principles of preventive psychiatry* (1st ed., 4th printing ed.). London: Tavistock Pubs., ix.

54. Huessy, H. R. (1966). Commentary. In G. Caplan (Ed.), *Principles of preventive psychiatry* (1st ed., 4th printing ed.). London: Tavistock Pubs., 91.

CHAPTER 4

1. Chittick, R. A., Brooks, G. W., Irons, F. N., & Deane, W. N. (1961). *The Vermont story: Rehabilitation of Chronic Schizophrenic Patients.* Queen City Printers, 17 (out of print).

2. Mesazaros, A. F. (1960). Principles of research in a therapeutic community. In H. C. B. Denber (Ed.), *Research conference on therapeutic community* (pp. 45–54). C. C. Thomas.

3. Boas, F.(Ed.). (1938). *General anthropology.* Heath & Co.

4. Malinowski, B. (1939). The group and the individual in functional analysis. *American Journal of Sociology, 44,* 938–964.

5. Meade, M. (1928). *Coming of age in Samoa.* William Morrow and Co.

6. Husserl, E. (1965). Philosophy as rigorous science (1910). In Q. Lauer (Ed.), *Phenomenology and the crisis of philosophy.* Harper.

7. Sonnemann, E. (1954). *Existence and therapy: An introduction to phenomenological psychology and existential analysis.* Grune and Stratton.

8. Lewin, K. (1951). *Field theory in social service: Selected theoretical papers.* Dorwin Cartwright (Ed.). Harpers.

9. Kohler, W. (1947). *Gestalt psychology: An introduction to new concepts in modern psychology.* Liveright.

10. Chittick et al. (1961), 42.

11. Ibid.

12. Ibid., 43.

13. Ibid., 44.

14. Raskis, H. A. (1960). Cognitive restructuring: Why research is therapy. *Archives of General Psychiatry, 2*(6), 612–621.

15. Chittick et al. (1961), 42.

16. Kidd, B. A., & Kral, M. J. (2005). Practicing participatory action research. *Journal of Counseling Psychology, 52*(2), 187–195.

17. Einstein, A., & Infeld, L. (1938). *The growth of ideas from early concepts to relativity and quanta: The evolution of physics.* Cambridge University Press.

18. Kidd & Kral (2005), 187.

19. Ibid., 188, 190.

20. Ibid., 189.

21. Chittick et al. (1961), 57–74.

22. Ibid., 57.

23. Ibid.

24. Jones, M., Baker, A., Freeman, T., Merry, J., Pomryn, S. J., & Tuxford, J. (1953). *The therapeutic community: A new treatment method in psychiatry* (1st ed.). Basic Books.

25. Freud, S. (1901). *Fragment of an analysis of hysteria.* Standard Edition, 7.3.157. Hogarth Press & Institute of Psycho-Analysis.

26. Chittick et al. (1961), 59.

27. Ibid., 61.

28. Ibid., 62.

29. Ibid., 62.

30. Bachrach, L. L. (1993). Continuity of care and approaches to case management for long-term mentally ill patients. *Hospital and Community Psychiatry, 14*(5), 465–468. https://doi.org/10.1176/ps.44.5.465

31. Chittick et al. (1961), 34.

32. Ibid., 64.

33. Meyerson, A. (1939). Theory and principles of the "total push" method in the treatment of chronic schizophrenia. *American Journal of Insanity, 95*(3), 1197–1204. https://doi.org/10.1176/ajp.95.5.1197

34. Chittick et al. (1961), 62.

35. Ibid., 70.

36. Ibid., 69.

37. Ibid., 70.

38. Ibid., 69.

39. Ridgway, P. (2008). Supported housing in Section IV. Psychosocial Treatment. In Kim T. Mueser & Dilip V. Jeste (Eds.), *Clinical handbook of schizophrenia.* Guilford Press.

40. Chittick et al. (1961), 71.

41. Ibid.

42. Ibid.

43. Ibid.

44. Gordon Neligh, Personal Communication, October, 17, 1991.

45. Chittick et al. (1961), 72.

46. Bleuler, M. (1979). On schizophrenia psychoses. *American Journal of Psychiatry, 136*(11), 1403–1409. doi:10.1176/ajp.136.11.1403 PMID: 495791

47. Mental Retardation Facilities and Community Mental Health Centers Construction Act of 1963.77 STAT U. S.C. PUBLIC LAW 88-164 [S. 1576].

48. Rodrigues, C. (2017, April 17). *The origin and iterations of "not in my backyard."'*. WNYC News.

49. Kincheloe, M. R., & Hunt, H. G. (1988). *Empty beds: A history of Vermont State Hospital.* Northlight Studio Press, 114. ISBN 0-9622832-07 HB

50. Galen. (172 CE/1884). *Day's collacon: An encyclopaedia of prose quotations* (p. 223).

51. Chittick et al. (1961), 33.

52. Ibid., 84–85.

53. Beard, J. H., Propst, R. N., & Malamud, T. J. (1982). The Fountain House model of psychiatric rehabilitation. *Psychosocial Rehabilitation Journal.*

54. Chittick et al. (1961), 84.

55. Ibid.

56. Ibid., 84–85.

57. Ibid., 85.

58. Ibid.

59. Ibid., 85–94.

60. Ibid., 95–96.

61. Ibid., 96–97.

62. Ibid., 53.

63. Ibid., 55–56.

64. Rakfeldt & Strauss (1989).

65. Chittick et al. (1961), 56.

66. Kincheloe & Hunt (1989), 114.

67. Chittick et al. (1961), 53.
68. Joint Commission for Mental Illness and Health. (1961). *Final Report: Summary of recommendations. Action for Mental Health.* Basic Books, xix.

CHAPTER 5

1. Deane, W. N., & Brooks, G. W. (1967). *The five-year follow-up study.* (Unpublished monograph). Vermont State Hospital, University of Vermont, 1–96.
2. Ibid., 7.
3. Chittick, R. A., Brooks, G. W., Irons, F. R., & Deane, W. N. (1961). *The Vermont story: Rehabilitation of schizophrenic patients.* Queen City Printers (out of print).
4. American Psychiatric Association (APA). (1952). *Diagnostic and statistical manual- mental disorders* (1st ed.). American Psychiatric Press.
5. Harding, C. M., Brooks, G. W., Ashikaga, T., Strauss, J. S., & Breier, A. (1987a). The Vermont longitudinal study of persons with severe mental illness: I. Methodology, study sample, and overall status 32 years later. *American Journal of Psychiatry, 144*(6), 718–726.
6. Deane & Brooks (1967), 6.
7. Ibid., 13.
8. Ibid., 6.
9. Ibid., 14.
10. Ibid., 9.
11. Ibid., 14.
12. Ibid., 2–3.
13. Ibid., 13.
14. Ibid., appendix A, 76–80.
15. Ibid., 16.
16. Ibid., 12–13.
17. Casey, Robert S. (Ed.). (1958/1951). *Punched cards: Their applications to science and industry* (2nd ed.). Reinhold.
18. Deane & Brooks (1967), 17–22.
19. Ibid., 22.
20. Ibid., i–iii.
21. Ibid., 26–29.
22. Ibid., 29.
23. Ibid., ii–iii.
24. Harding, C. M. (1995). The interaction of biopsychosocial factors, time, and the course of schizophrenia: Time is the critical co-variate. In C. L. Shriqui & H. A. Nasrallah (Eds.), *Contemporary issues in the treatment of schizophrenia* (pp. 653–681). APA Press.
25. Harding, C. M., Zubin, J., & Strauss, J. S. (1992). Chronicity in schizophrenia revisited. *British Journal of Psychiatry, 161*(Suppl. 18), 27–37.

26. Galioni, E. F. (1960). *Evaluation of a treatment program for chronically ill schizo-phrenic patients--a six-year program.* In L. Appleby, J. M. Scher, & J. Cumming (Eds.), *Chronic schizophrenia: Explorations in theory and treatment* (pp. 303–324). Free Press. doi.org/10.1037/10778-015

27. Goldstein, H., Israel, R. H., Johnson, N. A., & Kramer, M. (1956). Application of life table methodology to the study of mental hospital populations. *Psychiatric Research Reports of the APA* (no. 5), 49–87.

28. Freeman, H. E., & Simmons, O. G. (1958). Mental patients in the community: Family settings and performance levels. *American Sociological Revue, 23*(2), 147–154.

29. Galioni (1960).

30. Goldstein et al. (1956).

31. Freeman & Simmons (1958).

32. Deykin, E. (1961). The reintegration of the chronic schizophrenic patient discharge to his family and community as perceived by the family. *Mental Hygiene, 45*(2), 235–246.

33. Evans A., Bullard, D., & Solomon, M. (1961). The family as a potential resource in the rehabilitation of the chronic schizophrenic patient: A study of sixty patients and their families. *American Journal of Psychiatry, 117*(12), 1075–1081.

34. Brown, G. W., Carstairs, G. M., & Topping, G. G. (1958). Post-hospital adjustment of chronic mental patients. *Lancet, 2,* 685–689.

35. Walker, R., & McCourt, J. (1965). Employment experience among two hundred schizophrenic patients in hospital and after discharge. *American Journal of Psychiatry, 122*(9), 3116–3119.

36. Wessler, M. M., & Kahn, V. L. (1963). Can the chronic schizophrenic patient remain in the community? A follow-up study of twenty-four long-term hospitalized patients returned to the community. *Journal of Nervous and Mental Disease, 136*(5), 455–463.

37. Wing, J. K. (1963). Rehabilitation of psychiatric patients. *British Journal of Psychiatry, 109,* 635–641.

38. Gruenberg, E., & Archer, J. (1979). Abandonment of responsibility for the seriously mentally ill. *The Milbank Memorial Fund Quarterly. Health and Society, 57*(4), 485–506. doi:10.2307/3349724

39. https://www.nimh.nih.gov/health/statistics/mental-illness

40. Tullis, P. (2019). When mental illness becomes a jail sentence. *The Atlantic.*

41. Kincheloe, M. R., & Hunt, H. G. (1989). *Empty beds: History of Vermont state hospital.* Northlight Studio Press, 116, 118.

42. Ibid., 116–118.

43. Ibid., 130.

44. Ibid., 130.

45. Ibid., 131.

46. Ibid., 130–131.

47. Ibid., 131.

48. Ibid.

49. Donoghue M., & Ryan, M. (2011, August 3). VT state hospital evacuated. *Burlington Free Press*, 1B & 7B.

50. Faher, M., & Hewitt, E. (2018, April 5). Vt. considers new psych hospital. *Valley News* (VtDigger).

51. Faher & Hewitt (2018).

52. Harding, et al. (1987a).

53. Harding, C. M., Brooks, G. W., Ashikaga, T., Strauss, J. S., & Breier, A. (1987b). The Vermont longitudinal study: II. Long-term outcome of subjects who retrospectively met DSM-III criteria for schizophrenia. *American Journal of Psychiatry, 144*(6), 727–735.

CHAPTER 6

1. Harding, C. M., Brooks, G. W., Ashikaga, T., Strauss, J. S., & Breier, A. (1987a). The Vermont longitudinal study of persons with severe mental illness: I. Methodology, study sample, and overall status 32 years later. *American Journal of Psychiatry, 144*(6), 718–726.

2. Harding, C. M., Brooks, G. W., Ashikaga, T., Strauss, J. S., & Breier, A. (1987b). The Vermont longitudinal study: II. Long-term outcome of subjects who retrospectively met DSM-III criteria for schizophrenia. *American Journal of Psychiatry, 144*(6), 727–735.

3. DeSisto, M. J., Harding, C. M., McCormick, R. J., Ashikaga, T., & Brooks, G. W. (1995a). The Maine-Vermont three-decade studies of serious mental illness: I. Matched comparison of cross-sectional outcome. *British Journal of Psychiatry, 167*, 331–338.

4. DeSisto, M. J., Harding, C. M., McCormick, R. J., Ashikaga, T., & Brooks, G. W. (1995b). The Maine-Vermont three- decade studies of serious mental illness: II. Longitudinal course comparisons. *British Journal of Psychiatry, 167*, 338–342.

5. Friedman, L. J. (1990). *Menninger: The family and the clinic.* Knopf.

6. The U. S.–Venezuela Collaborative Research Project & Wexler, N. S. (2004, March 9). Venezuelan kindreds reveal that genetic and environmental factors modulate Hunting's disease age of onset. *Proceedings of the National Academy of Sciences of the United States of America, 101*(10), 3498–3503. https://doi.org/10.1073/pnas.0308679101

7. Wexler, A. (2010, June 30). The art of medicine. *Stigma, history, and Huntington's disease.* www.the lancet.com. doi:101016/S0140-6736(10)60957-9

8. Merton, R. K. (1957). *Social theory and social structure.* Free Press.

9. Heller, J. (1961). *Catch 22.* Simon & Schuster.

10. Sartorius, N., Shapiro, R., & Jablensky, A. (1974). The International Pilot Study of Schizophrenia. *Schizophrenia Bulletin, 1*(11), 21–34, https://doi.org/10.1093/schbul/1.11.21

11. Strauss, J. S., & Carpenter, W. T., Jr. (1972). The prediction of outcome in schizophrenia. I. Characteristics of outcome. *Archives of General Psychiatry*, 27(Suppl 6), 739–746. doi:10.1001/archpsyc.1972.01750300011002

12. Strauss, J. S., & Carpenter, W. T. Jr. (1974). The prediction of outcome in schizophrenia. II. Relationships between predictor and outcome variables. *Archives of General Psychiatry*, 31(1), 37–42. doi:10.1001/archpsyc.1974.01760130021003

13. Daum, C. M., Brooks, G. W., Albee, G. W. (1977). Twenty-year follow-up of 253 schizophrenic patients originally selected for chronic disability: Pilot study. *Psychiatric Journal of the University of Ottawa*, 2, 129–132.

14. Spitzer, R. L., & Endicott, J. DIAGNO II: Further developments in a computer program for psychiatric diagnosis. *American Journal of Psychiatry*, 125(75), 12–21.

15. Spitzer, R. (1992). The Structured Interview for DSM-III-R (SCID: I. History, rationale, and description. *Archives of General Psychiatry*, 49(8), 624–629.

16. American Psychiatric Association (APA). (1987). *Diagnostic and Statistical Manual of Mental Disorders* (DSM-III-R) (3rd ed. rev.). American Psychiatric Press.

17. Daum et al. (1977), 130.

CHAPTER 7

1. Skinner, B. F. (1976). *Walden two* (2nd ed.). Hackett.

2. Maher, B. A. (1966). *Principles of psychopathology.* McGraw-Hill.

3. Maher, B. A. (1978). A reader's, writer's, and reviewer's guide to assessing research reports in clinical psychology. *Journal of Consulting and Clinical Psychology*, 46(4), 835–838. https://doi.org/10.1037/0022-006X.46.4.835

4. Murphy, J. M., Laird, N. M., Monson, R. R., Sobol, A. M., & Leighton, A. H. (2000). A 40-year perspective on the prevalence of depression: The Stirling county study. *Archives of General Psychiatry*, 57(3), 209–215. doi:10.1001/archpsyc.57.3.209

5. Leighton, A. H., & Leighton, D. C. (1949). Gregorio, the hand-trembler: A psychobiological personality study of a Navaho Indian. Report no. 1 of the Ramah Project. Peabody Museum of American Archaeology and Ethnography XL (1). Harvard University Press.

6. Meyer, A. (1919/1951). The life chart and the obligation of specifying positive data in psychopathological diagnosis. In *Contributions to medical and biological research*, Vol. 2. Hoeber. Reprinted in E. E. Winters (Ed.), *The collected papers of Adolf Meyer*. Johns Hopkins University Press.

7. Harding, C. M., McCormick, R. V., Strauss, J. S., Ashikaga, T., & Brooks, G. W. (1989). Computerised life chart methods to map domains of function and illustrate patterns of interactions in the long-term course trajectories of patients who once met the criteria for DSM-III schizophrenia. *British Journal of Psychiatry*, 155(55), 100–106. https://doi.org/10.1192/S0007125000296062

8. Ragins, M. (2002). *Recovery with severe mental illness: Changing from a medical model to a psychosocial rehabilitation model.* The Village, Long Beach, California

9. DeSisto, M. J., Harding, C. M., McCormick, R. V., Ashikaga, T., & Brooks, G. W. (1995). The Maine-Vermont three-decade studies of serious mental illness: I. Matched comparison of cross-sectional outcome. *British Journal of Psychiatry*, *167*, 331–338.

10. DeSisto, M. J., Harding, C. M., McCormick, R. J., Ashikaga, T., & Brooks, G. W. (1995). The Maine-Vermont three-decade studies of serious mental illness: II. Longitudinal course comparisons. *British Journal of Psychiatry*, *167*, 338–342.

11. Robins, L. N. (1966). *Deviant children grown up: A sociological and psychiatric study of sociopathic personality*. Williams & Wilkins.

12. Zubin, J., & Spring, B. (1977). Vulnerability: A new view of schizophrenia. *Journal of Abnormal Psychology*, *86*(2), 103–126. https://doi.org/10.1037/0021-843X.86.2.103

13. Sartorius, N., Shapiro, R., & Jablensky, A. (1974). The International Pilot Study of Schizophrenia, *Schizophrenia Bulletin*, *1*(11), 21–34, https://doi.org/10.1093/schbul/1.11.21

14. Sartorius et al. (1974).

15. Fleiss J. L., & Cohen J. (!973). The equivalence of weighted kappa and the intraclass correlation coefficient as measures of reliability. *Educational and Psychological Measurement*, *33*(3), 613–619. doi:10.1177/001316447303300309

16. Herr, S. S., Gostin, L. O., & Koh, H. H. (2003). *The human rights of persons with intellectual disabilities*. Oxford University Press.

17. Geisel, T. S. (known as Dr. Seuss). (1954). *Horton hears a who*. Random House.

18. National Commission for the Protection of Human Subjects of Biomedical and Behavioral Research. (1976). *The Belmont report: Ethical principles and guidelines for the protection of human subjects of research*. Office of Human Research Protection.

19. Gilman, S. L., Conolly, J., & Diamond, H. W. (2014). *The face of madness: Hugh W, Diamond and the origin of psychiatric photography*. Echo Point Books.

20. Hogarty, G. E., Goldberg, S. C., Schooler, N. R., & The Collaborative Study Group. (1974). Drug and sociotherapy in the aftercare of schizophrenic patients: III. Adjustment of nonrelapsed patients. *Archives of General Psychiatry*, *31*(5), 609–618. doi:10.1001/archpsyc.1974.01760170011002

21. Spitzer, R. L., Williams, J. B. W., Gibbon, M., & First, M. B. (1992). The Structured Clinical Interview for DSM-III-R (SCID): I: History, rationale, and description. *Archives of General Psychiatry*, *49*(8), 624–629. doi:10.1001/archpsyc.1992.01820080032005

22. Kopelman, Michael D. T. (1995). The Korsakoff syndrome. *British Journal of Psychiatry*, 154–173. doi:10.1192/bjp.166.2.154

23. Kety, S. (1959). Biochemical theories of schizophrenia. *Science*, *129*(3363), 1590–1596.

24. Williams J. (2016). Conformity in the academy. In *Academic freedom in an age of conformity*. Palgrave Critical University Studies. Palgrave Macmillan. https://doi.org/10.1057/9781137514790_3

CHAPTER 8

1. Fleming, I., Marbaum, R., & Dehn, P. (1964). *Goldfinger*. United Artists.
2. American Psychological Association. (2019, August 7). The Commission for the Recognition of Specialties and Proficiencies in Professional Psychology (CRSPPP) recommended the Serious Mental Illness Psychology Specialty to the Council of Representatives and was approved.
3. Kuhn, T. S. (1962). *The structure of scientific revolutions*. University of Chicago Press.
4. Harding, C. M., Brooks, G. W., Ashikaga, T., Strauss, J. S., & Breier, A. (1987a). The Vermont longitudinal study of persons with severe mental illness: I. Methodology, study sample, and overall status 32 years later. *American Journal of Psychiatry, 144*(6), 720–21.
5. Harding et al. (1987a), 721.
6. American Psychiatric Association (APA). (1980). *Diagnostic and statistical manual of mental disorders* (3rd ed..). American Psychiatric Press.
7. Meyer, A. (1919/1951). The life chart and the obligation of specifying positive data in psychopathological diagnosis. In *Contributions to medical and biological research* (Vol. 2). Hoeber. Reprinted in E. E. Winters (Ed.), *The collected papers of Adolf Meyer*. Johns Hopkins University Press.
8. Leighton, A. H., & Leighton, D. C. (1949). Gregorio, the hand-trembler: A psychobiological personality study of a Navaho Indian. Report NO. 1 of the Ramah Project. Peabody Museum of American Archaeology and Ethnography XL (1). Harvard University Press.
9. Harding, C. M., McCormick, R. V., Strauss, J. S., Ashikaga, T., & Brooks, G. W. (1989). Computerized life chart methods to map domains of function and illustrate patterns of interaction in the long-term course trajectories of patients who once met the criteria for DSM-III schizophrenia. *British Journal of Psychiatry, 155*(Suppl. 5), 100–106.
10. Vaillant, G. E. (1980). Adolf Meyer was right: Dynamic psychiatry needs the Life Chart. *Journal of the National Association of Private Psychiatric Hospitals, 11*, 4–14.
11. Britannica. (2020). Monopoly board game. www.britannica.com/sports/monopoly-board-game. Accessed September 17, 2020.
12. World Health Organization. (1978). *WHO collaborative study of the determinants of outcome in severe mental disorders*. WHO.
13. Test, M. A., Burke, S. S., & Wallisch, L. S. (1990). Gender differences of young adults with schizophrenic disorders in community care. *Schizophrenia Bulletin, 16*(2), 331–344, https://doi.org/10.1093/schbul/16.2.331

CHAPTER 9

1. Bhattacharya, P. K., & Burman, P. (2016). *Theory and methods of statistics*. Academic Press.

2. Myers, D. G., & De Wall, C. N. (2018). *Psychology* (12th ed.). Worth.

3. Chittick, R. A., Brooks, G. W., Irons, F. S., & Deane, W. N. (1961). *The Vermont story: Rehabilitation of chronic schizophrenic patients*. Queen City Printers (out of print), 27.

4. McGlashan, T. H. (1988). A selective review of recent North American long-term follow-up studies of schizophrenia. *Schizophrenia Bulletin, 14*(4), 515–542. https://doi.org/10.1093/schbul/14.4.515

5. Chittick et al. (1961), 30.

6. US Census Bureau. (1954). *Vermont population*. US Government Printing Office.

7. Achenbach, T. M., McConaughy, S. H., & Howell, C. T. (1987). Child/adolescent behavioral and emotional problems: Implications of cross-informant correlations for situational specificity. *Psychological Bulletin, 101*(2), 213–232. https://doi.org/10.1037/0033-2909.101.2.213

8. Morton, N. E. (1955). Sequential tests for the detection of linkage. *American Journal of Human Genetics, 7*(3), 277–318.

9. Clayton, P., Desmarais, L., & Winokur, G. (1968). A study of normal bereavement. *American Journal of Psychiatry, 125*(2), 168–178. doi.org/10.1171/ajp.125.2.168

10. DeSisto, M., Harding, C. M., McCormick, Ashikaga, T., & Brooks, G. W. (1999). The Maine and Vermont three-decade studies of serious mental illness: Longitudinal course comparisons. In P. Cohen, C. Slomkowski, & L. N. Robins (Eds.), *Historical and geographical influences on psychopathology* (pp. 331–349). Erlbaum.

11. Harding, C. M. (1994). An examination of the complexities in the measurement of recovery in severe psychiatric disorders. In R. J. Ancill, S. Holliday, & G. W. MacEwan (Eds.), *Schizophrenia: Exploring the spectrum of psychosis* (pp. 153–169). Wiley.

12. http://isdn.modemhelp.net/g/gandalftechnologies.shtml

13. www.ibm.com › ibm › history › ibm100 › icons › punchcard

14. Cohen, J. (1968). Weighted kappa: Nominal scale agreement provision for scaled disagreement or partial credit. *Psychological Bulletin, 70*(4), 213–220. https://doi.org/10.1037/h0026256

15. Harding, C. M., Brooks, G. W., Ashikaga, T., Strauss, J. S., & Breier, A. (1987a). The Vermont longitudinal study of persons with severe mental illness: I. Methodology, study sample, and overall status 32 years later. *American Journal of Psychiatry, 144*(6), 718–726.

16. Abnormal Involuntary Movement Scale (AIMS). AAcAP. www.aacap.org › docs › member_resources › monitoring.

17. Fleiss J. L., & Cohen J. (1973). The equivalence of weighted kappa and the intraclass correlation coefficient as measures of reliability. *Educational and Psychological Measurement, 33*(3), 613–619. doi:10.1177/001316447303300309

CHAPTER 10

1. Harding, C. M., Brooks, G. W., Ashikaga, T., Strauss, J. S., & Breier, A. (1987a). The Vermont longitudinal study of persons with severe mental illness: I. Methodology, study sample, and overall status 32 years later. *American Journal of Psychiatry*, *144*(6), 718–726.

2. Harding, C. M., Brooks, G. W., Ashikaga, T., Strauss, J. S., & Breier, A. (1987b). The Vermont longitudinal study: II. Long-term outcome of subjects who retrospectively met DSM-III criteria for schizophrenia. *American Journal of Psychiatry*, *144*(6), 727–735.

3. Harding et al. (1987b).

4. Harding et al. (1987a).

5. Ibid., 720.

6. Vermont Department of Education. (1940). *History of education during the Great Depression.* Vermont Department of Education.

7. Aas, I. H. M. (2011). Guidelines for rating Global Assessment of Functioning (GAF). *Annals of General Psychiatry*, *20*(10), 2. doi:10.1186/1744-859X-10-2

8. Endicott, J., Spitzer, R. L., Fleiss, J. L., & Cohen, J. (1976). The Global Assessment Scale: A procedure for measuring overall severity of psychiatric disturbance. *Archives of General Psychiatry*, *33*(6), 766–771. doi:10.1001/archpsyc.1976.01770060086012

9. Spitzer, R. L., Gibbon, R., & Endicott, J. (1975). *The Global Assessment Scale (GAS).* New York State Psychiatric Institute.

10. Ibid.

11. Ibid.

12. Ibid.

13. Harding et al. (1987a), 722.

14. Ibid., 722–723. It should be noted that even with this split, statistically there were no significant differences between the sexes in levels of function using a 2×2 chi square analysis (GAS by sex); ($2X2 = 0.13$, df = 1, p = .72).

15. Chiders, S. E., & Harding, C. M. (1990). Gender, premorbid social functioning, and long-term outcome in DSM-III schizophrenia. *Schizophrenia Bulletin*, 1990, *16*(2), 309–318.

16. Strauss, J. S., & Carpenter, W. T., Jr. (1977). Prediction of outcome in schizophrenia. III. Five-year outcome and its predictors. *Archives of General Psychiatry*, *34*, 159–163.

17. Harding et al. (1987a), 723.

18. Ibid.

19. Ibid.

20. American Psychiatric Association (APA). (1968). *Diagnostic and statistical manual of mental disorders* (2nd ed.). American Psychiatric Press.

21. American Psychiatric Association (APA). (1980). *Diagnostic and statistical manual of mental disorders* (3rd ed.). American Psychiatric Press.

22. Harding et al. (1987a), 722.

23. Ibid.

24. Ibid.

25. Ibid.

26. Mechanic, D., Bilder, S., & McAlpine, D. D. (2002). Employing persons with serious mental illness. *Health Affairs*, *21*(5), 242–253. https://doi.org/10.1377/hlthaff.21.5.242

27. Harding et al. (1987a), 723.

28. Ibid., 722.

29. Ibid.

30. Schwartz, C., Mueller, C., & Spitzer, R. L. (1977). *The Community Care Schedule (CCS)*. New York State Psychiatric Institute.

31. Schwartz et al. (1977).

32. Harding et al. (1987a), 722.

33. Ibid., 723.

34. Ibid., 723.

35. Kraepelin, E. (1902). Dementia praecox. In A. B. Diefendorf (Trans.), *Clinical psychiatry: A textbook for students and physicians* (6th ed.). Macmillan.

36. Sacks, O. (1973). *Awakenings* (1st ed.). Duckworth.

37. Zubin, J. (1985). General discussion. In M. Alpert (Ed.), *Controversies in schizophrenia: Changes and constancies*. Guilford. 407.

CHAPTER 11

1. Harding, C. M., Brooks, G. W., Ashikaga, T., Strauss, J. S., & Breier, A. (1987a). The Vermont longitudinal study of persons with severe mental illness: I. Methodology, study sample, and overall status 32 years later. *American Journal of Psychiatry*, *144*(6), 718–726.

2. Harding, C. M. (2016). The doctor who saw through psychiatric labels to find the real person underneath. *American Journal of Psychiatric Rehabilitation*, *19*(1), 17–22. doi:10.1080/15487768.2016.1136175

3. Chittick, R. A., Brooks, G. W., Irons, F. S., & Deane, W. N. (1961). *The Vermont story: Rehabilitation of chronic schizophrenic patients*. Queen City Printers (out of print).

4. U. S. Census (1980). Rutland City population.

5. American Psychiatric Association (APA). (2013). *Diagnostic and statistical manual* (5th ed.). American Psychiatric Press. https://doi.org.org/10.org1176/appi.books.9780890425596; Chittick et al. (1961).

6. Harding, C. M., & Keller, A. B. (1998). Long-term outcome of social functioning in schizophrenia. In K. T. Mueser & N. Tarrier (Eds.), *The handbook of social functioning* (p. 139). Allyn & Bacon.

7. Harding et al. (1987a).

8. Harding, C. M., Brooks, G. W., Ashikaga, T., Strauss, J. S., & Breier, A. (1987b). The Vermont longitudinal study: II. Long-term outcome of subjects who

retrospectively met DSM-III criteria for schizophrenia. *American Journal of Psychiatry, 144*(6), 727–735.

9. Harding, C. M., Zubin, J., & Strauss, J. S. (1992). Chronicity in schizophrenia: Revisited. *British Journal of Psychiatry, 161*(S18), 27–37. https://doi:10.1192/S0007125000298887

10. Harding, C. M. (1984, April 18). Long-term outcome functioning of subjects rediagnosed as meeting the DSM-II criteria for schizophrenia. Dissertation presented to the Department of Psychology, University of Vermont.

11. Bleuler, M. (1978). *The schizophrenic disorders: Long-term patient and family studies.* S. M. Clemens (Trans.) Yale University Press.

12. Schooler, N. R., & Kane, J. M. (1982). Research diagnoses for tardive dyskinesia. *Archives of General Psychiatry, 39*(4), 486–487. https://doi:10.1001/archpsyc.1982.04290040080014

13. Pompili, M., Amador, X. F., Girardi, P., Harkavy-Friedman, J., Harrow, M., Kaplan, K., Krausz, M., Lester, D., Meltzer, H.Y., Modestin, J., Montross, L. P., Mortensen, P. B., Jørgensen, P. M., Nielsen, J., Nortentoff, M., Saarinen, P. I., Zisook, S. Wilson, S. T., & Tatarelli, R. (2007). Suicide risk in schizophrenia: Learning from the past to change the future. *Annals of General Psychiatry, 6*, 10. https://doi.org/10.1186/1744-859X-6-10

14. Harding, C. M., McCormick, R. V., Strauss, J. S., Ashikaga, T., & Brooks, G. W. (1989). Computerized life chart methods to map domains of function and illustrate patterns of interaction in the long-term course trajectories of patients who once met the criteria for DSM-III schizophrenia. *British Journal of Psychiatry, 155*(Suppl. 5), 100–106.

15. Spaniol, L., Gagne, C., & Koehler, M. (1999). Recovery from serious mental illness: What it is and how to support people in their recovery. In R. P. Marinellis & A. E. Dell Orto (Eds.), *The psychological & social impact of disability.* Springer.

16. Harding, C. M. (2002). *Lifeline: A way to engage people early in the course of working together.* Center for Psychiatric Rehabilitation, Boston University.

17. Harrow, M., Jobe, T. H., & Tong, L. (2021). Twenty-year effects of antipsychotics in schizophrenia and affective psychotic disorders. *Psychological Medicine*, 1–11. https://doi.org/10.1017/S0032017200004778

18. Hollingshead, A. B., & Redlich, F. C. (1958). *Social class and mental illness: Community study.* Wiley.

CHAPTER 12

1. Daniels, J. (1946). *The Wilson era: Years of war and after 1917–1923.* University of North Carolina Press, 624.

2. Ciompi, L., & Müller, C. (1976). *Lebensweg und Alter der Schizophrenien: Eine katamnestische Langzeitstudies bas in senium.* Springer Verlag.

3. Winokur, G. (1975). The Iowa 500: Heterogeneity and course in manic-depressive illness (bipolar). *Comprehensive Psychiatry, 16*(2), 125–131. https://doi.org/10.1016/0010-440X(75)90057-7

4. Schooler,N.R.(2006).GerardE.Hogarty,1935–2006.*Neuropsychopharmacology*,*11*, 2565–2566.

5. Sabshin, M. (2006). John A.Talbott, M. D. One hundred thirteenth President, 1984–1985. *American Journal of Psychiatry*, *142*(9), 1014–1016. https://doi.org/ 10.1176/ajp.142.9.1014

6. Bleuler, M. (1978). *The schizophrenic disorders: Patient and family studies.* S. M. Clemons (Trans).Yale University Press.

7. Ibid., 413.

8. Harding, C. M., Zubin, J., & Strauss, J. S. (1987). Chronicity in Schizophrenia: Fact, partial fact, or artifact? *Hospital and Community Psychiatry*, *38*(5), 477–486.

9. Harding et al. (1987).

10. Harding, C. M., Zubin, J., & Strauss, J. S. (1992). Chronicity in schizophrenia: Revisited. *British Journal of Psychiatry*, *161*(18S), 27–37. https://doi.org/ 10.1192/ S0007125000298887

11. Lidz,T., Cornelison,A. R., Fleck, S., & Terry, D. (1957).The intrafamilial environment of the schizophrenic patient. *Psychiatry*, *20*(4), 329–350.

12. Andreasen, N. C. (1984). *The broken brain: The biological revolution in psychiatry.* Harper & Row.

13. Gershon, E. S., & Cloninger, R. (1994). *Genetic approaches to mental disorders.* American Psychopathological Association Series. American Psychiatric Press.

14. Weinberger, D. R. (2017). Future of days past: Neurodevelopment and schizophrenia, *Schizophrenia Bulletin*, *43*, 6, 1164–1168, https://doi.org/ 10.1093/sch bul/sbx118

15. Ban, T. A., Healy, D., & Shorter, E. (Eds.). (2010). *The history of psychopharmacology and the CINP, as told in autobiography: The rise of psychopharmacology and the story of CINP.* Collegium Internationale Neuro-Psychopharmacologicum.

16. Chittick, R. A., Brooks, G.W., Irons, F. S., & Deane,W. N. (1961). *The Vermont story: Rehabilitation of chronic schizophrenic patients.* Queen City Printers (out of print).

17. Piaget, J. (1964). Cognitive development in children: Piaget development and learning. *Journal of Research in Science Teaching*, *6*, 176–186.

18. Breier,A., & Strauss, J. S. (1984). Social relationships in the recovery from psychiatric disorder. *American Journal of Psychiatry*, *141*(8), 949–955.

19. Rakfeldt, J., & Strauss, J. S. (1989). The low turning point: A control mechanism in the course of mental disorder. *Journal of Nervous and Mental Disease*, *177*(1), 32–37. https://doi.org/10.1097/00005053-198901000-00005

20. Chittick et al. (1961).

21. Strauss, J. S. (1985). Negative symptoms: Future developments of the concept. *Schizophrenia Bulletin*, *11*(3), 457–460. https://doi.org/10.1093/schbul/ 11.3.457

22. Strauss, J. S., & Harding, C. M. (1990). Relationships between adult development and the course of mental disorder. In A. S. Masten, J. Rolf, J., D. Cicchetti, K. Nuechterlein, K., & S.Weintraub (Eds.), *Risk and protective factors in the development of psychopathology.* Cambridge University Press.

23. Holstein, A. R., & Harding, C. M. (1992). Omissions in assessment of work roles: Implications for evaluating social functioning in mental illness. *Journal of Orthopsychiatry, 62*(3), 469–474.

24. Strauss, J. S., Hafez, H., Lieberman, P., & Harding, C. M. (1985). The course of psychiatric disorder: III. Longitudinal principles. *American Journal of Psychiatry, 142*(3), 289–296.

25. Strauss, J. S. (1989). Subjective experiences of schizophrenia: II. Toward a new dynamic psychiatry. *Schizophrenia Bulletin, 15*(2), 179–187.

26. Zigler, E. F., & Glick, M. (2001). *A developmental approach to adult psychopathology.* J. Wiley.

27. Zigler, E. F., & Muenchow, S. (1992). *Head Start: The inside story of America's most successful educational experiment.* Basic Books.

28. https://news.yale.edu/2019/02/08/edward-f-zigler-eminent-psychologist

29. Hogan, M. F. (2003). New Freedom Commission Report: The President's New Freedom Commission: Recommendations to transform mental health care in America. *Psychiatric Services, 54*(11), 1467–1474. https://doi.org/10.1176/appi.ps.54.11.1467

30. Vaillant, G. E. (1984). The disadvantages of the DSM-III outweigh its advantages. *American Journal of Psychiatry, 141*(4), 542–545.

31. American Psychiatric Association (APA). (1980). *Diagnostic and statistical manual of mental disorders* (3rd ed). American Psychiatric Press.

32. American Psychiatric Association (APA). (1987). *Diagnostic and statistical manual of mental disorders* (3rd ed. rev.). American Psychiatric Press.

33. American Psychiatric Association (APA). (1994). *Diagnostic and statistical manual of mental disorders* (4th ed.). American Psychiatric Press.

34. American Psychiatric Association (APA) (2000). *Diagnostic and statistical manual of mental disorders* (4th ed. text rev.). American Psychiatric Press.

35. American Psychiatric Association (APA). (2013). *Diagnostic and statistical manual of mental disorders* (5th ed.). American Psychiatric Press. https://doi.org/10.1176/appi.books.9780890425596

36. American Psychiatric Association (APA). (2022). *Diagnostic and statistical manual of mental disorders* (5th ed. TR). American Psychiatric Press.

37. APA (2013). *Schizophrenia Spectrum and Other Psychotic Disorders.* American Psychiatric Press.

CHAPTER 13

1. American Psychiatric Association (APA). (1980). *Diagnostic and statistical manual of mental disorders* (3rd ed.). American Psychiatric Press.

2. American Psychiatric Association (APA). (1952). *Diagnostic and statistical manual of mental disorders* (1st ed.). American Psychiatric Press.

3. American Psychiatric Association (APA). (1968). *Diagnostic and statistical manual of mental disorders* (2nd ed.). American Psychiatric Press.

4. Cooper, J. E. (1972). *Psychiatric diagnosis in New York and London: A comparative study of mental hospital admissions*. Oxford University Press.

5. APA (1952), v–viii.

6. Weckowicz, T. E., & Liebel-Weckowicz, H. P. (Eds.). (1990). Chap 12. The psychobiology and commonsense psychiatry of Adolf Meyer. In: *Advances in psychology*. Elsevier. *66*, 283–291. ISBN 9780444883919, doi.org/10.1016/S0166-4115(08)61450-8

7. Worthington, J. F. (2008, Winter). When psychiatry was very young. *Hopkins Medicine*. http://www.hopkinsmedicine.org/hmn/W08/annals.cfm

8. APA (1980), 1.

9. Leighton, A. H., & Leighton, D. C. (1949). Gregorio, the hand-trembler: A psychobiological personality study of a Navaho Indian. Report no. 1 of the Ramah Project. Peabody Museum of American Archaeology and Ethnography XL (1). Harvard University Press.

10. APA (1968), ix.

11. Ibid.

12. APA (1952), 26–28.

13. Ibid., 28.

14. APA (1968).

15. World Health Organization. (1968). *International classification of diseases* (8th ed., ICD-8). WHO.

16. APA (1968), 33–36.

17. Ibid., 33.

18. Ibid., 34.

19. Ibid., viii.

20. Ibid.

21. Ibid.

22. Ibid., ix.

23. APA (1980), 181–193.

24. APA (1980), 1.

25. World Health Organization. (1979). *International classification of diseases* (9th ed., ICD-9). WHO, 2.

26. APA (1980), 2.

27. Spitzer, R. L., Forman, J. B., & Nee, J. (1979). DSM-III field trials: I. Initial interrater diagnostic reliability. *American Journal of Psychiatry*, *136*(6), 815–817. https://doi.org/10.1176/ajp.136.6.815

28. APA (1980), 188–189.

29. Ibid.

30. Ibid., 6.

31. Kessler, R. C. (2002). The categorical versus dimensional assessment controversy in the sociology of mental illness. *Journal of Health and Social Behavior*, 171–188.

32. APA (1980), 185.

33. Harding, C. M., Brooks, G. W., Ashikaga, T., Strauss, J. S., & Breier, A. (1987b). The Vermont longitudinal study: II. Long-term outcome of subjects who retrospectively met DSM-III criteria for schizophrenia. *American Journal of Psychiatry, 144*(6), 727–735, at 730.

34. Ibid., 729.

35. Ibid., 730.

36. Ibid., 730.

37. Vaillant, G. E. (1984). The disadvantages of the DSM-III outweigh its advantages in The Debate on DSM-III with Klerman, G. L., Vaillant, G. E., Spitzer, R. L. and Michaels, R. *American Journal of Psychiatry, 141*(4), 539–553.

38. APA (1980), 185.

39. Strauss, J. S., & Harder, D. W. (1981). The Case Record Rating Scale. *Psychiatric Research, 4,* 333–345.

40. World Health Organization. (1978). Research protocols: Psychiatric and Personal History Schedule. Collaborative Project on Determinants of Outcome of Severe Mental Disorders (1977–79). WHO.

41. World Health Organization. (1973). *International Pilot Study of Schizophrenia (ISPSS),* vol. 1. WHO.

42. Spitzer, R. L., Endicott, J., & Robins, E. (1978). Research diagnostic criteria: Rationale and reliability. *Archives of General Psychiatry, 35*(6), 773–782.

43. Overall, J. E., & Gorham, D. R. (1962). The Brief Psychiatric Rating Scale. *Psychological Reports, 10*(3), 799–812. https://doi.org/10.2466/pro.1962.10.3.799

44. Folstein, M. F., Folstein, S. E., & McHugh, P. R. (1975). "Mini-Mental State": A practical method for grading the cognitive state of patients for the clinician. *Journal of Psychiatric Research, 12,* 189–198.

45. Endicott, J., Spitzer, R. L., Fleiss, J. L., & Cohen, J. (1976). The Global Assessment Scale: A procedure for measuring overall severity of psychiatric disturbance. *Archives of General Psychiatry, 33*(6), 766–771. doi:10.1001/archpsyc.1976.01770060086012

46. Strauss & Harder (1981).

47. Harding et al. (1987b), 728–729.

48. Cohen, J. (2013). *Statistical power analysis for the behavioral sciences.* Academic Press.

49. Vaillant (1984).

50. Harding et al. (1987b), 728.

51. Chittick, R. A., Brooks, G. W., Irons, F. S., & Deane, W. N. (1961). *The Vermont story: Rehabilitation of chronic schizophrenic patients.* Queen City Printers (out of print).

52. Harding et al. (1987b), 728–729.

53. APA (1980), 187.

54. American Psychiatric Association (APA). (2013). Diagnostic and (5th ed.). American Psychiatric Press..

55. Malaspina, D., Owen, M. J., Heckers, S., Tandon, R., Bustillo, J., Schultz, S., Barch, D. M., Gaebel, W., Gur, R. E., Tsuang, M., Van Os, J., & Carpenter, W. (2013). Schizoaffective disorder in the DSM-5. *Schizophrenia Research, 150*(1), 21–25. https://doi.org/10.1016/j.schres.2013.04.026

56. Harding et al. (1987b), 728.

57. Ibid.

58. APA (1980), 188–193.

59. Harding, C. M. (1984, May) Long-term functioning of subjects rediagnosed as meeting the DSM-III criteria for Schizophrenia. Dissertation, Department of Psychology, University of Vermont, 40.

60. Harding et al. (1987b), 727.

61. Harding et al. (1987a), 721.

62. Harding (1984).

63. Harding et al. (1987b), 730.

64. Ibid.

65. Ibid.

66. Ibid.

67. Herz, M. I., Glazer, W. M., Mostert. M, A., et al. (1991). Intermittent vs maintenance medication in schizophrenia: Two-year results. *Archives of General Psychiatry*, *48*(4), 333–339. doi:10.1001/archpsyc.1991.01810280049007

68. Carpenter Jr, W.T., & Heinrichs, D.W. (1983). Early intervention, time-limited, targeted pharmacotherapy of schizophrenia. *Schizophrenia Bulletin*, *9*(4), 533.

69. Black, D. W., & Nasrallah, A. (1989). Hallucinations and delusions in 1,715 patients with unipolar and bipolar affective disorders. *Psychopathology*, *22*(1), 28–34.

70. Goldstein, G., Shemansky, W. J., & Allen, D. N. (2005). Cognitive function in schizoaffective disorder and clinical subtypes of schizophrenia. *Archives of Clinical Neuropsychology*, *20*(2), 153–159.

71. Harding et al. (1987b), 731–732.

72. Ibid., 732–733.

73. Manderscheid R. W. (1987). Long-term perspectives on persons with chronic mental disorder. *American Journal of Psychiatry*, *144*(6), 783–784. doi:10.1176/ajp.144.6.783. PMID: 3592001

74. Cohen, J. (2013). *Statistical power analysis for the behavioral sciences*. Academic Press.

75. Cohen, P., & Cohen, J. (1984). The clinician's illusion. *Archives of General Psychiatry*, *41*(12), 1178–1182.

76. American Psychiatric Association. (APA). (1987). *Diagnostic and statistical manual of mental disorders* (3rd ed. rev.). American Psychiatric Press..

77. Ibid., xvii.

78. Ibid., xix–xx.

79. Ibid., 191.

80. Ibid.

CHAPTER 14

1. Jablensky A. (2010). The diagnostic concept of schizophrenia: Its history, evolution, and future prospects. *Dialogues in Clinical Neuroscience*, *12*(3), 271–287. https://doi.org/10.31887/DCNS.2010.12.3/ajablensky

2. American Psychiatric Association (APA). (2013). *Diagnostic and statistical manual of mental disorders* (5th ed). American Psychiatric Press. https://doi.org/10.1176/appi.books.9780890425596

3. Harding, C. M., Brooks, G. W., Ashikaga, T., Strauss, J. S., & Breier, A. (1987a). The Vermont longitudinal study of persons with severe mental illness: I. Methodology, study sample, and overall status 32 years later. *American Journal of Psychiatry*, *144*(6), 718–726.

4. Harding, C. M., Brooks, G. W., Ashikaga, T., Strauss, J. S., & Breier, A. (1987b). The Vermont longitudinal study: II. Long-term outcome of subjects who retrospectively met DSM-III criteria for schizophrenia. *American Journal of Psychiatry*, *144*(6), 727–735.

5. DeSisto, M. J., Harding, C. M., McCormick, R. V., Ashikaga, T., & Brooks, G. W. (1995a). The Maine-Vermont three-decade studies of serious mental illness. I. Matched comparison of cross-sectional outcome. *British Journal of Psychiatry*, *167*, 331–338.

6. DeSisto, M. J., Harding, C. M., McCormick, R. J., Ashikaga, T., & Brooks, G. W. (1995b). The Maine-Vermont three-decade studies of serious mental illness. II. Longitudinal course comparisons. *British Journal of Psychiatry*, *167*, 338–342.

7. Bowers, M. B., Jr., Harding, C. M., & Ashikaga, T. (1993, May 23). *Benign and/or Malignant Catatonia?* Symposium 27, "Vermont and Maine's Follow-up Studies of Psychoses" at the 146th Annual Meeting, American Psychiatric Association, San Francisco, CA.

8. Sledge, W. (2008). Malcolm Baker Bowers Jr, 1934–2008. *Neuropsychopharmacology*, *33*, 3248. https://doi.org/10.1038/npp.2008.26

9. APA (2013), 810.

10. Kahlbaum, K. L. (1874/1973). *Die katatonie oder das Spannungsirresein*. In Hirschwald (Trans.) *Catatonia*. Verlag von August/Johns Hopkins University Press.

11. Carroll B. T. (2001). Kahlbaum's catatonia revisited. *Psychiatry Clinical Neuroscience*, *55*(5), 431–436. https://doi:10.1046/j.1440-1819.2001.00887.x

12. Kraepelin. E. (1909/1915). *Psychiatrie: Ein Lehrbuch für Studierende und Aerzte*, 8th ed. Barth.

13. Fink, M., Shorter, E., & Taylor, M. A. (2010). Catatonia is not schizophrenia: Kraepelin's error and the need to recognize catatonia as an independent syndrome in medical nomenclature. *Schizophrenia Bulletin*, *36*, 2, 314–320. https://doi.org/10.1093/schbul/sbp059

14. Bleuler, E. (1911). *Dementia praecox oder Gruppe der Schizophrenien*. Deuticke.

15. Gazdag, G., Takács, R., & Ungvari, G. S. (2017). Catatonia as a putative nosological entity: A historical sketch. *World Journal of Psychiatry*, *7*(3), 177–183. https://doi.org/10.5498/wjp.v7.i3.177

16. APA (2013).

17. Fink et al. (2010).

18. American Psychiatric Association (APA). (1952). *Diagnostic and statistical manual of mental disorders* (1st ed.). American Psychiatric Press.

19. APA (1952), 26.

20. American Psychiatric Association (APA). (1968). *Diagnostic and statistical manual of mental disorders* (2nd ed.). American Psychiatric Press.

21. APA (1968), 33–34.

22. Ibid., 33.

23. Ibid., 34.

24. Ibid., 36.

25. Ibid., 40.

26. American Psychiatric Association (APA). (1980). *Diagnostic and Statistical Manual of Mental Disorders* (3rd ed.). American Psychiatric Press.

27. APA (1980), 191.

28. Ibid., 202–203.

29. Kahlbaum (1874/1973).

30. Gelenberg. A. J. (1976). The catatonic syndrome. *Lancet, 19*(1), 1339–1341.

31. Bowers et al. (1993).

32. Strauss, J. S., & Carpenter, W. T., Jr. (1974). The prediction of outcome in schizophrenia: II. Relationships between predictor and outcome variables: A report from the WHO International Pilot Study of Schizophrenia. *Archives of General Psychiatry, 31*(1), 37–42. https://doi:10.1001/archpsyc.1974.0176013 0021003

33. APA (1980), 192.

34. Ibid., 191.

35. Ibid.

36. Moskowitz, A. K. (2004). "Scared stiff": Catatonia as an evolutionary-based fear response. *Psychological Review, 111*(4), 984–1002. https://doi.org/10.1037/0033-295X.111.4.984

37. Strauss & Carpenter (1974).

38. DeSisto et al. (1995a).

39. Schwartz, C. L. M., Muller, C., Spitzer, R. L., Goldstein, J., & Serrano, O. (1977). *The Community Care Schedule (CCS)*. New York State Psychiatric Institute.

40. Overall, J. E., & Gorham, D. R. (1962). The Brief Psychiatric Rating Scale. *Psychological Reports, 10*(3), 799–812. https://doi.org/10.2466/pro.1962.10.3.799

41. Endicott, J., Spitzer, R., L., Fleiss, J., L., & Cohen, J. (1976). The Global Assessment Scale: A procedure for measuring overall severity of psychiatric disturbance. *Archives of General Psychiatry, 33*(6), 766–771. https://doi:10.1001/archpsyc.1976.01770060086012

42. Strauss, J. S., & Carpenter, W. T., Jr. (1972). The prediction of outcome in schizophrenia: I. Characteristics of outcome. *Archives of General Psychiatry, 27*, 739–746.

43. Harding et al. (1987b).

44. American Psychiatric Association (APA). (1987). *Diagnostic and classification manual of mental disorders* (3rd ed.). American Psychiatric Press, 189–190.

45. American Psychiatric Association (APA). (1994). *Diagnostic and statistical manual of mental disorders* (4th ed.). American Psychiatric Press, 288–289.

46. APA (1994), 288–289.

47. American Psychiatric Association (APA). (2000). *Diagnostic and statistical manual of mental disorders* (4th ed, text. rev.). American Psychiatric Press, 418.

48. APA (2000), 418.

49. Caroff, S. N., Mann, S. C., Francis, A., & Fricchione, G. L. (Eds.). (2007). *Catatonia: From psychopathology to neurobiology.* American Psychiatric Press.

50. Bräunig, P., Krüger, S., & Shugar, G. (1998). Prevalence and clinical significance of catatonic symptoms in mania. *Comprehensive Psychiatry, 39*(1), 35–46.

51. Philbrick, K. L., & Rummans, T. A. (1994). Malignant catatonia. *Journal of Neuropsychiatry and Clinical Neurosciences, 6*(1), 1–13. https://doi.org/10.1176/jnp.6.1.1

52. Philbrick, K. L., Bush, G., Fink, M., Petrides, G., Dowling, F., & Francis, A. (1996). Catatonia. I: Rating scale and standardized examination. *Acta Psychiatrica Scandinavica, 93*(2), 129–136.

53. Fricchione, G. L., Cassem, N. H. Hooberman, D., & Hobson, D. (1983). Intravenous lorazepam in neuroleptic-induced catatonia. *Journal of Clinical Psychopharmacology, 12*, 338–342.

54. Philbrick & Rummans (1994).

55. APA (2013), 810.

56. Ibid.

57. Ibid., 119.

58. World Health Organization (2015). *The International Classification of Diseases* (10th rev.) WHO, 877.

59. Mann, S. C, Caroff, S. N., Bleier, H. R., Welz, W. K. R., Kling, M. A., & Hayashida, M. (1986). Lethal catatonia. *American Journal of Psychiatry, 143*(11), 1374–1381. https://doi.org/10.1176/ajp.143.11.1374

60. Greenfeld, D., Conrad, C., Kincare, P., & Bowers, M. B. (1987). Treatment of catatonia with low-dose lorazepam. *American Journal of Psychiatry, 144*(9), 1224–1225. https://doi.org/10.1176/ajp.144.9.1224

61. APA (2013), 810.

62. Ibid., concerning catatonia in other medical disorders.

63. B each, S. R., Gomez-Bernal, F., Huffman, J. C., & Fricchione, G. L. (2017). Alternative treatment strategies for catatonia: A systematic review. *General Hospital Psychiatry, 48*, 1–19.

64. Rogers. J. P., Pollak, T. A., Blackman, G., David A. S. (2019, July). Catatonia and the immune system: A review. *Lancet Psychiatry, 6*(7), 620–630. doi:10.1016/S2215-0366(19)30190-7. Epub 2019 Jun 10. PMID: 31196793; PMCID: PMC7185541.

65. Breier et al. (1993). Validity of paranoid subtype: Long-term outcome. Symposium 27, "Vermont and Maine's Follow-up Studies of Psychoses." 146th

Annual Meeting, American Psychiatric Association, San Francisco, CA. May 24, 1993.

66. Strauss, J. S., & Carpenter, W. T., Jr. (1972). The prediction of outcome in schizophrenia: I. Characteristics of outcome. *Archives of General Psychiatry*, *27*(6), 739–746. https://doi:10.1001/archpsyc.1972.01750300011002

67. Strauss, J. S., & Carpenter, W. T. (1974). The prediction of outcome in schizophrenia: II. Relationships between predictor and outcome variables: A report from the WHO International Pilot Study of Schizophrenia. *Archives of General Psychiatry*, *31*(1), 37–42.

68. Lake, C. C. (2008). Hypothesis: Grandiosity and guilt cause paranoia: Paranoid schizophrenia is a psychotic mood disorder: A review. *Schizophrenia Bulletin*, *34*(6), 1151–1962. http://doi.org/10.1093/schbul/sbm132

69. Cheniaux, E., Landeira-Fernandez, J., Telles, L. L., Lessa, J. L. M., Dias, A., Duncan, T., & Versiani, M. (2008). Does schizoaffective disorder really exist? A systematic review of the studies that compared schizoaffective disorder with schizophrenia or mood disorders. *Journal of Affective Disorders*, *106*(3), 209–217.

70. Freeman, D., Dunn, G., Fowler, D., Bebbington, P., Kuipers, E., Emsley, R., Jolley, S., & Garrety, P. (2013). Current paranoid thinking in patients with delusions: The presence of affective biases. *Schizophrenia Bulletin*, *39*(6), 1281–1287. http://doi.org/10.1093/schbul/sbs145

71. APA (2013), 810.

72. Ibid., 121.

73. DeSisto et al. (1995a).

74. Ibid.

75. DeSisto, M. J., Harding, C. M., McCormick, R. V., Ashikaga, T., & Brooks, G. W. (1995b). The Maine-Vermont three-decade studies of serious mental illness. II. Longitudinal course comparisons. *British Journal of Psychiatry*, *167*, 338–242.

76. Cohen, P., Slomkowski, C., & Robins, L. N. (Eds.). (1999). *Historical and geographical influences on psychopathology*. Erlbaum.

CHAPTER 15

1. Maher, B. A. (1966). *Principles of psychopathology: An experimental approach*. McGraw-Hill.

2. Murphy, J., Laird, N., Monson, R., Sobol, A., & Leighton, A. (2000). Incidence of depression in the Stirling County Study: Historical and comparative perspectives. *Psychological Medicine*, *30*(3), 505–514. doi:10.1017/S0033291799002044

3. Zubin, J., & Spring, B. (1977). Vulnerability: A new view of schizophrenia. *Journal of Abnormal Psychology*, *86*(2), 103.

4. Robins, L. N. (1996). Deviant children grown up. *European Child & Adolescent Psychiatry*, *5*(1), 44–46.

5. DeSisto, M. J., Harding, C. M., McCormick, R. J., Ashikaga, T., & Brooks, G. W. (1999). The Maine and Vermont three- decade studies of serious mental

illness. II. Longitudinal course comparisons. In P. Cohen, C. Slomkowski, & L. N. Robins (Eds.), *Historical and geographical influences on psychopathology* (pp. 331–349). Erlbaum.

6. Ridgway, P. (2001). ReStorying psychiatric disability: Learning from first person recovery narratives. *Psychiatric Rehabilitation Journal, 24*(4), 335–343. https://doi.org/10.1037/h0095071

7. Harding, C. M., Brooks, G. W., Ashikaga, T., Strauss, J. S., & Breier, A. (1987a). The Vermont longitudinal study of persons with severe mental illness: I. Methodology, study sample, and overall status 32 years later. *American Journal of Psychiatry, 144*(6), 718–726.

8. Harding, C. M., Brooks, G. W., Ashikaga, T., Strauss, J. S., & Breier, A. (1987b). The Vermont longitudinal study: II. Long-term outcome of subjects who retrospectively met DSM-III criteria for schizophrenia. *American Journal of Psychiatry, 144*(6), 727–735.

9. https://www.maine.gov/dhhs/sites/maine.gov.dhhs/files/inline-files/History-Six-Eras.docx

10. Parry M. S. (2006). Dorothea Dix (1802–1887). *American Journal of Public Health, 96*(4), 624–625.1. https://www.maine.gov/dhhs/riverview/about-us

11. https://www.maine.gov/dhhs/sites/maine.gov.dhhs/files/inline-files/History-Six-Eras.docx

12. Ibid.

13. Ibid.

14. Ibid.

15. Ibid.

16. DeSisto, M. J., Harding, C. M., McCormick, R. V., Ashikaga, T., & Gautam, S. (1995a). The Maine-Vermont three-decade studies of serious mental illness: I. Matched comparison of cross-sectional outcome. *British Journal of Psychiatry, 167*, 331–338.

17. https://www. c.gov/quickfacts/ME (and VT)

18. Ibid., 334

19. Ibid., 333.

20. Harding et al. (1987a), 720.

21. DeSisto et al. (1995a), 333.

22. Harding et al. (1987a), 721.

23. https://www.nytimes.com/2015/02/15/business/behind-monopoly-an-inventor-who-didnt-pass-go.html

24. Harding et al. (1987a), 721.

25. DeSisto et al. (1996a), 333.

26. World Health Organization. (1978, August). *Collaborative project on determinates of outcome of severe mental disorders (1977–1979). Research protocols.* WHO.

27. Harding et al. (1987a), 721.

28. DeSisto et al. (1995a), 332.

29. Ibid.

30. Ibid.

31. Ibid., 334.

32. Yung, N. C. L., Wong, C. S. M., Chan, J. K. N., Chen, E. Y. H., & Chang, W. C. (2012). Excess mortality and life-years lost in people with schizophrenia and other non-affective psychoses: An 11-year population-based cohort study, *Schizophrenia Bulletin*, 47(2), 474–484. https://doi.org/10.1093/schbul/sbaa137

33. DeSisto et al. (1995a), 336.

34. Ibid.

35. Ibid., 334.

36. https://www.google.com/search?q=maine+state+archives+

37. DeSisto et al. (1995a), 336.

38. Cannon-Spoor, E., Potkin, S., & Wyatt, R. J. (1982). Measurements of pre-morbid adjustment in chronic schizophrenia. *Schizophrenia Bulletin*, 8, 470–484.

39. DeSisto et al. (1995a), 336.

40. McGorry, P. D., Nelson, B., Goldstone, S., & Yung, A. R. (2010). Clinical staging: A heuristic and practical strategy for new research and better health and social outcomes for psychotic and related mood disorders. *Canadian Journal of Psychiatry*, 55(8), 486–497. https://doi.org/10.1177/070674371005500803

41. Folstein, M. F., Robins, L. N., & Helzer, J. E. (1983). The Mini-Mental State Examination. *Archives of General Psychiatry*, 40(7), 812. doi:10.1001/archpsyc.1983.01790060110016

42. Gold, J. M., & Harvey, P. D. (1993). Cognitive deficits in schizophrenia. *Psychiatric Clinics*, 16(2), 295–312.

43. DeSisto et al. (1995a). 336.

44. https://www.ted.com/talks/sandrine_thuret_you_can_grow_new_brain_cells_here_s_how?language=en

45. Medalia, A., & Choi, J. (2009). Cognitive remediation in schizophrenia. *Neuropsycholology Review*, 19, 353 https://doi.org/10.1007/s11065-009-9097-y

46. Rund, B. R., & Borg, N. E. (1999). Cognitive deficits and cognitive training in schizophrenic patients: A review. *Acta Psychiatrica Scandinavica*, 100, 85–95. doi:10.1111/j.1600-0447.1999.tb10829.x

47. Bleuler, M. (1978). *The schizophrenic disorders: Long-term patient and family studies*. S. M. Clemens (trans.) Yale University Press.

48. DeSisto, M. J., Harding, C. M., McCormick, R. J., Ashikaga, T., & Brooks, G. W. (1995b). The Maine-Vermont three-decade studies of serious mental illness: II. Longitudinal course comparisons. *British Journal of Psychiatry*, 167, 338–342.

49. DeSisto et al. (1995b), 339.

50. Ibid.

51. Ibid., 340.

52. Ibid.

53. Ibid.

54. DeSisto, M., Harding, C. M., Howard, M. A., & Brooks, G. W. (1991). *Perspectives in rural mental health: A comparison of mental health system policy and program development in Maine and Vermont*. Maine Dept. of Mental Health and Mental Retardation.

55. DeSisto et al. (1991).

56. Harding et al. (1987a), 721.

57. DeSisto et al. (1995b), 341.

58. DeSisto et al. (1991).

59. DeSisto et al. (1995b), 339.

60. Deane, W. N., & Brooks, G. W. (1963). Chronic schizophrenics' view recovery. *Journal of Existential Psychiatry*, 4(14), 121–130.

61. Cousins, N. (1979). *The anatomy of an illness as perceived by the patient*. Norton.

62. Mead, S., & Copland, M., E. (2000). What recovery means to us: Consumers' perspectives. *Community Mental Health Journal*, 36(3), 315–328.

63. DeSisto et al. (1995b), 340.

64. Ibid., 336.

65. Hebb, D., O. (1949), *The organization of behavior: A neuropsychological theory*. Wiley.

66. Brown, R., & Milner, P. (2003). The legacy of Donald O. Hebb: More than the Hebb synapse. *National Review of Neuroscience*, 4, 1013–1019. https://doi.org/10.1038/nrn1257

67. Ibid.

68. Andreasen, N. C. (1984). *The broken brain: The biological revolution in psychiatry*. Harper and Row

69. Andreasen, N. C. (2001). *Brave new brain: Conquering mental illness in the era of the genome*. Oxford University Press, 31.

70. Ibid., 31.

71. Harding, C., M. (2003). Changes in schizophrenia across time: Paradoxes, patterns, and predictors. In Carl Cohen (Ed.), *Schizophrenia into later life: Treatment, research and policy* (pp. 19–42). APPI Press.

72. https://www.cdc.gov/genomics/disease/epigenetics.htm

CHAPTER 16

1. Cohen, P., Slomkowski, C., & Robins, L. N. (Eds.). (1999). *Historical and geographical influences on psychopathology*. Erlbaum.

2. DeSisto, M. J., Harding, C. M., McCormick, R. V., Ashikaga, T., & Brooks, G. W. (1995a). The Maine-Vermont three-decade studies of serious mental illness. I. Matched comparison of cross-sectional outcome. *British Journal of Psychiatry*, 167, 331–338.

3. DeSisto et al. (1995a), 334.

4. Paramount Pictures. (1954). *White Christmas*.

5. Klyza, C. M., & Trombulak, S. C. (2015). *The story of Vermont: A natural and cultural history*. University Press of New England.

6. Haviland, W. A., & Power, M. W. (1994). *The original Vermonters: Native inhabitants, past and present*. University Press of New England, 1–16.

7. Frost, R. (1914). Mending wall. In *North of Boston*. David Nutt.

8. *The Proceedings of the Vermont Historical Society*. (1965, January). The Vermont Sheep Industry: 1811–1880.

9. Allbee, R. (2017, March 14). A history of Vermont dairy. *Bennington Banner*.

10. https://www.fpr.Vermont.gov>forest>history-forestry-Vermont

11. https://www.census.gov

12. Ibid.

13. Ibid.

14. Wickman, D. (2005, September 1). Vermont firsts: Vt's pioneering spirit has left a proud legacy (updated October 17, 2018). *The Rutland Herald*.

15. Harding, C. M., Brooks, G. W., Ashikaga, T., Strauss, J. S., & Breier, A. (1987a). The Vermont longitudinal study of persons with severe mental illness: I. Methodology, study sample, and overall status 32 years later. *American Journal of Psychiatry, 144*(6), 718–726.

16. Division of Planning and Rehabilitation Services. (1982). *Statistics*. Vermont Department of Human Services.

17. Vermont State Health Department (1982). *Statistics*.

18. U. S. Census Data (2019). Vermont per capita income. https://www.census.gov/quickfacts/VT

19. https://www.mainememory.net/sitebuilder/site/895/page/1306/display?page=2

20. https://www.smithsonianmag.com/history/maines-lost-colony-106323660/

21. http://publications.americanalpineclub.org/articles/13198505302/Avalanche-Weather-Maine-Baxter-State-Park-Mount-Katahdin

22. https://www.maine.gov/msl/meorigin.htm

23. https://www.maineanencyclopedia.com/timeline-of-maine-history

24. https://statesymbolsusa.org/symbol-official-item/national-us/uncategorized/states-size

25. https://www.census.gov/quickfacts/ME

26. Ibid.

27. https://www.mainepotatoes.com/

28. https://coast.noaa.gov/data/docs/states/shorelines.pdf

29. Roorbach, B. (2014, November 21). Carolyn Chute's "Treat Us Like Dogs and We Will Become Wolves." *New York Times Book Review*

30. https://www.maine.gov/DACF/mfs/publications/reports/maine_assessment_and_strategy_final.pdf

31. https://acadiamagic.com/Downeast.html

32. https://www.acadiavisitor.com/downeast-dictionary-a-guide-to-maines-native-language/

33. https://www.Maine.gov/sos/kids/about

34. https://health.gov/healthypeople/objectives-and-data/social-determinants-health

CHAPTER 17

1. Harding, C. M. (2003). Changes in schizophrenia across time: Paradoxes, patterns, and predictors. In C. I. Cohen (Ed.), *Schizophrenia into later life: Treatment, research, and policy.* American Psychiatric Press.

2. Strauss, J. S., & Carpenter, W. T. Jr. (1974). Characteristic symptoms and outcome in schizophrenia. *Archives of General Psychiatry, 30*(1), 429–434.

3. Wunderink, L., Nieboer, R. M., & Wiersma, D. (2013). Recovery in remitted first episode psychosis at 7 years of follow-up of an early dose reduction/discontinuation or maintenance treatment strategy. *JAMA Psychiatry, 70*(9), 913–920.

4. Bleuler, M. (1972/1978) Die schizophrenien Geistesstörungen im Lichte langjähriger Kranken-und Familiengeschichten, Georg Thieme. In S. M. Clemens (Trans)., *The Schizophrenic disorders: Long-term patient and family studies* (p. 438). Yale University Press.

5. Harrow. M., & Jobe, T. H. (2013). Does long-term treatment of schizophrenia with antipsychotic medications facilitate recovery? *Schizophrenia Bulletin, 39,* 962–965.

6. Ciompi, L., & Müller, C. (1976). *Lebensweg und Alter Schizophrenen Eine Katamnestic Longzeitstudie bis ins Senium.* Springer-Verlag.

7. Ogawa, K., Miya, M., Wataral, A., Nakazawa, M., Yuasa, S., & Utena, H. (1987). A long-term follow-up study of schizophrenia in Japan with special reference to the course of social adjustment. *British Journal of Psychiatry, 151*(6), 758–765.

8. Huber, G., Gross, G., & Schüttler, R. (1979). *Schizophrenie. Verlaufs-und sozialpsychiatrische Langzeitunter-suchungen an den 1945–1959 in Bonn hospitalisierten schizophrenen Kranken.* Monographien aus dem Gesamtgebiete der Psych der Psychiatrie. Bd.21, Springer-Verlag.

9. Hinterhuber, H. (1973). Catamnestic studies on schizophrenia. *Fortschritte der Neurologie, Psychiatrie und ihrer Grenzgebiete, 41*(10), 527–558

10. Tsuang, M. T., Woolson, R. F., & Fleming, J. A. (1979). Long-term outcome of major psychoses: I. Schizophrenia and affective disorders compared with psychiatrically symptom-free surgical conditions. *Archives of General Psychiatry, 36*(12), 1295–1301. doi:10.1001/archpsyc.1979.01780120025002

11. Marinow, A. (1974). Klinisch-statistische und katamnestische Untersuchugen und chronisch Schizophrenen 1951–1960 und 1961–1970. *Archives für Psychiatrie und Nervenkrankheiten, 218*(2), 115–124.

12. Kreditor, D. Kh. (1977). Late katamnesis of recurrent schizophrenia with prolonged remissions (according to an unselected study). *Zh Nervopatol Psikaitr Im SS Korsakova, 77*(1), 110–113.

13. Bleuler, E. (1911/1950). *Dementia praecox oder Gruppe der Schizophrenien* (Vol. 12). Deuticke. In J. Zinkin (Trans.), *Dementia praecox or the group of schizophrenias.* International Universities Press.

14. McNeely, J. D. (1998, April 14). *The Burghölzli Clinic: Cradle of western psychiatry.* Paper presentation to Innominate Society, Louisville, KY.

15. Palmai, G., & Blackwell, B. (1966). The Burghölzli centenary. *Medical History, 10*(3), 257–265, at 260. doi:https://doi.org/10.1017/S0025727300011121
16. Bleuler (1972/1978), 413.
17. Cohen, P., & Cohen, J. (1984). The clinician's illusion. *Archives of General Psychiatry, 41*(12), 1178–1182.
18. Bleuler (1972/1978), 5.
19. Ibid., 16.
20. Boyle, M. (1990). Is schizophrenia what it was? A re-analysis of Kraepelin's and Bleuler's population. *Journal of the History of the Behavioral Sciences, 26*(4), 323–333.
21. Kraepelin, E. (1899). *Psychiatrie: Ein Lehrbuch für Studierende und Aerzte.* Barth.
22. Kraepelin, E (1903–1904). *Psychiatrie: Ein Lehrbuch für Studierende und Aerzte,* 7. Auflage, 2 Bände (A. Ross Diefendorf, Trans.). 1907. *Clinical psychiatry: A textbook for students and physicians,* 2 vols. MacMillan.
23. Bleuler (1972/1978), 438.
24. Ibid., 68/53
25. American Psychiatric Association (APA). (2013). *Diagnostic and statistical manual of mental disorders* (5th ed.). American Psychiatric Association. https://doi.org/10.1176/appi.books.937089045596
26. World Health Organization. (2022). International Classification of Disease (11th rev.). WHO.
27. American Psychiatric Association (2013), 3.
28. Harding, C. M., & Keller, A. B. (1998). Long-term outcome of social functioning in schizophrenia. In K. T. Mueser & N. Tarrier (Eds.), *The handbook of social functioning.* Allyn & Bacon.
29. Bleuler (1972/1978), 424.
30. Ibid.
31. Ibid., 425.
32. Bleuler, M. (1984). The old and new picture of the schizophrenic patient. *Schweizer Archiv fur Neurologie, Neurochirurgie und Psychiatrie, 135,* 135–149.
33. Bleuler (1972/1978), 414.
34. Csikszentmihalyi, M. (1997). *Finding flow.* Basic Books.
35. Huber, G., Gross, G., & Schüttler, R. (1979). Schizophrenie. Verlaufs-und socialpsychiatrische Langzeitunter-suchgen an den 1945 bis 1959 in Bonn hospitalisierten schizophrenen Kranken. In *Monographien aus dem Gesamtgebiete der Psychiatrie.* Bd. 21. Springer
36. Huber, G. Gross, G., Schüttler, R., & Linz, N. (1980). Longitudinal studies of schizophrenic patients. *Schizophrenia Bulletin, 8*(4), 592–603.
37. Ibid., 593–594.
38. Ibid., 595.
39. Ibid.
40. Ibid., 598.
41. Ibid., 596.

42. Ciompi, L (1980a). Catamnestic long-term study on the course of life and aging of schizophrenics (S. Clemens Trans.). *Schizophrenia Bulletin, 6*(4), 606–618 at 608.

43. Ibid., 607.

44. Ibid., 613.

45. Ibid., 610–611.

46. Ibid., 614.

47. Ibid., 616.

48. Hinterhuber (1973).

49. Ibid.

50. Kreditor (1977).

51. Marinow, A. (1981). Uber Verlauf, Ausgang, und Prognose bei Schizophrenien. In G. Huber (Ed.), *Schizophrenic: Stand und Entwicklungstendenzen der Forschung* (pp. 85–95). Schattauer.

52. Marinow, A. (1986). Prognostication in schizophrenia. *Psychopathology, 19,* 192–195.

53. Ibid., 193.

54. Strauss, J. S., & Carpenter, W. T. (1974). The prediction of outcome in schizophrenia. II. Relationships between predictor variables and outcome variables. *Archives of General Psychiatry, 31,* 37–42.

55. Marinow, 194.

56. Ibid., 195.

57. World Health Organization (1979–1998). *The International Classification of Diseases* (9th rev.). WHO.

58. Ogawa, K., Miya, M., Wataral, A., Nakazawa, N., Yuasa, S., & Utena, H. (1987). A long-term follow-up study of schizophrenia in Japan with special reference to the course of social adjustment. *British Journal of Psychiatry, 151,* 758–765.

59. Ogawa et al. (1987), 758.

60. Ibid.

61. Eguma, Y. (1962). The prevention of failure in the rehabilitation of discharged schizophrenic patients (in Japanese). *Psychiatrie et Neurologia, 64,* 921–927.

62. WHO (1979–1998).

63. Ogawa et al. (1987), 759.

64. Ibid., 760.

65. World Psychiatric Association. (2002). *Schizophrenia: Open the doors. The WPA Global Programme against stigma and discrimination because of schizophrenia.* WPA.

66. Sato, M. (2006). Renaming schizophrenia: A Japanese perspective. *World Psychiatry, 5*(1), 53–55.

67. Takahashi, H., Ideno, T., Okubo, S., Matsui, H., Takemura, K., Matsuura, M., Kato, M., & Okubo, Y. (2009). Impact of changing the Japanese term for "schizophrenia" for reasons of stereotypical beliefs of schizophrenia in Japanese youth. *Schizophrenia Research, 112*(1–3), 149–152.

68. Lee, Y. S., & Kwon, J. S. (2011). Renaming of schizophrenia. *Journal of Korean Neuropsychiatric Association, 50,* 16–19.

69. Chiu, C. P., Lam, M. M., & Chan, S. K. (2010). Naming psychosis: The Hong Kong experience. *Early Intervention Psychiatry, 4*, 53–54.

70. Sartorius, N., Chiu, H., Heok, K. E., Lee, M. S., Ouyang, W. C., Sato, M., Yang, Y. K., & Yu, X. (2014). Name change for schizophrenia. *Schizophrenia Bulletin, 40*(2), 255–258.

71. Carpenter, W. T. (2016). Shifting paradigms and the term schizophrenia. *Schizophrenia Bulletin, 42*(4), 863–864. https://doi.org/10.1093/schbul/sbw050

72. Feighner, J. P., Robins, E., Guze, S. B., Woodruff, R. A., Winokur, G., & Munoz, R. (1972). Diagnostic criteria for use in psychiatric research. *Archives of General Psychiatry, 26*(1), 57–63.

73. American Psychiatric Association (APA). (1968). *Diagnostic and statistical manual of mental disorders* (2nd ed.). American Psychiatric Press.

74. Harding, C. M., Brooks, G. W., Ashikaga, T., Strauss, J. S., & Breier, A. (1987a). The Vermont longitudinal study of persons with severe mental illness: I. Methodology, study sample, and overall status 32 years later. *American Journal of Psychiatry, 144*(6), 718–726.

75. Harding, C. M., Brooks, G. W., Ashikaga, T., Strauss, J. S., & Breier, A. (1987b). The Vermont longitudinal study: II. Long-term outcome of subjects who retrospectively met DSM-III criteria for schizophrenia. *American Journal of Psychiatry, 144*(6), 727–735

76. Winokur, G., & Tsuang, M. T. (1996). Follow-up of untreated patients. In *The natural history of mania, depression, and schizophrenia* (pp. 131–142). American Psychiatric Press.

77. Mental Hospital Survey Committee, New York, NY. (1937). A Survey of the state hospitals of Iowa (50, 51). http://publications.iowa.gov/26294/1/Survey%20of%20the%20State%20Hospital%20or%20Iowa%201937.pdf

78. Ibid.

79. Tsuang, M. T., Woolson, R. F., & Fleming, J. A. (1979). Long-term outcome of major psychoses: I. Schizophrenia and affective disorders compared with psychiatrically symptom-free surgical conditions. *Archives of General Psychiatry, 36*(12), 1295–1301.

80. Tsuang, T., & Winokur, G. (1975). The Iowa 500: Field work in a 35-year follow-up of depression, mania, and schizophrenia. *Canadian Psychiatric Association Journal. 20*(5), 359–365. (360)

81. Tsuang et al. (1979), 1296.

82. Winokur, G., & Tsuang, M. T. (1996). *The natural history of mania, depression, and schizophrenia.* American Psychiatric Publishers, 50.

83. Ibid., 183.

84. Ibid., 205.

85. Ibid., 206–207.

86. Harrow, M., Grossman, L. S., Jobe, T. H., & Herbener, E. S. (2005). Do patients with schizophrenia ever show periods of recovery? A 15-year multi-follow-up study. *Schizophrenia Bulletin, 31*(3), 723–734. https://doi.org/10.1093/schbul/sbi026

87. Harrow, M., Jobe, T. H., & Faull (2014). Does treatment of schizophrenia with antipsychotic medications eliminate or reduce psychosis? A 20 -year multi-follow-up study. *Psychological Medicine*, *44*(14), 1–11. doi:10.1017/S0033291714000610

88. Harrow, M., Jobe, T. H., Faull, R. N., & Yang, J. (2017). A twenty-year multi-followup longitudinal study assessing whether antipsychotic medications contribute to work functioning in schizophrenia. *Psychiatry Research*, *256*, 267–274, at 271. doi:10.1016/psychres.2017.06069

89. Harrow, M., & Jobe, T. H. (2007). Factors involved in outcome and recovery in schizophrenia patients not on antipsychotic medications: A 15-year multifollow-up study. *Journal of Nervous and Mental Disease*, *195*(5), 406–414, at 406.

90. Ibid., 407–408.

91. Harrow et al. (2014), 8

92. Harrow & Jobe (2007), 410.

93. Lewin, K. (1951). *Field theory in social science: Selected theoretical papers*. D. Cartwright (Ed.). Harper & Row.

94. Harrow et al. (2005), 723.

95. Harrow, M., Jobe, T. H., & Tong, L. (2021). Twenty-year effects of antipsychotics in schizophrenia and affective psychotic disorders. *Psychological Medicine*, *1*(11), 1, 4. https://doi.org/10.1017/S0032017200004778

96. Harrow et al. (2021), 5–6.

97. Insel, T. (2010). Rethinking schizophrenia. *Nature*, *468*(7321), 187–193. doi:10.1038/nature09552

98. Harrow et al. (2021), 2.

99. Moncrieff, J., Lewis, G., Freemantle, N., Johnson, S., Barnes, T. R. E., Morant, N., Pinfold, V., Hunter, R., Kent, L. J., Smith, R., Darton, K., Horne, R., Crellin, N. E., Cooper, R. E., Marston, L., & Priebe, S. (2019). Randomised controlled trial of gradual antipsychotic reduction and discontinuation in people with schizophrenia and related disorders: The RADAR trial (Research into Antipsychotic Discontinuation and Reduction). *British Medical Journal*, *9*(11), e030912. doi:10.1136/bmjopen-2019-030912. Erratum in: BMJ Open. 2020 Jul 28;10(7), e030912corr1. PMID: 31780589; PMCID: PMC6887002.

100. Steingard, S. (2019). Clinical implications of the drug-centered approach. In Sandra Steingard (Ed.), *Critical psychiatry: Controversies and clinical implications* (pp. 113–135). Springer.

CHAPTER 18

1. Harding, C. M. (2003). Changes in schizophrenia across time: Paradoxes, patterns, and predictors. In C. I. Cohen (Ed.), *Schizophrenia into later life: Treatment, research, and policy*. American Psychiatric Press.

2. Harding, C. M. &., & Keller, A. B. (1988). Chapter 9: Long-term outcome of social functioning. In K. T. Mueser & N. Tarrier (Eds.), *The handbook of social functioning* (pp. 134–148). Allyn & Bacon.

3. Bleuler, M. (1972/1978). Die schizophrenien Geistesstörungen im Lichte langjähriger Kranken-und Familiengeschichten, Georg Thieme. In S. M. Clemens (Trans.), *The schizophrenic disorders: Long-term patient and family studies* (p. 438). Yale University Press.

4. Hinterhuber, H. (1973). Catamnestic studies on schizophrenia. *Fortschritte der Neurologie, Psychiatrie und ihrer Grenzgebiete, 41*(10), 527–558.

5. Ciompi, L., & Müller, C. (1976). *Lebensweg und Alter Schizophrenen Eine Katamnestic Longzeitstudie bis ins Senium.* Springer-Verlag.

6. Kreditor, D. Kh. (1977). Late katamnesis of recurrent schizophrenia with prolonged remissions (according to an unselected study). *Zh Nervopatol Psikaitr Im SS Korsakova, 77*(1), 110–113.

7. Huber, G., Gross, G., & Schüttler, R. (1979). *Schizophrenie. Verlaufs-und sozialpsychiatrische Langzeitunter-suchungen an den 1945–1959 in Bonn hospitalisierten schizophrenen Kranken.* Monographien aus dem Gesamtgebiete der Psych der Psychiatrie, Bd.21. Springer-Verlag.

8. Tsuang, M. T., Woolson, R. F., & Fleming, J. A. (1979). Long-term outcome of major psychoses: I. Schizophrenia and affective disorders compared with psychiatrically symptom-free surgical conditions. *Archives of General Psychiatry, 36*(12), 1295–1301. doi:10.1001/archpsyc.1979.01780120025002

9. Marinow, A. (1974). Klinisch-statistische und katamnestische Untersuchugen und chronisch Schizophrenen 1951–1960 und 1961–1970. *Archives für Psychiatrie und Nervenkrankheiten. 218*(2), 115–124.

10. Harding, C. M., Brooks, G. W., Ashikaga, T., Strauss, J. S., & Breier, A. (1987b). The Vermont longitudinal study: II. Long-term outcome of subjects who retrospectively met DSM-III criteria for schizophrenia. *American Journal of Psychiatry, 144*(6), 727–735.

11. Ogawa, K., Miya, M., Wataral, A., Nakazawa, M., Yuasa, S., & Utena, H. (1987). A long-term follow-up study of schizophrenia in Japan-with special reference to the course of social adjustment. *British Journal of Psychiatry, 151*(6), 758–765.

12. DeSisto, M. J., Harding, C. M., McCormick, R. J., Ashikaga, T., & Brooks, G. W. (1995b). The Maine-Vermont three-decade studies of serious mental illness: II. Longitudinal course comparisons. *British Journal of Psychiatry, 167*, 338–342.

13. Harrow, M., Grossman, L. S., Jobe, T. H., & Herbener, E. S. (2005). Do patients with schizophrenia ever show periods of recovery? A 15-year multi-follow-up study. *Schizophrenia Bulletin, 31*(3), 723–734. https://doi.org/10.1093/schbul/sbi026

14. Harrow, M., Jobe, T. H., & Faull, R. N. (2014). Does treatment of schizophrenia with antipsychotic medications eliminate or reduce psychosis? A 20-year multi-follow-up study. *Psychological Medicine*, 1–10.

15. Harding et al. (1987b).

16. Rosen, K., & Garety, P. (2005). Predicting recovery from schizophrenia: A retrospective comparison of characteristics at onset of people with single and multiple episodes. *Schizophrenia Bulletin, 31*(3), 735–750.

17. Seeman, M. V. (1986). Current outcome in schizophrenia: Women vs men. *Acta Psychiatrica Scandinavica, 73*(6), 609–617.

18. Angermeyer, M. C., Kühn, L., & Goldstein, J. M. (1990). Gender and the course of schizophrenia: Differences in treated outcomes. *Schizophrenia Bulletin, 16*(2), 293–307.

19. American Psychiatric Association (APA). (2013). *Diagnostic and statistical manual of mental disorders* (5th ed). American Psychiatric Press. https://doi.org/10.1176/appi.books.9780890425596

20. Harrow, M., Jobe, T. H., & Tong, L. (2021). Twenty-year effects of antipsychotics in schizophrenia and affective psychotic disorders. *Psychological Medicine, 1*(11) 1, 4. https://doi.org/10.1017/S0032017200004778

21. Deegan, P. E. (2010). A Web application to support recovery and shared decision making in psychiatric medication clinics. *Psychiatric Rehabilitation Journal, 34*(1), 23–28. https://doi.org/10.2975/34.1.2010.23.28

22. Solomon, P. (2004). Peer support/peer provided services underlying processes, benefits, and critical ingredients. *Psychiatric Rehabilitation Journal, 27*(4), 392–401. https://doi.org/10.2975/27.2004.392.401

23. Engstrom, E. J., & Kendler, K. S. (2015). Emil Kraepelin: Icon and reality. *American Journal of Psychiatry, 172*(12), 1190–1196.

24. Insel, T. (2022). *Healing: Our path from mental illness to mental health.* Penguin Random House.

25. Kapur, S., Phillips, A. G., & Insel, T. R. (2012). Why has it taken so long for biological psychiatry to develop clinical tests and what to do about it? *Molecular psychiatry, 17*(12), 1174–1179.

26. Moncrieff, J., Lewis, G., Freemantle, N., Johnson, S., Barnes, T. R.E., Morant, N., Pinfold, V., Hunter, R., Kent, L. J., Smith, R., Darton, K., Horne, R., Crellin, N. E., Cooper, R. E., Marston, L., & Priebe, S. (2019). Randomised controlled trial of gradual antipsychotic reduction and discontinuation in people with schizophrenia and related disorders: The RADAR trial (Research into Antipsychotic Discontinuation and Reduction). *British Medical Journal, 9*(11), e030912. doi:10.1136/bmjopen-2019-030912. Erratum in: BMJ Open. 2020 Jul 28;10(7), e030912corr1. PMID: 31780589; PMCID: PMC6887002.

27. Milani, R. M., Nahar, K., Ware, D., Butler, A., Roush, S., Smith, D., Perrino, L., & O'Donnell, J. (2020). A qualitative longitudinal study of the first UK Dual Diagnosis Anonymous (DDA), an integrated peer-support programme for concurrent disorders. *Advances in Dual Diagnosis, 13*(4), 151–167.

28. Roush, S., Monica, C., Carpenter-Song, E., & Drake, R. E. (2015). First-person perspectives on dual diagnosis anonymous (DDA): A qualitative study. *Journal of Dual Diagnosis, 11*(2), 136–141.

29. Mosher, L. R. (1999). Soteria and other alternatives to acute psychiatric hospitalization. *Journal of Nervous & Mental Disease, 187*(3), 142–149.

30. Marrone, J., & Golowka, E. (1999). If work makes people with mental illness sick, what do unemployment, poverty, and social isolation cause? *Psychiatric Rehabilitation Journal, 23*(2), 187.

31. DeSisto, M., Harding, C. M., Howard, M. A., et al. (1991). *Perspectives on rural mental health: A comparison of mental health services and program development in Maine and Vermont.* Kennebec Press.

32. Slade, M., Amering, M., Farkas, M., Hamilton, B., O'Hagan, M. Panther, G., Perkins, R., Shepherd, G., Tse, S., & Whitley, R. (2014). Uses and abuses of recovery: Implementing recovery-oriented practices in mental health systems. *World Psychiatry, 13*(1), 12–20. doi:10.1002/wps.20084

33. Ibid.

34. Ibid.

35. Spaniol, L., Gagne, C., & Koehler, M. (1999). Recovery from serious mental illness: What it is and how to support people in their recovery. In R. P. Marinelli & A. E. Dell Orto (Eds.), *The psychological & social impact of disability* (pp. 409–422). Springer.

36. Chittick, R. A., Brooks, G. W., Irons, F. S., & Deane, W. N. (1961). The Vermont Story: Rehabilitation of chronic schizophrenic patients. Queen City Printers (out of print)..

37. Kidd, B. A., & Kral, M. J. (2005). Practicing participatory action research. *Journal of Counseling Psychology, 52*(2),187–195.

38. Joint Commission for Mental Illness and Health. (1961). *Final Report: Summary of recommendations. Action for Mental Health.* Basic Books, xix.

39. https://www.nimh.nih.gov/health/topics/schizophrenia

40. Anthony, W. A. (993). Recovery from mental illness. The guiding vision of the mental health system in the 1990s. *Psychosocial Rehabilitation Journal, 16*(4), 11–23, at 15. https://doi.apa.org/doi/10.1037/h0095655

41. Deegan, P. E. (1988). Recovery: The lived experience of rehabilitation. *Psychosocial Rehabilitation Journal, 11*(4), 11.

42. Ridgway, P. (2008). Supported housing. In K. T. Mueser & D. V. Jeste (Eds.), *Clinical handbook of schizophrenia* (pp. 287–297). Guilford.

43. Vine, P. (2022). *Fighting for recovery: An activists' history of mental health reform.* Beacon Press.

44. The 2009 Resolution on APA Endorsement of the Concept of Recovery for People with Severe Mental Illness was completed by the Task Force on Serious Mental Illness and Severe Emotional Disturbance (TFSMI/SED) and approved by APA Council of Representatives om August 5, 2009.

45. American Psychological Association & Jansen, M. A. (2014). *Recovery to practice initiative curriculum: Reframing psychology for the emerging healthcare environment.* American Psychological Association.

46. Ibid.

47. The British Psychological Society & Cooke, A. (Ed.). (2017). *Understanding psychosis and schizophrenia.* A report by the Division of Clinical Psychology. Canterbury Christ Church University.

48. Torgalsbøen, A., K. (2001). Nye forskrifter i psykisk helsevern: gjennombrudd for psykologene. Intervju. *Tidsskrift for Norsk psykologforening, 38*(1), 49–51.

49. APA (2014).

50. Insel, T. (2012). *The Director's Blog: Words matter.* National Institute of Mental Health, October 2, 2012. Accessed January 10, 2013. http://www.nimh.nih.gov/about/director/index.shtml#p143631

51. Breier, A., & Strauss, J. S. (1984). Social relationships in the recovery from psychiatric disorder. *American Journal of Psychiatry, 141*(8), 949–955.

52. Brooks, G. W. (1960). Rehabilitation of hospitalized chronic schizophrenic patients. In L. Appleby, J. Scher, & J. Cumming (Eds.), *Chronic Schizophrenia.* Free Press.

53. Vine (2022).

CHAPTER 19

1. Warner, R. (2013). *Recovery from schizophrenia: Psychiatry and political economy.* Routledge.

2. Rapp, C. A., & Goscha, R. J. (2006). *The strengths model: Case management with people with psychiatric disabilities.* Oxford University Press.

3. de Girolamo, G., Barale, F., Politi, P., & Fusar-Poli, P. (2008). Franco Basaglia, 1924–1980. *American Journal of Psychiatry, 165*(8), 968–968.

4. Mezzina, R. (2014). Community mental health care in Trieste and beyond: An "open door–no restraint" system of care for recovery and citizenship. *Journal of Nervous and Mental Disease, 202*(6), 440–445.

5. Frances, A. (2021). Save Trieste's mental health system. *Lancet Psychiatry, 8*(9), 744–746. https://doi.org/10.1016/S2215-0366(21)00252-2

6. Barbato, A., D'Avanzo, B., D'Anza, V., Montorfano, E., Savio, M., & Corbascio, C. G. (2014). Involvement of users and relatives in mental health service evaluation. *Journal of Nervous and Mental Disease, 202*(6), 479–486.

7. Anttinen, E. E., Jokinen, R., & Ojanen, M. (1985). Progressive integrated system for the rehabilitation of long-term schizophrenic patients. *Acta Psychiatrica Scandinavica, 71*(319), 51–59.

8. Alanen, Y. O. (2009). Towards a more humanistic psychiatry: Development of need-adapted treatment of schizophrenia group psychoses. *Psychosis, 1*(2), 156–166. http://doi.org/10.10801/1752243090295667

9. Ibid.

10. Seikkula, J., & Olson, M. E. (2003). The open dialogue approach to acute psychosis: Its poetics and micropolitics. *Family Process, 42*(3), 403–418.

11. Olson, M., Seikkula, J., & Ziedonis, D. (2014). *The key elements of dialogic practice in Open Dialogue.* University of Massachusetts Medical School. http://www.umassmed.edu/globalassets/psychiatry/open-dialogue/keyelementsv1.109022014.pdfGoogle Scholar

12. Cullberg, J., Levander, S., Holmqvist, R., Mattsson, M., & Wieselgren, I. M. (2002). One-year outcome in first episode psychosis patients in the Swedish Parachute project. *Acta Psychiatrica Scandinavica, 106*(4), 276–285.

13. Ibid., 277.

14. Strålin, P., Skott, M., & Cullberg, J. (2019). Early recovery and employment outcome 13 years after first episode psychosis. *Psychiatric Research, 271*(1), 374–380. doi:10.1016/j.psychres.2018.12.013

15. Hopper, K., Van Tiem, J., Cubellis, L., & Pope, L. (2020). Merging intentional peer support and dialogic practice: implementation lessons from Parachute NYC. *Psychiatric Services, 71*(2), 199–201.

16. Ciompi, L. (1994). Affect logic: An integrative model of the psyche and its relations to schizophrenia. *British Journal of Psychiatry, 164*(S23), 51–55.

17. Ciompi, L. (2017). Soteria Berne: 32 years of experience. *Swiss Archives of Neurology, Psychiatry and Psychotherapy, 168*(01), 10–13.

18. Mosher, L. R. (1999). Soteria and other alternatives to acute psychiatric hospitalization: A personal and professional review. *Journal of Nervous and Mental Disease, 187*(3), 142–149.

19. Diaz, E., Fergusson, A., & Strauss, J. S. (2004). Innovative care for the homeless mentally ill in Bogota, Colombia. *Cambridge Studies in Medical Anthropology*, 219–237.

20. Fergusson, A. (2012). *Accompanied self-rehabilitation*. Editorial Universidad del Rosario.

21. Romme, M. A. J., Honig, A., Noorthoorn, E. O., & Escher, A. D. M. A. C. (1992). Coping with hearing voices: An emancipatory approach. *British Journal of Psychiatry, 161*(1), 99–103.

22. https://www.hearing-voices.org/

23. Dillon, J., & Longden, E. (2012). Hearing voices groups: Creating safe spaces to share taboo experiences. In M. Romme & S. Escher (Eds.), *Psychosis as a personal crisis: An experience-based approach* (pp. 129–139). Routledge.

24. Hornstein, G. A., Putnam, E. R., & Branitsky, A. (2020). How do hearing voices peer-support groups work? A three-phase model of transformation. *Psychosis*. https://doi.org/10.1080/17522439.2020.174987

25. Longdon, E., Read, J., & Dillon, J. (2018). Assessing the impact and effectiveness of hearing voices network self-help groups. *Community Mental Health Journal, 54*, 184–188. https://doi.org/10.1007/s10597-017-0148

26. https://www.ted.com/talks/eleanor_longden_the_voices_in_my_head?language=en

27. Hornstein, G. A., Branitsky, A., & Putnam, E. R. (2021). The diverse functions of hearing voices peer-support groups: Findings and case examples from a US national study. *Psychosis*, 1–11. doi:10.1080/17522439.2021.1897653

28. Hornstein, G. A. (2009/2019). *Agnes's jacket: A psychologist's search for the meaning of madness*. 1st ed., Transaction Publishers; 2nd ed, Routledge. https://doi.org/10.4324/9781315083728

29. Brown, G. W., & Birley, J. (1968). Crises and life changes and the onset of schizophrenia. *Journal of Health and Social Behavior, 9*, 203–214.

30. Leff, J., Williams, G., Huckvale, M., Arbuthnot, M., & Leff, A. P. (2014). Avatar therapy for persecutory auditory hallucinations: What is it and how does it work? *Psychosis, 6*(2), 166–176. https://doi.org/10.1080/17522439.2013.773457

31. Perkins, D. O., Gu, H., Boteva, K., & Lieberman, J. A. (2005). Relationship between duration of untreated psychosis and outcome in first-episode schizophrenia: A critical review and meta-analysis. *American Journal of Psychiatry*, *162*(10), 1785–1804.

32. McGorry, P. D., Edwards, J., Mihalopoulos, C., Harrigan, S. M., & Jackson, H. J. (1996). EPPIC: An evolving system of early detection and optimal management, *Schizophrenia Bulletin*, *22*(2), 305–326, https://doi.org/10.1093/schbul/22.2.305

33. McGorry, P. D., Yung, A., & Phillips, L. (2001). Ethics and early intervention in psychosis: Keeping up the pace and staying in step. *Schizophrenia Research*, *51*(1), 17–29.

34. Dixon, L. B., Goldman, H. H., Bennett, M. E., Wang, Y., McNamara, K. A., Mendon, S. J., Goldstein, A. B., Chien-Wen, J. C., Rufina, J. L., Lieberman, J. A., & Essock, S. M. (2015). Implementing coordinated specialty care for early psychosis: The RAISE Connection Program. *Psychiatric Services*, *66*(7), 691–698.

35. Rosen, A., Gill, N. S., & Salvador-Carulla, L. (2020). The future of community psychiatry and community mental health services, *Current Opinion in Psychiatry*, *33*(4), 375–390. doi:10.1097/YCO.0000000000000620

36. Rosen, A., & Holmes, D. J. (2023). Co-leadership to co-design in mental health-care ecosystems: What does it mean to us? *Leadership in Health Services*, *36*(1), 59–76.

37. Rosen, A. (2006). The Australian experience of deinstitutionalization: Interaction of Australian culture with the development and reform of its mental health services. *Acta Psychiatrica Scandinavica*, *113*, 81–89.

CHAPTER 20

1. Beels, C. C., & McFarlane, W. R. (1982). Family treatments of schizophrenia: Background and state of the art. *Psychiatric Services*, *33*(7), 541–550.

2. Newmark, M., & Beels, C. (1994). The misuse and use of science in family therapy. *Family Process*, *33*(1), 3–17. https://doi.org/10.1111/j.1545-5300.1994.00003.x

3. LeMelle, S., Arbuckle, M. R., & Ranz, J. M. (2013). Integrating systems-based practice, community psychiatry, and recovery into residency training. *Academic Psychiatry*, *37*(1), 35–37.

4. McFarlane, W. R., Dunne, E., Lukens, E., Horton, B., Newmark, M., & McLaughlin-Toran, J. (1993). From research to clinical practice: Dissemination of New York State's Family Psychoeducation Project. *Hospital and Community Psychiatry*, *44*(3) 265–270. https://doi.org/10.1176/ps.44.3.265

5. Anderson, C. M., Reiss, D. J., & Hogarty, G. E. (1986). *Schizophrenia and the family: A practitioner's guide to psychoeducation and management*. Guilford.

6. Anthony, W. A., Cohen, M., & Farkas, M. (1999). The future of psychiatric rehabilitation. *International Journal of Mental Health*, *28*(1), 48–68. doi:10.1080/00207411.1999.11449446

7. Rogers, C. R. (1977). *Carl Rogers on personal power*. Delacorte.

8. Frankl, V. E. (1985). *Man's search for meaning*. Simon and Schuster.

9. Maslow, A. H. (1954). The instinctoid nature of basic needs. *Journal of Personality*, *22*, 326–347. https://doi.org/10.1111/j.1467-6494.1954.tb01136.x

10. Davidson, L., Rakfeldt, J., & Strauss, J. S. (2011). *Roots of the recovery movement in psychiatry: Lessons learned*. Wiley-Blackwell, 17.

11. Farkas, M., & Anthony, W. A. (1989). *Psychiatric rehabilitation programs: Putting theory into practice*. Johns Hopkins University Press.

12. Anthony, W. A. (1993). Recovery from mental illness: The guiding vision of the mental health service system in the 1990s. *Psychosocial Rehabilitation Journal*, *16*(4), 15.

13. Frost, R. (1914). Mending wall. In *North of Boston*. D. Nutt.

14. Wang, C., & Burris, M. A. (1997). Photovoice: Concept, methodology, and use for participatory needs assessment. *Health Education & Behavior*, *24*(3), 369–387. https://doi.org/10.1177/109019819702400309

15. Brown, E. O. (Autumn, 1984). The Diner by the Falls: Serving up smiles in Springfield. *Vermont Life Magazine*, 2–4.

16. https://www.courtinnovation.org/programs/brooklyn/mental-health-court. Reaccessed July 1, 2021.

17. https://ww2.nyccourts.gov/mental-health-courts-overview-27066. Reaccessed July 1, 2021.

18. https://www.csgjusticecenter.org/projects/mental-health-courts/. Reaccessed July 1, 2021.

19. Beard, J. H., Propst, R. N., & Malamud, T. J. (1982). The Fountain House model of psychiatric rehabilitation. *Psychosocial Rehabilitation Journal*, *5*(1), 47–53.

20. https://clubhouse-intl.org

21. Harding, C. M. (2009). Star Chart: Measuring social network supports.

22. MHA Village Long Beach, California. (2000). Gold Award: A comprehensive treatment program helps persons with severe mental illness integrate into the community. *Psychiatric Services*, *51*(11), 1436–1438. https://doi.org/10.1176/appi.ps.51.11.1436

23. http://presstelegram.com/2021/03/18/martha-long-creator-of-the-village

24. Ragins, M. (2002). *Road to recovery*. Mental Health of America Los Angeles. http://www.village-isa/ragins

25. Ragins, M. (2021). *Journeys beyond the frontier: A rebellious guide to psychosis and other extraordinary experiences*. Amazon.

26. Fisher, D. G., Pilon, D., Hershberger, S. L., Reynolds, G. L., LaMaster, S. C., & Davis, M. (2009). Psychometric properties of an assessment for mental health recovery programs. *Community Mental Health Journal*, *45*(4), 246–250.

27. https://www.villlage cookieshoppe.com. Re-accessed July 3, 2021.

28. https://www.lbpost.com/hi-lo/mha-village-recognizes-those-recovering-from-mental-illness/. ReAccessed July 1, 2021.

29. Neligh, G., Shore, J. H., Scully, J., Kort, H., Willett, B., Harding, C. M., & Kawamura, G. (1991). The program for public psychiatry: State-university collaboration in Colorado. *Psychiatric Services*, *42*(1), 44–48.

30. Plante, T. G., &. Sharma, N. K. (2001). Religious faith and mental health outcomes. In T. G. Plante & A. C. Sherman (Eds.), *Faith and health: Psychological perspectives* (pp. 381–402). Guilford.

31. Smith, S., & Beitzel, T. (Eds.). (2014). *One hundred years of service through community: A Gould Farm reader.* University Press of America.

32. Monica, C., Nikkel, R. E., & Drake, R. E. (2010). Dual Diagnosis Anonymous of Oregon. *Psychiatric Services, 61*(8), 738–740.

33. Milani, R. M., Nahar, K., Ware, D., Butler, A., Roush, S., Smith, D., Perrino, L., & O'Donnell, J. (2020). A qualitative longitudinal study of the first UK Dual Diagnosis Anonymous (DDA), an integrated peer-support programme for concurrent disorders. *Advances in Dual Diagnosis, 13*(4), 151–167. ISSN 1757-0

34. Roush, S., Monica, C., Carpenter-Song, E., & Drake, R. E. (2015). First-person perspectives on dual diagnosis anonymous (DDA): A qualitative study. *Journal of Dual Diagnosis, 11*(2), 136–141.

35. https://www.wellnessrecoveryactionplan.com

36. Cook, J. A., Copeland, M. E., Jonikas, J. A., Hamilton, M. M., Razzano, L. A., Grey, D. D., Floyd, C. B., Hudson, W. B., Macfarlane, R. T., Carter, T. M., & Boyd, S. (2012). Results of a randomized controlled trial of mental illness self-management using wellness recovery action planning. *Schizophrenia Bulletin, 38*(4), 881–891. https://doi.org/10.1093/schbul/sbr012

37. Deegan, P. E. (2010). A Web application to support recovery and shared decision making in psychiatric medication clinics. *Psychiatric Rehabilitation Journal, 34*(1), 23–28. https://doi.org/10.2975/34.1.2010.23.28

38. info@patdeegan.com

39. Ridgway, P. (2008). Chapter 10—Supported housing. In K. T. Mueser & D. V. Jeste (Eds.), *Clinical Handbook of Schizophrenia* (pp. 287–297). Guilford.

40. Ridgway, P. (2010). Recovery in Mental Health: Reshaping Scientific and Clinical Responsibilities. *Psychiatric Services, 62*(5), 567–568. doi:10.1176/appi.ps.62.5.567-a

41. Davidson, L., Ridgway, P., Wieland, M., & O'Connell, M. (2009). A capabilities approach to mental health transformation: A conceptual framework for the recovery era. *Canadian Journal of Community Mental Health, 28*(2), 35–46. https://doi.org/10.7870/cjcmh-2009-00212

Index

For the benefit of digital users, indexed terms that span two pages (e.g., 52–53) may, on occasion, appear on only one of those pages.

Tables are indicated by *t* following the page number